MW01611204

Innovations in Deaf Studies

Perspectives on Deafness

Series Editors
Marc Marschark
Harry Knoors

Innovations in Deaf Studies

The Role of Deaf Scholars

Edited by
Annelies Kusters
Maartje De Meulder
Dai O'Brien

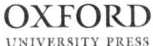
OXFORD
UNIVERSITY PRESS

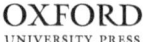

OXFORD
UNIVERSITY PRESS

Oxford University Press is a department of the University of Oxford. It furthers
the University's objective of excellence in research, scholarship, and education
by publishing worldwide. Oxford is a registered trade mark of Oxford University
Press in the UK and certain other countries.

Published in the United States of America by Oxford University Press
198 Madison Avenue, New York, NY 10016, United States of America.

Library of Congress Cataloging-in-Publication Data
Names: Kusters, Annelies, editor. | De Meulder, Maartje, editor. | O'Brien, Dai, editor.
Title: Innovations in deaf studies : the role of deaf scholars /
[edited by] Annelies Kusters, Maartje De Meulder, Dai O'Brien.
Description: New York : Oxford University Press, [2017] |
Series: Perspectives on deafness Identifiers: LCCN 2016038696 |
ISBN 9780190612184 (jacketed hardcover : alk. paper)
Subjects: LCSH: Deaf—Education. | Deaf—Study and teaching. |
Sign language—Study and teaching. Classification: LCC HV2430 .I526 2017 |
DDC 371.91/2—dc23
LC record available at https://lccn.loc.gov/2016038696

To the pioneers in Deaf Studies who inspired and motivated us,
and to all emerging Deaf Studies scholars who wait to be inspired in
their turn.

Contents

Foreword

This book offers deaf voices that reflect deaf people's inquiry into their lived experiences. Each writer is interested in how deaf people understand, how they position themselves in their worlds, how they negotiate meaning, and how they connect themselves to others. It seems we have a hunger to know deaf people's hearts and minds more than ever before. The chapters in this book are food for both the heart and the mind.

We have many unresolved conflicts in our individual and collective lives: recognition of our unique needs, our language rights, our socioeconomic situations, and our schooling, to mention just some of them. The deaf scholars we hear from in this book do not look to non-deaf people to illuminate or improve how we live; they are taking the problems into their own hands. This is as it should be.

We hear from researchers who had much to say about the complexity of how deaf people live, but we also hear from some who describe and explain how complicated are the situations of deaf people throughout the world. More sharply focused research places the power in our own hands. We have the ability to promote understanding and light the way where the next step is not always easy or clear.

Listening carefully to each scholar in these chapters, we hear personal journeys both as individuals and as scholars. These chapters are about the humanity of deaf people and their concern that research and scholarship have not been as centered as they should be in a *deaf authority*. The academy where much of the formal knowledge about deaf people's lives has been produced has refracted the light to the outside rather than to the inside. The essays in this book converge on a single thought; they amount to a maturing from *assisting* in the examination of deaf people's lives to *authoring* them. However, even as we study ourselves, we realize we are not insiders in other deaf worlds.

A basic truth of cultural studies is that culture ceaselessly circulates through people and their worlds. It is in a state of constant construction. So, too, is the study of it. This book is a discussion about the state of Deaf Studies. As two researchers who have had long careers in cultural study, we say with a great deal of experience that there has been growth and change in our discipline and there will continue to be. This is as it should be. Deaf people have succeeded, in ways we could not have conceived of a generation ago, in projecting ourselves into public culture and influencing the lives of others. We are moving into new spaces, not just geographically, but mentally, where describing the texture of our lives is a work in progress.

We have written elsewhere that the future of sign languages and "deaf culture" is not imprisoned and locked in the places and spaces of our past. As scholars who were there when sign languages started to be named, and cultures started to be described, we often are asked whether there is a future for sign languages and our ways of life. One prediction we often encounter is that as deaf schools vanish, sign languages will vanish with them. But we see a different outcome today: sign languages are now learned in more places and by more people than ever before. We also see how new rhetoric about deafness and deaf lives has positively influenced a younger generation of deaf people.

We are excited about the possibilities for Deaf Studies. Technology and social media are raising issues faster than we can write about them. Even as we try to understand the past and present, the future is already upon us. Our language and cultural heritages are challenged by the rapidity of cultural change. High tech accessibility is changing us, especially in communities where there used to be no connectivity to the wider world. YouTube is filled with the diversity of deaf people's expressions of culture: poetry, blogging, dancing, acting, and teaching. There are more paths to being deaf than ever before. Increasingly, our sign languages are detaching and floating away from their roots. Once known almost exclusively to deaf people and their friends and relatives, our sign languages are being studied and learned by children and adults who are not deaf. What does it mean to become so public that we hardly recognize our roots? The discipline of Deaf Studies is how we can better understand the present.

There is a concern expressed in these chapters regarding the effect we as researchers have on the communities we study. And we question whether our research methods alter the landscapes that we visit, just by our having entered them. Only good can come from this kind of self-examination. It is an important contribution of these authors that they are self-aware, because, quite honestly, in the early days of research on a "culture" of deaf people, we were flying by the seat of our pants. There were few, if any, models. Now we see a multiplicity of models, each complementing the other. Several authors in this book raise moral and ethical arguments in these pages. You will find much to think about in regard to getting it right. Deaf people everywhere have a vested interest in *doing no harm,* with respect to medical treatment, child rearing, schooling, *and research.* This is a responsibility we take seriously.

We now have had over 40 years of introspection about our languages and cultures. This book represents that very rich heritage of language and cultural studies. It is very nice to have been there at the beginning, to have written for a different generation, and to be invited to read, in these pages, the thoughts of the next generation of deaf scholars. We appreciate the invitation.

Tom Humphries and Carol Padden
April 2016

Contributors

Maartje De Meulder
Department of Languages
University of Jyväskylä
Jyväskylä, Finland

Michele Friedner
School of Health Technology and
    Management
Stony Brook University
New York, New York

Hilde Haualand
Institute of Sign Language and
    Interpreter Education
Department of Language and
    Literature
Norwegian University of Science
    and Technology
Trondheim, Norway

Lynn Y-S Hou
Department of Communication
University of California,
    San Diego
La Jolla, California

Tom Humphries
Department of Education Studies
Department of Communication
University of California,
    San Diego
La Jolla, California

Annelies Kusters
Department of Languages &
    Intercultural Studies
Heriot-Watt University
Edinburgh, Scotland, UK

Marieke Kusters
Federation of Flemish Deaf
    Organisations (Fevlado)
Ghent, Belgium

Paddy Ladd
Bristol, England, UK

Hannah Lewis
Church of England
Diocese of Liverpool
Liverpool, England, UK

Rachel Mazique
Department of Liberal Studies
Rochester Institute of Technology
Rochester, New York

Rezenet Moges
Department of Linguistics
California State University,
    Long Beach
Long Beach, California

Erin Moriarty Harrelson
Department of Anthropology
Gallaudet University
American University
Washington, DC

Joseph J. Murray
Department of ASL and Deaf
    Studies
Gallaudet University
Washington, DC

Dai O'Brien
School of Languages and
   Linguistics
York St. John University
York, England, UK

Noel O'Connell
Research and Graduate School—
   Mary Immaculate College
University of Limerick
Limerick, Ireland

Carol Padden
Department of Communication
University of California,
   San Diego
La Jolla, California

Rebecca Sanchez
Department of English
Fordham University
New York, New York

Kirk VanGilder
Department of History,
   Philosophy, Religion, and
   Sociology
Gallaudet University
Washington, DC

1

Innovations in Deaf Studies: Critically Mapping the Field

Annelies Kusters, Maartje De Meulder, and Dai O'Brien

What does it mean to do Deaf Studies and who gets to define the field? What would a truly deaf-led[1] Deaf Studies look like? What are the research practices of deaf scholars in Deaf Studies, and how do they relate to deaf research participants and communities? What innovations do deaf scholars deem necessary in the field of Deaf Studies? A desire to ask, and to attempt to answer, these questions was a prime motivator for us to start editing this volume and writing this introduction. We do not ask these questions just for the sake of asking them: Our common background at the (now defunct) Centre for Deaf Studies (CDS) at the University of Bristol taught us that "doing Deaf Studies" is an inherently political activity, because of the history of both the field and of deaf communities in general. This legacy of the CDS inspired us as we engaged in developing this long overdue volume.

The present volume foregrounds deaf ontologies, defined as "deaf ways of being," and how the lived experience of being deaf is central not only to the research participants' ontologies but also to researchers' ontologies, positionalities, and theoretical framings. The authors of this volume also make a number of suggestions as to how new research, ideas, and methods have the potential to develop Deaf Studies in a way which meets the challenges of the present.

The imperative for exploring deaf scholars' research practices in Deaf Studies is strengthened by a gradual increase in the number of Deaf Studies scholars who are deaf.[2] This development is important because the historical and current situation in the academic hierarchies in Deaf Studies and sign language departments is one in which hearing

---

[1] See page 14 for an explanation of d/D use in this introduction.
[2] In addition, there are increasing numbers of deaf academics in the humanities, social sciences (e.g., Zehnter 2014), and hard sciences whose work does not explicitly engage with deafness: There are thus more spaces opening up for deaf people to be able to research whatever they want—not merely to be experts in matters concerning deaf people, deaf communities, and sign languages.

1

academics outnumber deaf academics (O'Brien & Emery 2014). When reviewing Deaf Studies publications and professorial positions, most publications in high-impact volumes/journals and the majority of the higher (Assistant Professor, Associate Professor, and Full Professor) positions in Deaf Studies are held by hearing scholars. This discrepancy has to be situated historically: sign languages have been (and to a certain extent still are) oppressed in educational settings, and spoken languages are not optimally accessible for deaf people (even if advanced hearing technology is used). Language deprivation resulted in generations of deaf people having obtained lower levels of formal education overall in comparison to hearing peers (Conrad 1979, Parasnis 2012, Knoors & Marschark 2014). Due to improvements in educational attainment outcomes (e.g., sign bilingual educational policies in some countries and access to the national curriculum), a growing number of deaf scholars are conducting research in Deaf Studies, and for many of them, this research is informed by their own experience of being deaf.

In the process of developing this book, we produced an academic "deaf space in print," in which Deaf Studies is discussed: All chapters in this book are written by deaf scholars and each chapter has been reviewed by at least four deaf scholars. Furthermore, the editors discussed this introduction during a three-day think tank; a subsequent draft was circulated to all authors to invite their feedback and suggestions; and we received and incorporated a large amount of productive and critical feedback (although we emphasize that we bear final responsibility for any perspectives shared in this introduction). There is something "deaf" about the process, which goes beyond everyone involved being deaf: Part of thinking about methodology involves (re)examining how we approach academic collaboration or interaction.[3] Thus, in the process of creating the book, we employed "deaf capital" (Hauser 2013), that is, we made productive use of a network of deaf peers.

Despite strategically and purposefully focusing on deaf scholars' work, we do not wish to downplay the importance of hearing scholars' contributions to the field of Deaf Studies. Our aim is to create a space for contributions from deaf researchers and to see what happens when deaf scholars enter into conversation. Indeed, particular themes and concerns come clearly to the foreground in this book. One of the recurring themes in the book is reflection on the way in which deaf researchers position themselves in their work, which is why our authors make use of concepts such as "positionality," "intersectionality," "reflexivity," and "reflexive meta-documentation" (Moges, Hou, Haualand, O'Brien & Kusters, this volume). Another theme that permeates the various chapters in this book is the investigation of collaborative and power

---

[3] Thanks to Rebecca Sanchez for pointing out this connection.

relationships between deaf scholars and deaf research participants, and between deaf scholars and deaf community members and activists (De Meulder, O'Brien, O'Brien & Kusters, Kusters, Murray, this volume). In short, this book demonstrates that research frameworks and methodologies built around the ontologies of deaf people offer suggestions for new ways forward for the discipline as a whole.

Innovations in Deaf Studies are not only spurred by the growing engagement of deaf scholars with deaf ontologies and with methodological processes, but also by a number of new theoretical trends. Several authors have stated that Deaf Studies is a field that has developed slowly and needs an updated, stronger, and more coherent theoretical foundation (Ladd 2003, Turner 2007, CDS 2008, Marschark & Humphries 2009, Fernandes & Myers 2010, Myers & Fernandes 2010, Friedner, this volume). The conceptual apparatus of Deaf Studies often was not updated (as discussed later) in a way that kept pace with developments in related fields. Furthermore, although Deaf Studies has been inspired by other disciplines such as anthropology, geography, sociology, and political theory, it has not had much interaction with, made contributions to, or offered critiques of those other disciplines. As set out later in this chapter, to innovate the field, we need to interrogate the foundation of Deaf Studies critically (see Friedner, this volume), to work in a more interdisciplinary fashion, and to intervene in other disciplines (see Sanchez, this volume).

Some approaches to Deaf Studies, such as O'Brien's (this volume) and Marschark and Spencer's (2011), have defined the field broadly to include the study of anything linked to deaf people, including research in neuropsychology, theoretical sign linguistics, deaf education, language acquisition, and sign language interpretation. This volume focuses, however, on certain specific strands within the field of Deaf Studies, particularly concentrating in areas around deaf people's ontologies (deaf ways of being) and epistemologies (deaf ways of knowing), communities, networks, ideologies, literature, histories, religion, language practices, political practices, and aspirations. Our aim is to contribute to the expansion of those areas in the field of Deaf Studies that have been underdeveloped and underfunded, in contrast to, for example, theoretical sign linguistics, which is generally better developed and funded.

Within these underdeveloped areas of study, the founding concepts of Deaf Studies, namely Deaf culture and Deaf community (see Murray, this volume) (and note their capitalization of "Deaf") often are still treated as a monolithic and static theoretical apparatus. There is a need for innovations in the conceptual apparatus of Deaf Studies, not only because the discipline is maturing, but also because deaf worlds have changed considerably since the birth of the discipline in the 1970s. Examples of such changes are the decline of deaf schools, the normalization of cochlear implants, the multiplication of pathways into deaf communities, increased virtual and transnational contact, a diversification of intersectional backgrounds, and a growing number of hearing people who learn and use sign language, to name but a few. To analyze what these processes mean for deaf people, there is a need to look beyond traditional concepts and frameworks and to break new ground.

In this introductory chapter, we first offer an overview of the field of Deaf Studies, and outline a number of theoretical trends. Central in this discussion is an exploration of investigated themes and a critical examination of the theoretical frameworks and concepts that have been used (such as Deaf culture and the d/D distinction). We identify a number of current trends in Deaf Studies, suggesting that they offer innovations to the field. Subsequently, we discuss the role of collaboration, dominance, and hegemony among deaf and hearing scholars, and among deaf scholars of various educational and national (privileged) backgrounds, and their research participants. Having thus established the theoretical, sociopolitical, and geographical contexts of the current state of the field of Deaf Studies, we then will introduce the main themes of the current volume and explicate the unifying threads that run through the following chapters.

THE INSTITUTIONAL BASIS OF DEAF STUDIES

Deaf Studies, as a multidisciplinary field of study, is conducted by scholars whose job, program, or institution title includes the words "Deaf Studies" *and* those who work in more "mainstream" programs or institutions and approach Deaf Studies not as a separate discipline but as a research focus within their respective disciplines (Fernandes & Myers 2010). Correspondingly, the authors in this book have varied backgrounds: Some of them (including the editors) studied and/or taught Deaf Studies as a separate subject, while others are doing Deaf Studies research while based in non-Deaf Studies institutions and disciplines, such as anthropology, sociology, education, rehabilitation sciences, theology, linguistics, and disability studies. Importantly, Deaf Studies (in the narrower sense outlined in our introductory paragraph) is geospatially predominantly located in the Anglophone west, mostly the United States and United Kingdom, where English is used as the academic lingua franca.

Although a wide range of institutions offer bachelor modules (including in summer schools) or bachelor degrees in Deaf Studies (in the United Kingdom, United States, and beyond), master's-level degrees in Deaf Studies are much rarer (e.g., Gallaudet University offers such a degree program). We (the editors) have studied Deaf Studies to the master's level (between 2004 and 2007) in the Centre for Deaf Studies

(CDS) at the University of Bristol, and Kusters has a PhD in Deaf Studies from the same center. The CDS was a formerly well-known cultural and academic landmark but was closed down in 2013 due to funding cuts. Within this program, we were submerged in the field of Deaf Studies in a sign-bilingual environment wherein both deaf and hearing staff (including Paddy Ladd, Jim Kyle, Rachel Sutton-Spence, and other eminent Deaf Studies scholars), used British Sign Language. For us, it was an extremely nurturing place both personally and academically. Indeed, the CDS was the most important place in Europe for nurturing and practicing the development of the underrepresented areas in Deaf Studies mentioned earlier. The fact that the CDS does not exist anymore means that Deaf Studies as a field has lost a very important centralized and internationally recognized place of teaching, research, and exchange.

The MSc degree program in Bristol was (and the BA and MA degree programs in Gallaudet University are) important given that in most other scholarly contexts, Deaf Studies subjects are offered within the context of a (degree) program for sign language interpreters/teachers/researchers, educators, or audiologists (e.g., at HU Berlin, University of Hamburg, Herriot Watt University, Boston University). When looking at these programs' curricula and staffing, it appears that the underdeveloped areas of Deaf Studies mentioned earlier (e.g., the study of deaf people's everyday lives, and their communities) receive only minor attention and often are taught by experts in sign-language teaching or sign linguistics rather than by experts in other fields. Indeed, within the current neoliberal market-driven climate, Deaf Studies in the aforementioned sense is given only very little space, time, and funding to develop.

In addition to these institutes and programs, there are a few Deaf Studies-specific publications, journals, and conferences. Deaf Studies-specific journals include *Sign Language Studies, Journal of Deaf Studies and Deaf Education,* and *American Annals of the Deaf.* The second of these mostly publishes research that falls outside the scope of the field of Deaf Studies as we focus on it in this volume. Deaf Studies conferences are scarce in comparison to international conferences that focus on sign linguistics and deaf education, for example; and are found mostly in the United States rather than on the international level. For example, a series of Deaf Studies conferences were held in the United States in the 1990s, and biennial Deaf Studies Today conferences were organized in Utah between 2004 and 2014.

THE THEORETICAL FOUNDATIONS OF DEAF STUDIES

Deaf Studies as an academic discipline emerged in the 1970s. The context of its emergence, more elaborately described in Murray (this volume), originates in the birth of sign linguistics as an academic discipline in the 1950s and 1960s (Tervoort 1953, Stokoe 1960, Stokoe et al. 1965). These early sign linguists proved that sign languages were genuine full-fledged languages with complex structures, deserving academic scrutiny. American Sign Language, British Sign Language, and other sign languages (previously just known as "signing," see Murray, this volume) became named as such and their parameters were explored. Crucial in the spirit of the age were the civil rights movements of the 1960s and 1970s in the United States, in which African Americans and later also Chicanos, people with disabilities, queer people, and women fought for equality (Bauman 2008a, Murray, this volume).

Within this broader academic and societal context, theory building on (and legitimization of the existence of) the American deaf community, and its culture, began (Padden 1980). Woodward (1975) suggested writing Deaf with capital D when referring to sociocultural aspects of deafness, analogous with national/ethnic group identities such as "Italians." These perspectives challenged the medical-pathological view that deaf/disabled people are "broken" and should be "cured." Concepts such as Deaf culture, Deaf pride, and Deaf identity were coined and explored. Padden (1980:92–93) defined Deaf culture as: a "set of learned behaviors of a group of people who have their own language, values, rules for behavior, and tradition, (. . .) Members of the Deaf culture behave as Deaf people do, use the language of Deaf people, and share the beliefs of Deaf people toward themselves and other people who are not Deaf." Later on, theory on biculturalism and cultural hybridity emerged, which meant that deaf people were said to be part of both deaf and hearing cultures, of minority and majority cultures (Padden 1998, Ladd 2003).

Important publications written by both deaf and hearing scholars in this period described and explored "the Deaf community," its history and culture, initially mostly in the United States and the United Kingdom (although a large number of brief accounts from all over the world were included in Erting et al. 1994). Seminal works published between 1980 and 2000 are Higgins (1980), Padden (1980), Baker and Battison (1981), Kannapell (1982), Kyle and Allsop (1982), Lane (1984b), Bienvenu and Columnos (1986, 1989), Van Cleve and Baker-Schenk (1987), Padden and Humphries (1988), Johnson and Erting (1989), Schein (1989), Wilcox (1989), Brien (1991), Carmel and Monaghan (1991), Gregory (1991), Taylor and Bishop (1991), Ladd (1992), Van Cleve and Crouch (1992), Fischer and Lane (1993), Erting et al. (1994), Cohen (1995), Lane, Hoffmeister, and Bahan (1996), Wrigley (1996), and the Deaf Studies Conference Proceedings (Washington DC, College of Continuing Education).

Murray (this volume) maps out how community activists interacting with academics jointly created the discipline of Deaf Studies in the United States, interactions that were particularly important in the work of the Linguistics Research Laboratory in Gallaudet University in the 1970s (Maher 1996). The Centre for Deaf Studies in Bristol was formally established in 1986 (but Deaf Studies research at the University of Bristol already had started in 1978); and initially also had a strong foundation within the local Bristol deaf community, by organizing certificate courses for the local deaf community and regular research dissemination events. The first decades of Deaf Studies thus featured a strong relationship among deaf communities, deaf people in academia, and hearing people in academia (also see Turner 2007).

Early Deaf Studies thus focused on overturning the dominant medical model in society, the educational system, and academia, including at Gallaudet University, where the medical-pathological perspective on deaf people was dominant (Murray, this volume, Turner 2007). The "culturo-linguistic model," proposed by Ladd (2003), is the perspective on deaf communities as collectivities, minority language communities with their own cultures. This model challenges the individual medical-pathological model and supplements the "social model" of disability; the latter posits that society disables people, that society has to adapt to accommodate a range of abilities, and that society also is focused on individuals rather than communities or groups (Oliver 1990). The culturo-linguistic model (Ladd 2003) and the related ethnic group-perspective on deaf people (Eckert 2010, Lane 2005, Lane et al. 2011) often are used to distinguish (the study of) deaf people and disabled people.

A focus on addressing oppression was central to the overturning of dominant views in this period. Some authors identified parallels with other oppressed groups such as First Nations and some African peoples (Lane 1992, Ladd 2003). To address hegemonies, power imbalances, and inequalities between passive, dominated, oppressed deaf subjects and hearing colonizers/oppressors (mostly pastors, educators, and administrators), scholars coined or used concepts such as audism, colonialism, phonocentrism, hegemony, and paternalism (Bauman 2004, Humphries 1975, Lane 1992, Ladd 2003, Wrigley 1996). Closely connected with this identifying and challenging of oppression is the theme of decolonization, liberation, and empowerment (Jankowski 1997, Ladd 2003). Central to many discussions of deaf liberation are the Deaf President Now protest at Gallaudet University in 1988 (Christiansen & Barnartt 1995), Ladd's (2003) discussion of "the Deaf Resurgence" in the United Kingdom, and his Deafhood concept, all of which aimed to challenge and overcome the oppressions experienced by deaf people.

THE CONCEPT OF DEAF CULTURE

The foundational concept of Deaf Studies is thus very much based upon a (monolithic/essentialist) dichotomy between "Deaf world/ Deaf culture" and (an often hostile, discriminatory, and inaccessible) "hearing world" (Murray 2007). The article "How is Deaf Culture?" by Turner (1994) and the responses in *Sign Language Studies* (volumes 83– 85, 1994), mark the surfacing of discourses that have become increasingly central to Deaf Studies during the past two decades. Turner (1994) criticized the fact that the understanding of "Deaf culture" hitherto had been dominated by Padden's (1980) "static" account of Deaf culture. The latter constituted a checklist with identifiable characteristics and emphasized unity and homogeneity, thus suggesting a unitary (and one-sided) view of "the" American deaf community. Turner argued in favor of an anti-essentialist, fluid, dynamic, and processual view of deaf culture rather than a static one that lists "Deaf features" and describes Deaf communities as having well-defined boundaries (such as comprising only fluently signing white deaf people). He argues for understanding Deaf culture as a verb (in which dominances are reproduced) rather than consolidating representations of dominant deaf groups.

The set of responses in *Sign Language Studies* displayed a number of perspectives, both in agreement and disagreement with Turner. Ladd (1994, 2003) for example, while on a par with Turner in recognizing hybridity and complexity in deaf cultures and communities, nonetheless defended and consolidated the "Deaf culture" concept (and engaged with its critics in the process of doing so). Ladd (2003) argued the need for *strategic essentialism* after a long period of oralism, stating that deaf communities and researchers should be allowed to use essentialist notions, as a necessary first step in reframing and understanding Deaf communities and cultures after a century of oralism in education (Ladd 2003).

After 2005, the concepts of Deaf culture/community/identity and the d/D distinction were questioned or critically explored by an increased number of Deaf Studies scholars (such as Baynton 2008, Leigh 2009, De Clerck 2010, Kusters & De Meulder 2013, Kusters 2015, Friedner 2015, Sanchez 2015, Friedner, this volume). In response to Turner (1994), Johnston (1994:138) argued that the Deaf culture concept "may already be doing far more work than it was ever intended to do." Indeed, "Deaf culture" has been used as an umbrella term to include embodied behavior such as waving or causing vibrations, the arts, technology, accessibility issues, and checklists of deaf "values" or "habits."

Today we see an increasing tendency to use more specific terms for these various elements of "deaf culture," rather than treating "deaf culture" as an overarching concept, even though there are authors, such as Mindess (2006) and Holcomb (2013), who perpetuate this perspective along with overviews of Deaf cultural traits and rules. Indeed, while Deaf culture could refer to the arts, other concepts such as deaf ontologies (this volume), deaf epistemologies (Paul & Moores 2012), Deaf Gain (Bauman & Murray 2014), Deafnicity (Eckert 2010), deaf sociality (Friedner 2014, Kusters 2015), and deaf space (Mathews 2007, Gulliver 2009, Bauman 2014, Kusters 2015) are all terms that are used in different contexts to refer to different aspects of deaf experiences and lives. In addition, some scholars suggested that the way forward for Deaf Studies' maturation, was to let go of deaf "identity politics" (Davis 2008), the "Deaf culture" concept (Baynton 2008), and the concepts of phonocentrism and colonialism (Myers & Fernandes 2010).

DEAF ONTOLOGIES AND EPISTEMOLOGIES

A second problem with the foundational terminology in Deaf Studies, such as "Deaf culture," "Deaf community," and "Deaf identity," is that such concepts have become *top-down concepts*, leading to "frozen" ways of thinking and structuring descriptions and analyses of deaf lives (Friedner, this volume). Because the foundation of Deaf Studies has, indeed, been largely "reactive" and driven by a social justice agenda (Turner 2007, De Clerck 2010), Humphries (2008:41) stated that Deaf Studies scholars "need to achieve a balance between the rhetoric of talking culture that too often seeks to 'prove' something and talking culture that is about the circulation and acceleration of culture." Humphries (2008) suggested that the way forward was to focus on deaf ontologies and epistemologies. We interpret this as a focus on "the whole picture"—both oppression/inequalities and positive experiences.

Although an exploration of deaf ontologies also was central to the first decades of Deaf Studies scholarship (Murray, this volume), later scholarship makes the need to create bottom-up accounts of deaf ontologies and epistemologies more explicit, and regards them as *embodied* ones. Indeed, central in deaf ontologies are corporeality and embodied subjectivity, which means that our bodies influence our experiences and thoughts. We could speak of a sensory turn, by which we mean the renewed focus in deaf epistemologies and ontologies on the role of the visual (Bahan 2008, Baynton 2008, Hauser et al. 2010, O'Brien & Kusters, this volume) and tactile senses (Napoli 2014, Edwards 2015, Friedner & Helmreich 2012) (and also in architecture: see Bauman 2014). Neuropsychological research corroborates this focus on the senses (Capek et al. 2013, Cardin et al. 2013, Emmorey 2002, Sacks 1989). This sensory turn is crucial, because in much of early Deaf Studies scholarship a focus on the (broken) body was associated with the medical perspective and thus was to be avoided. It was exactly this early scholarship, however, (which established the foundations of the field as *not* being about "deafness") that allowed this return to the body from secure foundations.

An important example of a deaf ontological theory is Ladd's (2003) Deafhood concept, a teleological open-ended essentialist concept centring on visual ontologies, deaf sameness, and liberation. It is essentialist because it states that deaf people are visual beings who should sign; liberating because it makes deaf people aware of, and helps them to cope with, detrimental effects of oppression; teleological because the ultimate aim is to become a signing deaf person who socializes with other deaf people; and open-ended because signing deaf people can develop in multiple ways. The concept resonated with many deaf people around the world, including many outside of academic contexts. It was discussed and explored in local deaf communities and applied in myriad ways (Kusters & De Meulder 2013).

Deaf epistemologies (Ladd 2003, De Clerck 2010, Paul & Moores 2012) are based on deaf ontologies. In response to Turner during the aforementioned debate in *Sign Language Studies*, Bahan (1994) pointed out that "Deaf culture" is an academic term, contrasting it with the signed concepts DEAF WORLD and DEAF WAY, and argued that it is important to investigate concepts used on the ground (further discussed in Murray, this volume; see Ladd 2003 for a similar argument). Another bottom-up investigation of deaf epistemologies is the exploration of the meaning of the widely used phrase "DEAF-SAME" in a variety of contexts, including international ones (Friedner & Kusters 2015). Friedner (2016) argues that valuing and checking for *understanding* together with other deaf people is a core feature of deaf ontologies and epistemologies. Authors in Bauman and Murray's (2014) edited volume on Deaf Gain argue that deaf epistemologies contribute to human diversity. Sanchez (2015, this volume) employs what she terms "deaf insight" to interpret mainstream (i.e., non-deaf related) texts such as Charlie Chaplin's work.

We argue that focusing on deaf epistemologies and ontologies is important because it acknowledges deaf people's ways of being without "locking" their experiences in top-down, essentializing, imposed concepts and theories. Indeed, such a focus on bottom-up ways of creating knowledge in Deaf Studies can liberate us from constraining academic concepts and theories (see, for example, Lewis 2007), in addition to allowing us to experiment with new concepts such as "deaf sociality," as mentioned earlier.

DIVERSITY AND INTERSECTIONALITY

Apart from the static theoretical apparatus of Deaf Studies, Deaf Studies scholars also have identified a second problem within the early Deaf Studies canon; although the cornerstones of the discipline have been and still are essential for its maturation, they exclude people, reduce rights, and create marginalized communities through oppressive and rigid definitions of deaf peoples' relationships with one another and with hearing people. For example, Fernandes and Myers (2010:22) state that Deaf Studies "scholars are engaged in perpetuating a maladaptive myth rather than studying the reality of a complex group," and argue in favor of an "inclusive Deaf Studies" studying a wide variety of deaf people and (sign) language use, including people with different racial, ethnic, and language backgrounds, as well as different preferences with regard to use of amplification and signed/spoken language. The initial (unpublished[4]) resistance against Fernandes and Myers' (2010) piece was perhaps caused by the aforementioned fact that many scholars feel that forms of strategic essentialism (Ladd 2003) and strong promotion of sign language use (Bauman 2008b) are still needed in the young field of Deaf Studies.

In any case, particularly from the 1990s onward, we see an increasing focus on diverse deaf lives in Deaf Studies publications. *Open Your Eyes* (Bauman 2008), which emerged from a Deaf Studies think tank held at Gallaudet University in 2002, amplifies marginalized voices and considers how ethnicity, gender, sexual orientation, class, family, and nationality shape the experience of being deaf. Other works that have addressed diversity within deaf communities are works on deafblind people (Clark 2014, Edwards 2015), deafdisabled people (Ruiz et al. 2015), CODAs (children of deaf adults) (Preston 1994, Bishop & Hicks 2009), deaf women (Brueggemann & Burch 2006, Fries 2013), class (Carmel 1997, Ladd 2003, Padden & Humphries 2005, De Meulder, this volume), deaf queer (Luczak 1993, 2007, Bienvenu 2008, Moges, this volume), deaf black/African Americans as minority (Dunn 1998, 2008, James & Woll 2004, Clark 2010, Stapleton 2014), deaf Latina/Latinos as minority (García-Fernandez 2014), deaf Asians as minority (Ahmad, Atkin & Jones 2002), deaf First Nations (Paris & Wood 2002), and so on. Such accounts are being increasingly, albeit slowly, incorporated into or discussed in mainstream Deaf Studies. In addition, scholars who are themselves members of such underrepresented groups are bringing their work into the spotlight (see Moges, this volume).

Paralleling this increasing diversity in Deaf Studies accounts, is a broader geographical coverage in edited volumes published after 2000 (although note that Erting et al., based on the *Deaf Way* [1989], was published in 1994), such as in *The Deaf Way II Reader* (Goodstein 2006), *Many Ways to Be Deaf* (Monaghan et al. 2003), *Deaf around the World* (Napoli & Mathur 2011), and Cooper and Rashid's (2015) edited volume on deaf

---

[4] An important example of deaf discourses not finding their way into print; see further in the chapter.

people and signed languages in sub-Saharan Africa. Monographs also have been published, most of them focusing on deaf people in Africa and Asia; for example, China (Callaway 2000), Thailand (Reilly & Reilly 2005), Japan (Nakamura 2006), South Africa (Morgan 2012), Zimbabwe (VanGilder 2012), India (Friedner 2015), Ghana (Kusters 2015), Nepal (Hoffmann-Dilloway 2016), Việt Nam (Cooper in press) and Uganda (Lutalo-Kiingi & De Clerck forthcoming). There has been an increased interest in deaf lives in shared signing communities, too, which are (mostly rural) communities with a high rate of hereditary deafness (Nonaka 2004, 2014, Kisch 2007, 2008, Marsaja 2008, Kusters 2010a, 2015, MacDougall 2012).

Significantly, an increasing number of Deaf Studies contributions are written by scholars, such as anthropologists and international development scholars, doing research *in the global South*, and their works no longer exist in the margin but rather in the center of social and cultural Deaf Studies. (See Friedner, this volume, for a description and analysis of Deaf Studies work based in the global South.) It is important to mention, though, that almost all these works are written by scholars coming from, or based in, the global North. Moriarty Harrelson (this volume) discusses what this means in terms of ownership, representation, and power.

This emerging body of work in the global South often has combined local fieldwork with a focus on international interactions among deaf people. Other authors have focused explicitly on these interactions. Breivik et al. (2002), Breivik (2005), and Murray (2007) set up the foundations for the study of deaf transnationalism. Their research is based mostly on international conferences and sports events. The edited volume *It's a Small World* (Friedner & Kusters 2015) assembles a number of articles exploring how deaf people meeting each other in a wide variety of international contexts (such as camps, missions, research, and tourism), experience sameness and difference; including a focus on interactions between deaf people from the global North and the global South. This volume is one of the first to explicitly explore intersectionality within deaf worlds.

The theoretical and analytical lens of intersectionality helps us understand the importance and meaning of variables such as nationality, gender, ethnicity, religion, migration status, educational background, disability, and class in deaf–deaf interactions and in deaf signers' everyday interactions with hearing people. Crenshaw (1989) coined the concept of intersectionality in order to draw attention to multiple inequalities experienced by working-class black women in the United States. Intersectionality scholars have focused mostly on a gender–race–class triumvirate, arguing that people are doubly or triply oppressed because of patriarchy, racism, and classism (Crenshaw 2002). More dimensions have been added recently, including sexual orientation, religion, age, and (dis)ability. A number of Deaf Studies scholars have focused on intersectionality (whether or not they employed the term) including Foster and Kinuthia (2003), Leigh (2009), Friedner and Kusters (2015), Ruiz et al. (2015), and, of course, the authors who worked on the aforementioned intersections (such as deaf and blind or deaf and part of an ethnic minority).

We think that for Deaf Studies, the definition of intersectionality as posited by Cho, Crenshaw, and McCall (2013:795, our emphasis) is helpful: "what makes an analysis intersectional (...) is its adoption of an intersectional way of thinking about the problem of *sameness and difference and its relation to power*. This framing—conceiving of categories not as distinct but as always *permeated* by other categories, *fluid and changing*, always in the process of creating and being created by dynamics of power—emphasizes what intersectionality *does* rather than what intersectionality *is*." This definition includes *both* the traditional focus on power, privilege, inequality, and oppression and attention to how intersections produce opportunities and/or empowerment.

An intersectional analysis examines how identities change one another's meaning and impact. For example, deaf and migrant, deaf and blind, or deaf and researcher cannot be seen as additive or mutually constitutive, but rather as *mutually shaped*: Each identity is transformed by engaging with the others (Walby et al. 2012). Identities also can be "subordinate in some times and places and more dominant in others" (Anthias 2012:106–107). Deaf people negotiating multiple intersections might be privileged in some situations and disadvantaged in others. We believe that it is crucial that Deaf Studies scholars pay attention to diversity and intersectionality, not as separate strands of study, but as central to the core of the field, and to its methodology (see discussion later in this chapter). In order to do this, it may be time to move beyond the slippery language of identity, which as an analytical concept can "mean too much (when understood in a strong sense), too little (when understood in a weak sense), or nothing at all (because of its sheer ambiguity)" (Brubaker & Cooper 2000:1).

THE d/D DISTINCTION

Related to the recognition of increasing diversity in deaf worlds, a number of researchers are moving away from the practice of using the term "Deaf" for signing deaf people and "deaf" for non-signing deaf people, instead preferring to use only "deaf". We think that there are multiple problems with the capitalization of "deaf", because "small d" (deaf) has come to mean "deaf people who do not sign and who affirm medicalized deafness and wear hearing aids" rather than just biologically deaf (as in not being able to hear). The d/Deaf distinction creates or perpetuates a *dichotomy* between deaf and Deaf people (even when trying to be inclusive by writing "d/Deaf"), and it has caused practices and experiences of exclusion. This dichotomy is, in fact, an *oversimplification* of what is an increasingly complex set of identities and language practices, and the multiple positionalities/multimodal language use shown is impossible to represent with a simplified binary.

These problems also are noted by Woodward, who originally used the d/D distinction in 1975 (Woodward 1975) and who points out that many Deaf Studies scholars, including Padden and Humphries in their influential work (1988), have been mis-citing him (Woodward & Horejes 2016). Woodward and Horejes (2016) state that "a rigid taxonomy of deaf/Deaf is dangerous, colonizing, ethnocentric, and reinforces tautological and spiral debates with no positive constructions to the understanding of what it means to be deaf/Deaf. It starts with the misunderstanding of the origins of deaf/Deaf and why this distinction was originally made." They point out that the distinction originally was made to emphasize that there is a sociocultural experience of being deaf, and that "deaf" was not meant to be connected to the "medical model" (which was Padden & Humphries' [1988] interpretation), being "oral," or as existing in opposition to "Deaf": Indeed, people could be Deaf and deaf at the same time. Woodward and Horejes (2016) deplore that "The notion of d/D has become an ideological battlefield that further creates rigid and static notions of what being deaf means."

Furthermore, we feel using "Deaf" is anachronistic when writing about deaf history and ethnocentric when applying it outside the Anglo-Saxon western context. As explained earlier, the use of "Deaf" was initiated in the early years of Deaf Studies, within a certain political and academic landscape that has changed and evolved considerably since then. Capitalizing groups and nationalities (such as "Italian") is customary in the English language; but the capital "D" makes little sense in many other languages. It is also paternalistic, obscuring, and imposing: the capitalized "Deaf" is often used to describe the self-affirmation and pride of a group. But a deaf person who signs is not necessarily thinking actively about these issues. We think it is potentially problematic for scholars (both deaf and hearing) to "label" deaf people as Deaf, if these deaf people do not label themselves as such.

There have been other suggestions for writing conventions, none of which has really gained ground: D/deaf (Eckert 2010), DeaF (McIlroy & Storbeck 2010), DEAF (Gulliver 2009), and DDBDDHH (Ruiz et al. 2015). In a research context, we believe that complex labels are not helpful or transparent and that a single inclusive term might be more beneficial. Senghas (2016) suggests not using terms/capitalizations that need to be seen in print, given that they are hard to use during spoken or signed discussion. Other concepts that have been used are those of Sign Language Peoples (SLPs) (Ladd, Batterbury & Gulliver 2007) and the Finnish term *viittomakielinen* (sign language person) (Jokinen 2001); but these are political and identity concepts respectively, rather than writing conventions, and there is discussion about whether and how these concepts include hearing people who sign.

If we hold that the d/Deaf dichotomy should cease being used within the community at large and within academic publications, we need to find a more inclusive term with more expansive possibilities. Is the way forward to use "Deaf" for every deaf person, or is it to use "deaf" for everyone (cf. most chapters in this book)? Many authors have used "deaf" for individuals and "Deaf" for sociocultural entities like "Deaf community" and/or established theoretical concepts, such as "Deaf culture" (e.g., Haualand 2012). In this case (which we for the most part have adopted in this introduction), "deaf" does not mean "oral/medical" but rather biologically/corporally deaf. We regard this term as the basis to which several layers can be added, such as "signers" (e.g., "deaf signers"). Note that the term "deaf signers" does not say anything about being able to use spoken language in addition to sign language or about variations in proficiency. Other categories or layers that could be attached to "deaf" are: use of speech, CI (cochlear implant), "Africans," "people of color" (as in DPOC: deaf people of color), "queer," "blind" (as in deafblind), "disabled" (as in deafdisabled) and so on. Thus, in this book, we define "deaf" as a term describing all kinds of deaf persons, including those who are hard of hearing. Yet, we want to emphasize that we acknowledge that there are benefits and values connected to capitalizing "Deaf", and concurrently, several authors in this book have opted for this even after considering the aforementioned arguments (Moges, this volume, Mazique, this volume).

CURRENT THEORETICAL ISSUES AND TRENDS IN DEAF STUDIES

Later in this chapter, we outline a number of current theoretical trends in Deaf Studies. This is a nonexhaustive list: We also note an interest in deaf education (Ladd & Gonçalvez 2012, O'Connell & Deegan 2014, Kusters, this volume, O'Connell, this volume, Ladd forthcoming), interest in Deaf and Disability Studies (Friedner, Moges, this volume, Sanchez 2015), and in art (Kochhar-Lindgren 2006, Schétrit 2016), for example. We also see a number of trends running through these different themes: increasing internationalization and attention to intersectionality.

Deaf Spaces and Networks

The study of deaf embodiment, as well as deaf ontologies, epistemologies, and histories is explicitly *spatialized* in the field of Deaf Geographies; that is, increasing attention is given to the spatial forms of social activities, social phenomena, and material things or locations (Gulliver & Kitzel 2016). The concept of "deaf space" emerged in the

2000s, around the time that a spatial turn was initialized in the social sciences in general, and several authors started to use the concept largely independently of one another (Heap 2003, Gulliver 2005, O'Brien 2005, Mathews 2007, Murray 2007, Valentine & Skelton 2008). Closely related to "deaf space" is the concept of "networks" (see, for example, Heap 2003, Kusters 2017). After these initial works, several scholars, mostly with backgrounds in architecture, geography, and anthropology, have picked up on "deaf space" and/or "deaf geographies" and used/ expanded them in their theories on historical geographies (Gulliver 2009, Kitzel 2014, Shaw 2015), architecture (Malzkuhn 2007, Sangalang 2012, Bauman 2014, Edwards & Harold 2014), urban and rural geographies (Kusters 2010b, 2015, 2017), international deaf spaces (Friedner & Kusters 2015), and mobilities (İlkbaşaran 2015, Kusters 2017).

Languaging and Language Ideologies

Current Deaf Studies research marks an increasing focus on everyday language use and language ideologies. Outside Deaf Studies, in the current sociolinguistics of diversity, scholars explore multimodality, multilingualism, and translanguaging (combining features of various languages in order to make oneself understood; see García & Wei 2014) in spoken languages. These scholars explore how visual–kinetic–spatial elements (e.g., gesture) are part of spoken languages. Similarly, fingerspelling and mouthing are part of most sign languages; and people often rapidly switch between language modalities (signing, writing, speech) when making themselves understood to (deaf or hearing) people who do not share the same first language. Indeed, today there is less need to defend sign languages as *languages*—this is now an established fact in Deaf Studies, although not in all other academic disciplines and not at a policy level.

The establishment of sign languages as languages (at least within Deaf Studies) allows scholars to explore more freely how everyday languaging works. This is not limited to national sign languages, but includes gesture (Kusters forthcoming), International Sign (Napier & Rosenstock 2015), and regional/local sign languages (Nyst 2012). An increasing number of scholars (both sign linguists and Deaf Studies scholars) explore languaging strategies in which various resources are selected and mixed, such as in deaf education (Swanwick 2015), customer interactions (Hoffmann-Dilloway 2016, Kusters forthcoming), villages (Nyst 2012, Green 2014a), within deaf communities (Palfreyman forthcoming), deaf international contacts (Green 2015, Zeshan 2015), and interpreting situations (Haualand et al. 2016, Napier 2016), in both the global North and in the global South.

We also see a growing interest in language ideologies (although the relationships between language ideologies and language practices are under-researched). Recent accounts on language ideologies include Schmaling (2003), Hoffmann-Dilloway (2011), Reagan (2011), Hill (2012), Green (2014a, 2014b), Kusters (2014), Safar (2014), Cooper (2015), Cooper and Nguyễn (2015), İlkbaşaran (2015), Krausneker (2015), Moges (2015a), Van Herreweghe et al. (2015), and Hou (this volume). Many of these works explore language ideologies not just of sign languages versus spoken languages but also of hierarchies of sign languages, again in both the global North and the global South.

Given the current climate of many hearing parents and deaf children being advised against using sign language (Humphries et al. 2012), we strongly believe that a distinction should be made between *studying* language practices and *promoting* them. We believe that although the study can include deaf people's fluid and hybrid language practices as they are, the promotion of language practices needs to focus on multilingualism and sign language rights rather than on the interrelationships among various modalities.

Citizenship and Rights

Increasing attention is being paid to deaf communities' political practices and aspirations. This knowledge and theory building happens in several domains. One is the recognition of sign languages. Previously, attention merely went to the need for this recognition and included overviews of which countries had recognition laws (Krausneker 2000, 2009, Timmermans 2005, Reagan 2006). Current scholarship marks an increasing number of researchers investigating deaf communities' aspirations for sign language recognition and how the communities work with their governments to achieve these goals, the outcomes and implementation of recognition legislation, and the disparity between deaf communities' expectations and governments' intentions during the drafting of legislation (McKee 2011, Quer 2012, De Meulder 2015, 2016, McKee & Manning 2015, Murray 2015, De Meulder & Murray in press).

Other researchers have investigated sign language policies from an equality perspective or compared (outcomes of) various pieces of sign language legislation (Conama 2010, Reffell & McKee 2009). Another strand of research to receive increasing attention, is that of (differentiated) citizenship and group rights, in which deaf communities seek to accommodate their particular group's needs and practices (Emery 2006, 2009, Cooper & Rashid 2015, De Meulder & Murray in press, Mazique, this volume). Although deaf communities generally do not resist their inclusion in society, they want to decide on the terms and conditions for this inclusion, and achieve it without the loss of their identities. This also has been termed "difference-aware equality," "substantive equality" (Conama 2013) or "co-equality" (Murray 2007). It requires a renegotiation of the social contract for deaf communities, namely, a process of renegotiation in policy arenas in order to reflect adequately deaf peoples' experience as citizens (Emery 2006). The claim for group rights also has been taken up in a more direct academic critique and reflection on policies and legislation, such as the discourse used by the World Federation of the Deaf and by the United Nations Convention on the Rights of Persons with Disabilities (De Meulder 2014, Kusters et al. 2015).

Value and Deaf Gain

The common belief that deafness limits a person in many ways is challenged by the perspective that deaf people contribute to wider society and human diversity. These perspectives are consolidated in the concept "Deaf Gain" (Bauman & Murray 2014). Deaf people contribute to human diversity in a myriad of ways: biodiversity (visucentrism), linguistic and cultural diversity (sign languages), design and architecture, and so on. In the same line, Friedner (2013, 2015) contends that in India, deafness actually becomes a source of (ambivalent) value for deaf people as they interact with nongovernmental organizations, with employers in the global information technology sector, and with the state, when these stakeholders embrace deafness as a source of productive labor and a way of making themselves look good to others. Cooper (2015) narrates how tourism agencies catering to the needs of deaf tourists are set up; thus making a profit out of providing signed guides. Such contributions make clear that the Deaf Gain concept is a double-edged sword, and can place deaf people in disadvantaged positions (also see Sanchez, this volume, for a criticism of only focusing on "the positive"). Friedner (2013, 2015), for example, points out that an uncritical focus on Deaf Gain can cover up class issues and the unhappiness and oppression of workers by seeing deaf workers as ideal and idealized diverse neoliberal "workers with disability," performing "productivity" and "contributing to society" while not making claims or engaging in contentious politics.

Deaf Futures and Sustainable Development

Last but not least, current Deaf Studies research demonstrates a growing concern regarding deaf communities' future existence, with research on the impact and ethics of genetic evolutions (Blankmeyer Burke 2011, Bryan & Emery 2014, Emery & Ladd forthcoming, Mazique, this volume), the future vitality of sign languages (Bickford et al. 2014, McKee & Vale 2014, De Meulder 2016, De Meulder & Murray in press), deaf communities' sustainable development (Cooper & Rashid 2015, De Clerck & Paul 2015, Lutalo-Kiingi & De Clerck 2015, VanGilder 2012), and a beginning of attempts to shape Deaf Legal Theory (Bryan & Emery 2014).

It could be argued that these forward-looking research projects are taking advantage of the security offered by previous work in Deaf

Studies, which established the viability of sign languages as languages in their own right, and of deaf communities as sociolinguistic groups. In this sense, newer research in Deaf Studies is building on the foundations laid by those who came before.

STRENGTHENING THE DISCIPLINE OF DEAF STUDIES

Although Deaf Studies certainly has been a *multi*disciplinary field, we believe that it has not been *inter*disciplinary. Indeed, Deaf Studies has been inspired by, and has borrowed and built on theories from other fields, but only seldom has made interventions into other fields. Ladd (2003) and Bechter (2008) already emphasized that Deaf Studies research can impact other disciplines, but we believe that only now are we effectively and increasingly making those contributions rather than only talking about them (Sanchez 2015, this volume). One of the obstacles to this has been that Deaf Studies' theoretical apparatus has not been as intensively updated as those of other disciplines in the social sciences and humanities. Awareness of, and participation in, current theoretical debates in other disciplines is crucial to making interventions in them.

Today, the contributions of scholars doing Deaf Studies are becoming more visible as they increasingly are published in mainstream journals and by mainstream presses. Perhaps this is one of the strengths of having a growing number of people focusing on Deaf Studies while having had training in other fields. Because publishing in international peer-reviewed journals (in addition to grant writing) is one of the most demanding and competitive academic activities, this is a significant achievement of scholars in the field. "Infiltrating the academy" in this way also means that we are claiming a space of authority as insiders and experts and thus creating conditions for change via research and teaching.[5]

In mainstream fields, for example, all theorizing is deeply grounded in (the assumption of) the use of spoken languages. By engaging with these fields, Deaf Studies not only questions compliance with hegemonic audiocentric and audist structures and authoritative voices but also includes and affirms the embodied "poiesis" ("making") (Calhoun et al. 2013) of deaf people by studying steadily complexifying communicative events and structures. Deaf Studies also can offer insights into wider research on sociality, social formations, ethics, spatiality, language policy and language planning, politics, and literature (Sanchez, this volume), to name but a few areas of potential contribution. These developments (i.e., engaging with, and contributing to, broader current

---

[5] Thanks to Joseph Murray for this insight.

debates) also mean that getting research funding will become more achievable, particularly in Europe, for example, where research is driven by the need for funding grants to a greater extent than it is in the United States.

Importantly, we believe that making these interventions and building these bridges can only be successful if the discipline has a stronger foundation as a field. Indeed, Deaf Studies does not consist of a unified, coherent, cohesive package (Turner 2007, CDS 2008). Turner (2007:11) states that "a carefully-textured, dovetailing program of scholarship was a luxury the field could not afford," because of external push-and-pull factors, such as availability of funding and certain governmental initiatives. The recent demise of *Deaf Worlds—International Journal of Deaf Studies*, along with the lack of specialized conferences, also has a deleterious effect on the future development and consolidation of the field. The Deaf Studies Today conferences in Utah were American rather than international and have been discontinued, and the International Deaf Academics and Researchers conference series is organized for deaf scholars working in all fields, rather than with a specific focus on Deaf Studies. A regularly scheduled international Deaf Studies conference would enable the field to be consistently deepened, expanded, and innovated.

HEARING HEGEMONY IN DEAF STUDIES

Having established a brief history of the field as well as several new trends, the remainder of this introduction will focus on the position of deaf and hearing scholars in Deaf Studies. In other words, we consider the question: "Who is doing Deaf Studies?" Several ground-breaking works in Deaf Studies were published by deaf scholars: Padden and Humphries' (1988) and Ladd's (2003) classics are by far the most cited in Deaf Studies, and many authors in *Open Your Eyes* (Bauman 2008) are deaf, too. They are exceptions, however, because most other authors and editors of Deaf Studies publications are hearing.

A particular traditional pattern in Deaf Studies is that deaf scholars were (and many still are) employed as assistants in the planning and conduct of research: They acted as language models, research assistants, and cultural guides (Baker-Schenk & Kyle 1990) rather than as lead researchers. (See Murray, this volume, however, for an extensive review of the role of deaf scholars in early Deaf Studies in the United States.) These deaf researchers often served as important bridges between deaf communities and hearing researchers who lacked a previous knowledge of sign language and of deaf cultural behaviors or expectations (Jones & Pullen 1992). Many deaf researchers have felt exploited because they did not receive adequate credit for or ownership of their work (Singleton et al. 2012, 2014). Deaf researchers or research assistants were often the only deaf persons on their research team (though there were exceptions, such as at Gallaudet University; see Murray, this volume), and their input and opinions were thus not monitored by other deaf people (Baker-Schenk & Kyle 1990, Ladd 2002). Therefore, the deaf researcher's "cultural representativeness" was sometimes called into question (Young & Ackerman 2001).

In their position as a bridge, deaf research assistants also had to explain/justify the project to their communities and participants, sometimes without having full knowledge/understanding of its theoretical frame, and they risked being regarded as betraying deaf communities in their association with hearing researchers (Baker-Schenk & Kyle 1990). Indeed, because of negative experiences with hearing professionals in deaf education and in other contexts, hearing researchers often were regarded with suspicion or mistrust, just as some of the deaf people who worked with them were regarded (Ladd 2003; De Meulder, this volume).

It must be acknowledged that hearing researchers have taken different positions. Baker-Schenk and Kyle (1990), both hearing themselves, classified hearing scholars in Deaf Studies, demonstrating their awareness of positionalities of, and differences among, hearing scholars. These included different rates of involvement with deaf researchers and issues in deaf communities, different levels of signing proficiency, different motivations for doing Deaf Studies, different positive and negative experiences in doing research on or with deaf people, differences in involvement in advocacy efforts, and different attitudes toward deaf researchers and deaf communities. Similarly, and focusing on hearing professionals in general, Hoffmeister and Harvey (1996) identify a number of ways in which these professionals became interested in working with deaf people; such as having deaf parents, having met a deaf person, having become fascinated by sign language, wanting to improve the quality of life of deaf people, and/or being convinced that deaf people need help, guidance, or religious salvation. Hoffmeister and Harvey also identify a number of different relational postures (which can combine, alternate and/or conflict in the same individual); such as being freedom fighters; blaming deaf people for their problems; idealizing deaf people (and feeling betrayed afterward); experiencing deep distress over deaf people's problems; or wanting to immerse themselves totally in deaf communities. They argue that hearing professionals have to work out their reasons for working with deaf people; and that "Deaf and hearing professionals must co-create a mechanism for exercising a shifting balance of power" (94).

Although such classifications and enumerations can be regarded as essentialist, awareness of the existence of these diverse experiences and attitudes helps us to avoid, for example, defining hearing academics in Deaf Studies as a monolithic "oppressor." However, Baker-Schenk and

Kyle's and Hoffmeister and Harvey's work are exceptions. As Sutton-Spence and West (2011:422) note, there is "almost no debate about the tricky epistemological and ontological ground navigated by hearing people who work in Deaf Studies." They continue that "[t]he problem of Hearingness remains the elephant in the room" and that "[a] productive, (de)constructive exploration of the place of Hearing people within Deaf Studies has yet to occur" (425). Turner (2007:12) wonders: "have we at all effectively uncovered the power relations and machinations of interest groups at work within our field? Too often, I suspect, the ways in which any one group may take advantage of its social position in relation to another pass without comment because it is considered politically unacceptable or inexpedient to make an issue of what is known and seen, but can't be admitted."

For a productive exploration of deaf–hearing relationships in academia, discussion cannot be reduced to a set of methodological, technical issues or attitudes of researchers, but has to be positioned within broader sociocultural patterns and power relations (Jones & Pullen 1992). O'Brien and Emery (2014) point out that this broader sociopolitical context was not discussed in Sutton-Spence and West's article (in contrast to Young & Ackerman's [2001], for example). O'Brien and Emery (2014:29) urge hearing academics within Deaf Studies to look at the big picture and write, "While the numbers of Deaf academics are increasing, their influence, cultural or otherwise, over the fields in which they work remains miniscule." They continue: "it is vital that hearing academics face up to the context within which Deaf Studies operates; that is, a sociocultural–political society in which d/Deaf people do not enjoy equality" (also see Ladd 2002).

In an attempt to face up to this context, Napier and Leeson (2016) state they want to acknowledge this "elephant in the room" up front at the beginning of their book, discussing several aspects in relation to their position as hearing researchers. They identify themselves "as 'Deaf (hearing)'; that is, as hearing people we align ourselves with deaf people and their values based on our long involvement in the community, and we bring that subjectivity to our writing" (6). They acknowledge that despite this long involvement and their strong philosophy of collaboration, they are not deaf and are allies of "the deaf community" and guests in it. They recognize the power they have as hearing people in the community and the historical backdrop of hearing researchers dominating the field of Deaf Studies. They acknowledge they have "hearing privilege," although they say this does not always entail a negative position, and that this privilege can be accepted and used positively "to broker engagement and educate inside and outside the community" (11).

While acknowledging and discussing their position honestly and openly, Napier and Leeson (2016) also in some way place themselves

outside the debate, by stating that "neither of us see ourselves as positioned only in Deaf Studies" (9). They see their work within a broader
context of applied linguistics and intercultural communication, "and
the languages that we work with happen to include sign languages"
(9). This volume demonstrates that virtually no so-called Deaf Studies
research is positioned solely in Deaf Studies and that in most cases it
increasingly entails interdisciplinary research. Drawing parallels with
Black Studies, Napier and Leeson (2016) further state that "the key difference, however, is that white people cannot become black but hearing
people can learn to sign. Thus our focus is on *sign language use*, not *deafness*" (9). This comparison with black people does not work because it is
comparing apples (skin color) with pears (language use), and the separation of sign language use from deafness does not take the aforementioned "big picture" (of power and hegemony in Deaf Studies and sign
language research) (Ladd 2002) into account. The comparison also is
reminiscent of Young and Temple's (2014) pointing at parallels between
Deaf people and women/feminism: "There may be people who find it
difficult to swallow the idea that two hearing women have written a
book about research with d/Deaf people. Is this because we are hearing
or women? Or is it both?" (187). They go on to argue that women *also*
experience discrimination and oppression in academic structures, an
argument that is similarly unhelpful.

In our eyes, the question is not whether particular (fluently signing)
hearing researchers *can* or *cannot* do research in Deaf Studies, indeed
many hearing researchers have done high quality research within Deaf
Studies. We believe that hearing researchers do not need to defend their
doing Deaf Studies work per se, but it's vital that they think and write
about their positionalities. The above mentioned hearing researchers'
discussions of positionality are an important first step. An increasing
number of hearing scholars within Deaf Studies (in the broad sense,
including sign language research and interpreting research) do work on
a par with deaf scholars and contribute towards enhancing deaf scholars' careers, challenging the existing patterns of hearing hegemony.

We believe, though, that increasing numbers of deaf scholars
holding PhDs and/or being in positions of lead researcher (rather
than assistants or coordinators), and thus having risen in academic
hierarchies, already should have contributed to a more extensive
extent to redressing the aforementioned sociopolitical/hierarchical
imbalances. In the past few years, a trend seems to have developed
for high-profile presses to publish *handbooks* and *textbooks* on sign
language (and to a lesser extent, Deaf Studies) theory and methodology—again, by hearing authors or editors working without deaf
coauthors or coeditors. This is problematic since textbooks and
handbooks carry a lot of authority and are often used for teaching
and referencing. Examples include Marschark and Spencer (2003,

2011, 2016), Brentari (2010), Pfau, Steinbach, and Woll (2012), Young and Temple (2014), Orfanidou, Woll, and Morgan (2015), Napier and Leeson (2016), Baker, van den Bogaerde, Pfau, and Schermer (2016)—contrasting with Gertz and Boudreault (2016) and Bakken Jepsen, De Clerck, Lutalo-Kiingi, and McGregor (2015) where all or some of the editors are deaf. Redressing the balance will happen only if the number of deaf (co-)editors and (co-)authors of textbooks and handbooks increases. This volume is an important step in that direction. Another example is that as of 2016, the editorial board of the Gallaudet University Press journal *Sociolinguistics in Deaf Communities* is headed by a deaf scholar (Dr. Jordan Fenlon), and the four new scholars who were subsequently added to the editorial board are all deaf. We also believe that the growing number of deaf scholars will further influence the course that Deaf Studies is taking. For example, we hope that the future will lead to more methodologies designed/adapted for and by deaf people; sustainable relationships with deaf communities; and research themes that are close to deaf people's everyday life experiences and concerns, indeed, to deaf ontologies. Authors in this volume demonstrate several examples, which are summarized here.

DEAF SCHOLARS IN DEAF STUDIES

Deaf Studies scholars who are deaf have increasingly explained and explored the links among ontologies, research practice, and positionality, and between research practice and relationships with deaf communities. Thus the role of deaf scholars is being (re)defined. In such explorations, a number of themes, concerns, and positive and negative observations were consistently present. Before commencing to summarize them here, it is important to recognize that deaf scholars usually have literacy and educational privileges as compared to most other deaf people, and that these are fundamental assets for advancing in academia. It also appears that many deaf scholars have been mainstreamed for all or most of their education (which is the case for almost all the authors of this book). This is unsurprising given that in the United States and Europe, many deaf children have been mainstreamed since the 1970s/1980s.

In addition, we observe that deaf scholars who pursue academic careers often have been privileged according to majority society perspectives, such as having more/better hearing (without or with technology such as cochlear implants) and/or being able to use/understand spoken language. Some also have had the advantage of being surrounded by deaf/signing family members. With many deaf scholars we observe a strong will to "survive (in) the system." As such, most deaf scholars of the current generation are not representative of wider deaf communities, do not necessarily identify with the "classic native deaf" model, and generally have very different backgrounds from the first generation of deaf scholars in Deaf Studies, as discussed in Murray's and De Meulder's chapters. The effects of (lacking) the aforementioned resources are poorly understood, or are debated and dismissed, as, for example, by Fernandez and Myers (2010). Indeed, this background calls into question what it means to produce deaf ontologies in a way that potentially could expand or rupture the native deaf narratives of the 1980s and 1990s (De Meulder, this volume).[6]

It is thus important to be aware of and transparent about the aforementioned privileges and resources, and it is equally important to be aware of intersectionality not only in research (as discussed earlier) but also in researcher positionality. In this book, for example, there is diversity with regard to authors' gender and sexual orientation, hearing status (including both deaf and hard-of-hearing people), being deafblind or deafdisabled, use of hearing technology, ethnicity/nationality, and location of research projects. Diverse life experiences and diverse forms of embodiment shape our perspectives, thus having authors of underrepresented backgrounds seemed crucial.

We encountered problems, however, in finding authors from these underrepresented groups. For example, we would have liked to see more diversity with regard to authors' national background or residence, given that all authors included here are based in the global North, more particularly in the United Kingdom, United States, Germany, Belgium, and Norway. Some deaf scholars from the global South study/work in Deaf Studies in the global North but very few conduct research in the global South, and very few pursue an academic career. Although there are a number of deaf scholars originating in the global South who are working as sign linguists, activists/lobbyists, or leading intervention-based work, we looked, in vain, for deaf people in the global South who worked in the underrepresented field of social, cultural, literary, and political Deaf Studies *and* could write for the book, in English. Indeed, there are a number of Deaf Studies scholars in, for example, Brazil, who do work in these areas of Deaf Studies, but who publish in Portuguese. Being unable to offer financial aid for translating their work to English, we could not include their contributions. This is all the more an indication that Deaf Studies, in the sense of the study of deaf ontologies and epistemologies is a very Western and English-dominated discipline (also see Friedner, this volume). We are well aware that deaf scholars in other scholarly traditions will have developed different interests and we do not claim that our accounts necessarily reflect broader perspectives of deaf communities or deaf scholars globally.

---

[6] Thanks to Joseph Murray and Paddy Ladd for pointing this out.

Because there is enormous diversity among deaf scholars, we want to emphasize that it is not our purpose to essentialize their experiences in the sections that follow. Some experiences could prove recognizable to hearing scholars in Deaf Studies, too, and some experiences could prove recognizable to some, but not to other deaf scholars. Rather, we aim to pay attention to "the big picture" (Ladd 2002) and to explore which issues deaf scholars encounter. In the first ever methodology textbook in Deaf Studies, Young and Temple (2014) defined methodology as not just about methods but about position, performance, identity, and associated epistemology; but they did not venture into implications for method or design from a deaf ontological perspective. Both of the authors are hearing, and one has, by her own admission, had little or no contact with deaf communities. There is a wealth of literature in other fields (such as Disability Studies, anthropology and sociology) on positionality, reflexivity, and the position of underrepresented researchers (such as migrants, women, people of color, or people with disabilities), and many of us have been inspired by texts from these fields (see, for example, De Meulder 2007, Haualand, this volume). Although discussing these works is outside of the scope of this chapter, it is important to acknowledge their influence on our work.[7]

Thus, what we want to do in the section that follows, is point out some experiences of deaf scholars in Deaf Studies, their positionality, and their methodologies. Most of these experiences are related to ethnographic research, because ethnography implies personal contact between researchers and research participants, which has caused reflections on positionality.

DEAF SCHOLARS AND RELATIONSHIPS WITH RESEARCH PARTICIPANTS

Generally, deaf scholars are more likely to get access to deaf ontologies and epistemologies in the communities they investigate compared with hearing scholars: Deaf people often open up more easily to a deaf researcher (Sutherland & Rogers 2014, Moges 2015b). Within international contexts, deaf ethnographers often are invited by deaf research participants to take part in, and thus gain insight into, the lives of research participants (Dikyuva et al. 2012, Kusters 2012, Boland et al. 2015, Haualand, this volume, Hou, this volume; and see Moriarty-Harrelson, this volume, for a longer discussion). In this context, deaf researchers also often make use of networks in the global deaf community to connect with research participants in other countries (Boland et al. 2015, Dikyuva et al. 2012). Deaf scholars also have reported that

---

[7] Thanks to Hilde Haualand for pointing this out.

they acquired access to marginalized or underrepresented *hearing* peoples' experiences, such as in Hauschildt's (2010) research on CODAs and Zehnter's (2014) research on homeless people in New York. Similarly, Sanchez (this volume) powerfully demonstrates how what she terms "deaf insight" (insights based on deaf epistemology) brings particular perspectives into literature that are not related to deaf people in the first place.

Connected with the previous point, deaf scholars often have the necessary linguistic capital (O'Brien & Emery 2014) through which to make these connections with other deaf people. They often have or acquire a better understanding/knowledge of national/regional/local sign languages and variants, as well as International Sign, used by research participants. These sign languages/variants might be known or unknown in advance of the research: Indeed, deaf scholars often quickly learn new sign languages or variants (Breivik et al. 2002, Dikyuva et al. 2012), although they also have made use of local interpreters who knew more than one sign language, such as ASL and another national sign language (Wilson & Wyniarckzyk 2014). Generally, deaf scholars are better able to suit specific communication needs, to interpret subtle body language (Sutherland & Rogers 2014), and to have insight in the meaning of particular idioms or concepts in sign languages (Young & Ackerman 2001). They also are more likely to have or attain access to discourses in informal deaf gatherings, which is very important because recording interviews (with or without an interpreter) is a much more formal activity that (ideally) is often complemented with participant observation.

Deaf scholars also are likely to understand certain experiences from the inside out (Sutherland & Rogers 2014) (even when they have enjoyed more privileges in comparison to their research participants), because they have had the same (or similar) experiences as their participants. Examples include being deaf signers, being the only deaf signer in their family, barriers and oppression in public places, lack of communication with family and colleagues, being offered wheelchairs in airports, and being provided menus in Braille. Indeed, Sutton-Spence and West (2011:423) observe that hearing scholars in Deaf Studies "can go up to the fence and look through, but we cannot cross." This could equally apply, however, to the current generation of often mainstreamed deaf scholars, who may not be able to understand fully or appreciate the ontologies following from a deaf-school background, often the background of people who are considered to be more traditional or core members of deaf communities.

Deaf scholars often experience emotional and personal involvement and personal curiosity in the communities where they do research, even in communities where they had no previous involvement (Dikyuva et al. 2012). Kusters (this volume) explains that she feels responsible for doing research into deaf pedagogies with the ultimate aim of improving conditions in deaf education. This personal involvement and investment is also true for deaf scholars in the humanities: Moges (this volume) expresses frustration at the fact that although there are many deaf queers in academia, the development of Deaf Queer theory is long overdue. This lack led her to undertake an analysis of Deaf Queer literature. Mazique (this volume) powerfully demonstrates how deaf literature analysis can contribute to greater social justice.

Many deaf scholars stated that they felt an urgent need to do something for the communities in which they researched, often in common effort with hearing scholars and professionals. This "something" could either be related or unrelated to the research. Examples include engaging in paid or (often) unpaid work to improve access and services for deaf communities; for example, using their position for advocacy efforts, interpreting on the news, investing time in the organization of activities in the deaf club, initiating or engaging in development projects, assisting in the setting up of a deaf school, strengthening deaf associations, and/or creating a sign language dictionary or DVD (Dikyuva et al. 2012, Boland et al. 2015, De Clerck & Paul 2015, Kusters 2015, De Meulder, this volume, Kusters, this volume). Yet, we observed that others have refrained from such activities following (or trying to prevent) the accusation of being biased, activist researchers.

Sometimes, deaf scholars are the first foreign deaf person and/or the first deaf researcher (or one out of very few) visiting a particular community, which can be surprising, inspiring (Boland et al. 2015, Dikyuva et al. 2012, Kusters 2012, Hou, this volume) or even disconcerting, such as in the case of a deaf researcher who is a person of color (Moges 2015b). Deaf scholars often play an important role in making deaf communities aware that they have their own language (Dikyuva et al. 2012, Murray, this volume), but this is also one of the actual and important achievements of hearing sign linguists.

Deaf scholars have experimented with methodology and writing styles to capture deaf ontologies. Examples include visual methodologies, in particular photography and filmmaking (O'Brien & Kusters, this volume) or "visually reliant tools" such as drawings, photographs, and video diaries (Sutherland & Rogers 2014, Sutherland & Young 2014). Other examples include tactile methodologies (Barnett 2014); a monolingual approach in a community using a signed language previously unknown to the researcher (immersing oneself in a particular language, not using an intermediary language) (Hou, this volume); and experiments with writing styles such as autoethnography (a method of research that connects the researcher's self with the theme under study using self-reflexive analysis) (O'Connell, this volume, Haualand 2012); and a dialogical style (Lewis & VanGilder, this volume).

There are also a few examples where deaf scholars' deafness and/or privileges can be counterproductive in research. Deaf scholars,

especially if carrying out research in their own communities, are sometimes perceived as knowing "too much," so that participants give less
in-depth explanations because they expect that deaf scholars "already
know" (Conama 2010, Haualand 2001, Sutherland & Rogers 2014,
Moges 2015b, Kusters, this volume). Some deaf scholars have reported
they had difficulties gaining insight into hearing people's perspectives,
especially in foreign countries, even when interpreters are present or
even when hearing people know how to sign (see Dikyuva et al. 2012,
Kusters 2012, Hou, this volume, Moges 2015b). In contexts of participant
observation, deaf scholars are also less likely to be able to observe spontaneous behavior between deaf and hearing people in their research
settings, because they are a magnet to deaf research participants who
expect them to interact with them (Hou, this volume, Kusters 2012).
Deaf ethnographers' interactions with hearing participants are sometimes actively prevented or limited by deaf research participants, who
tell them "how to behave" toward hearing people in their research settings (such as ignoring them: Kusters 2012; or not interrupting them:
Hou, this volume).

Privileges of the deaf researcher (such as privilege as an academic,
privileged access to financial resources) can get in the way of constructive relationships in the field, and also can lead to misunderstandings (De Meulder, this volume, Dikyuva et al. 2012, Hou this volume,
Kusters 2012, Moges 2015b, Moriarty Harrelson, this volume). In international contexts, it sometimes happens that deaf scholars unintentionally impose their (Western) deaf perceptions/presumptions on research
participants, based on perceptions of deaf sameness. This happens
particularly when scholars do not yet have a deep understanding of
a different culture in a different country (Boland et al. 2015, VanGilder
2015). Because of the perceived "DEAF-SAME" feeling by informants and
the privileged position of deaf scholars (such as in terms of finance,
position of power), deaf scholars sometimes encounter high expectations in deaf communities they do research in; for example, informants
expecting them to provide information, material or financial resources,
or medical advice. Failure to respond to such requests can result in distrust and disappointment (Kusters 2012, Boland et al. 2015, De Meulder,
this volume).

A related problem is that of representation: deaf scholars doing Deaf
Studies "speak for" deaf communities and yet are part of a privileged
elite (Moriarty Harrelson, this volume). Deaf scholars can claim that
their work purely represents their own perspective. But still, doing
research and disseminating findings (whether through blogs, books,
articles, presentations, or vlogs) means that their perspective is powerful, arguably more powerful than the voices of their informants, particularly if the respective community counts few literate deaf people with
opportunities or tools at their disposal to react to research that they

do not endorse. This discrepancy can lead to resistance against deaf scholars' position, as Moriarty Harrelson (this volume) has discussed. Important power dimensions need to be addressed, and the question of who or what is an "outsider" needs to be nuanced (Moriarty Harrelson, this volume). This is not only the case with regard to the global South, as in Moriarty Harrelson's chapter, but also in western countries.

DEAF SCHOLARS IN ACADEMIC SETTINGS

Having discussed deaf scholars' relations with research participants and their personal involvement in the field, we now move on to a discussion of deaf scholars' positions within academic institutions such as universities and research centers, which are hearing-dominant spaces (Stapleton 2015). This section is not specific to Deaf Studies: Many of the experiences listed here are also true for deaf scholars in fields other than Deaf Studies.

To begin with, deaf scholars in academic settings often are pushed into categories such as "disabled," "to be included" (Haualand, this volume), or "to be rehabilitated" (McDermid 2009). They sometimes are perceived or labeled as "too native" (Haualand 2012), "(too) activist," too "radical" (Trowler & Turner 2002), or too impolite and indiscrete (McDermid 2009). Faculty, staff, and students might underestimate deaf scholars' (whether they are students or lecturers) skills, competence, intelligence, or authority (Brueggemann & Moddelmog 2002, Blankmeyer Burke & Nicodemus 2013, Stapleton 2014, 2015). Deaf scholars might have different (deaf-centric) values (Trowler & Turner 2002, McDermid 2009) compared with hearing scholars, including visual–tactile orientations.

Deaf scholars in academic settings often lack access to university discourses, such as non-signing colleagues' work (in sharp contrast with their vibrant and often life-changing international deaf academic networks; see, for example, Blankmeyer Burke & Nicodemus 2013), and they often work in isolation from the wider university (such as in other departments, or in higher levels of hierarchy in the university) (Trowler & Turner 2002, McDermid 2009). They often work in physical isolation from their deaf peers and, as such, lack deaf capital (Hauser 2013, Stapleton 2015). They often recharge their batteries by socializing with deaf peers in their leisure time (Trowler & Turner 2002). Deaf or hard-of-hearing students, faculty, and staff have to "come out," either to fellow students, colleagues, to lecturers (Blankmeyer Burke & Nicodemus 2013), or to their own students (Brueggemann & Moddelmog 2002). They may experience multiple intersections, such as deafness intersecting with gender and ethnicity, which further shape the discrimination and oppression they experience (including aggression and distorted expectations). These intersections, however, also can be sources of cultural capital and peer support (Blankmeyer Burke & Nicodemus 2013, Stapleton 2014, Moges, this volume).

Deaf scholars are less likely to have access to conferences in both Deaf Studies and non-Deaf Studies fields where spoken languages are the main conference languages. Instead, they are dependent on reasonable accommodations for the provision of highly qualified sign language interpreters (who have to be able to work with specialized academic vocabulary) and/or palantypists (see, for example, Hauser, Finch & Hauser 2008, Blankmeyer Burke & Nicodemus 2013). They also have less access to the informal information sharing and networks created and maintained during such events (Woodcock et al. 2007). Lack of access during conferences led to the Amsterdam Manifesto authored by a group of deaf academics after they experienced a lack of access at TISLR (Theoretical Issues in Sign Language Research) in Amsterdam in 2000[8] and some 15 years later to the Athens Declaration on Access for Deaf Participants at ICED (International Conference on the Education of the Deaf) in 2015. In addition, in their everyday lives, deaf scholars often have to spend a great amount of time organizing access, such as booking interpreters or other language/communication support which eats into their work time (Woodcock et al. 2007, Stapleton 2015, Haualand, this volume).

Deaf scholars also often have additional commitments in the deaf communities outside their academic work and take on diverse (voluntary) roles (for example, in national deaf associations or political activities), which again eats into their time. Sometimes, such responsibilities take so much time from deaf scholars that they pull out of the academy or find it difficult to balance their professional and other commitments (see also De Meulder, this volume). Indeed, deaf professionals are scarce and their efforts are thus in high demand in many different areas. At the same time, Deaf Studies scholars who are deaf are generally more likely than hearing scholars to remain in Deaf Studies for the entire course of their careers, either through choice and commitment and/or because of perceived or actual barriers that prevent them from accessing non-deaf research communities/participants (see Woodcock et al. 2007).

In the academic culture of referring to other people's work, deaf scholars often are faced with very few academic written-language publications by deaf people and with deaf people (Harris et al. 2009), because deaf communities and scholars' discourses (epistemologies) and interests are less likely to find their way into print (Young & Ackerman 2001, Ladd 2002). In this respect, it is important to consider that there are vibrant transnational networks of deaf scholars

---

[8] http://www.deafacademics.org/conferences/amsterdam_manifesto.pdf

where International Sign, ASL, and written English are used as lingua franca, and where discourses about methodology, ethics, "giving back" to the communities under study, ownership of data, theory-building, and academic criticism do occur. This happened during a series of international gatherings in Europe and the United States in the 1980s and 1990s; the first of these was organized in Bristol in 1985. Their main focus was to bring together members of deaf communities involved in education, sign language teaching, and research, a strategy by which they would then spread the new info throughout their communities. These workshops were more egalitarian and more in touch with deaf communities than is their successor, the biennial International Deaf Academics and Researchers conferences that began in Austin in 2002 and were organized in Europe, Brazil and the United States.[9] These conferences and workshops have been enormously important resources for deaf scholars in order to create and build upon deaf capital (Blankmeyer Burke & Nicodemus 2013, Hauser 2013).

Such conferences often are video-recorded (and the presentations of the 2015 International Deaf Academics and Researchers conference are available online), but presentations and discourses often do not find their way into print, and they are not always accessible for hearing scholars. Also, many deaf scholars cease their research work after receiving their PhD, never publish their PhD dissertation in articles or books, and whether by choice or not, end up teaching sign language and Deaf Studies rather than investing their time into research and publishing. Furthermore, many deaf scholars in Deaf Studies have difficulty finding a forum in mainstream publishing venues, because Deaf Studies themes often are regarded as too specialized.

Another barrier is language: Writing grant applications and publications in written English is a barrier for many deaf scholars, especially for deaf scholars for whom English is a third or fourth language and who publish in French, Portuguese, Chinese, or German, for example. Publication in signed languages (such as in the online Deaf Studies Digital Journal or on DVD published by Ishara Press) is not always the solution, because even those deaf scholars who are fluent in sign languages do not always master and often have not been trained in using the appropriate academic register. Furthermore, the academic impact of these appearances is lower than for printed journals, which is a concern for many scholars (especially when applying for grants or tenure). In addition, publishing in English is necessary in order to contribute to other disciplines.

---

[9] Personal communication, Paddy Ladd (March 2, 2016).

ETHICAL RESEARCH PRACTICE IN DEAF STUDIES

Throughout the discussion of Deaf Studies scholarship in the first half of this introduction, it has become clear that there is a tension between rigorous scholarship and activism, that is, the need for defending and maintaining "Deaf culture" as a concept and as an entity versus theoretical development of the field. We believe that this tension continues to be present, but that current scholarship suggests some new ways forward, and that these are voiced within ethical debates. Singleton et al. (2015) state that although "researchers undertake research primarily for theoretical reasons, [...] when carrying out sign language work in the Deaf community, we should always bear in mind that the social impact of doing so is great" (18). In the search for new ways for deaf and hearing scholars to collaborate on the one hand, and for scholars and communities to collaborate on the other, several scholars have offered critiques of unethical research practice and suggestions for ways to move forward. Most of these critiques were written by deaf scholars, or were coauthored by deaf and hearing scholars (which is a departure from previous Deaf Studies scholarship, where the majority of authors or editors were hearing).

A very important study on ethical conduct in deaf-related research, undertaken by Singleton et al. (2012, 2014) identified myriad ethical problems in studies with deaf research participants, including distrust toward non-signing or not fluently signing researchers. In addition, deaf research participants found that consent forms were not translated; had incorrect ideas about how data would be used; and were concerned about anonymization when they were video-recorded, even when pseudonyms were used. Other researchers have faced similar concerns and have come up with a range of solutions, such as gaining consent in sign languages, gaining consent in groups, and, through constant evaluations, conducting ongoing and repeated conversations about research ethics (Dikyuva et al. 2012, Kusters 2012, McKee, Schlehofer & Thew 2013, Singleton et al. 2012, 2014, Sutherland & Young 2014). They also introduced anonymization of video-recorded data by using a deaf relay interpreter (Fries 2015), and by constituting "composite counter-narratives" written like a play, in order to avoid identifying individual participants (not even through pseudonyms) (Stapleton 2014). In autoethnography, as well, a number of ethical issues arise when writing about people who can be identified, which are addressed by O'Connell (this volume).

Rather than come up with a checklist of suggestions, some authors have devised new overarching frameworks for ethical research. In this context, Harris, Holmes and Mertens (2009) propose a Sign Language Communities' Terms of Reference, based on the Indigenous Terms of Reference, which later was applied by Hochgesang (2015) in the Kenyan deaf community. Singleton, Martin, and Morgan (2015) suggest "deaf friendly community-engaged research" (CEnR). Lutalo-Kiingi and De Clerck (2015) promote an interactive model of partnership among nongovernmental organizations (NGOs), academia, governments, and deaf communities. Similarly, Boland et al. (2015) reflect on the relationship between research and sustainable development. O'Brien (this volume) explores Kaupapa Māori research frameworks for Deaf Studies research. All these authors emphasize that research must be endorsed by deaf/sign language communities before, during, and after the research. Given that a few individual people cannot speak for entire communities, advisory boards consisting of experts and community members could be installed and could function as ethics committees, too. Furthermore, long-term relations with deaf communities are important. Ownership of research findings should be the communities', and data should be published in accessible ways.

Related to publication and dissemination is the question of how to get this information back to deaf communities, and how to deliver it to important stakeholders such as doctors, teachers, and educators. Scholars have experimented with several different methods. One example, already mentioned, is publication in signed languages: Emery (2011) published his book on deaf citizenship together with a full translation in British Sign Language, on DVD. Other venues are *Deaf Studies Digital Journal* and ASLize. Harris (2009) suggests seeking ways to disseminate findings in signed language *before* publishing them in written languages in academic journals, even though there is pressure to publish in written English. Alternative ways of dissemination in sign languages are through documentary film (O'Brien & Kusters, this volume), blogs/vlogs (Moriarty-Harrelson, this volume), or an accessible website (Adam 2015).

A second example is dissemination during events: Adam (2015), for example, narrates the efforts of the Deafness, Cognition and Language Research Centre (University College London) to engage with the deaf public by organizing workshops or Open Days with hands-on interactive sessions, presentations in the national signed language, and a cultural event with performances and short films, along with a roadshow to local deaf clubs in the country. He concludes that "given the bidirectional process of the public engagement process, the Deaf community will be able to have a greater stake in research, and researchers, Deaf or hearing ones alike, will have a greater awareness of what is high on the agenda for Deaf people, be that a social, cultural, political or linguistic agenda" (50). In a number of universities in the United Kingdom, a new series of events, Bridging the Gap, have been organized during since 2014. These not only aim to disseminate research findings and engage local deaf communities in Deaf Studies research, but also to act as consultation events to discuss these communities' own priorities and hopes for Deaf Studies research.

Dissemination during events also can be an important means of reaching hearing stakeholders: Cooper and Nguyễn (2015) described and analyzed how they did effective advocacy work in Việt Nam by disseminating research findings to stakeholders such as teachers for the deaf and the media, and how they recognized the role of highly skilled interpreters in this process. Another direct use of academic knowledge is targeted dissemination of research findings in mainstream journals, with the aim of making the public aware of certain practices, such as the lack of linguistic rights for deaf children (Kushalnagar et al. 2010, Humphries et al. 2012, 2013, 2015).

STRUCTURE OF THE BOOK

The chapters in this volume are organized into three sections, each addressing a different element of Deaf Studies. The first, "Developments and Directions in Deaf Studies," reflects upon the history, current state, and future of the field, including how perspectives gained in Deaf Studies can be used to contribute to and intervene in other academic disciplines and fields. The second section, "Deaf Ontologies," takes a more in-depth look at how the ontologies of deaf people and deaf researchers can inform and influence research practice in Deaf Studies. The third and final section, "Ethnographic Methodologies," explores how deaf ontologies have informed the way in which our contributors conduct their research, whether this be this the choice of method, their positionalities in the field, or how they choose to disseminate their research.

The first section, "Developments and Directions in Deaf Studies," begins with a chapter written by Dai O'Brien, who offers a potential research framework for Deaf Studies academics. Using this framework, academics can ensure that their research is ethical and that they can connect with deaf communities and deaf individuals through an ontologically informed approach: O'Brien argues that this approach should be rooted in the identities and communities of those involved in the research. Through O'Brien's engagement with the Māori concept of Kaupapa Māori research, this chapter also suggests ways in which engagement with other fields of study can broaden the horizons of Deaf Studies.

In the next chapter, Murray describes the beginnings of the discipline of Deaf Studies in the United States and the way in which the growth of this field shone a spotlight on the ontologies of the deaf researchers working within it. He also draws out some of the "growing pains" associated with the development of Deaf Studies out of the field of sign linguistics, exploring how the field, through the nature of those who worked in it, and its location within the academy, lent legitimization to deaf community members' claims for an understanding of deaf people and their lives outside the medical model.

Maartje De Meulder continues the theme begun in Murray's chapter by shifting focus to the United Kingdom and exploring the emergence of a deaf academic professional class during the "Deaf Resurgence." She analyzes their positionalities as emerging "professionals" during a time when most deaf people in the United Kingdom worked in blue collar jobs. She goes on to explore the consequences of this status for their relationships with both the wider academy and the deaf communities of which they are a part. She ends by discussing what all of this means for the current generation of deaf scholars.

Deaf Studies in the global South is the topic of the following chapter, in which Michele Friedner problematizes the discipline of "Deaf Studies" and the construct of the "global South" and explores how both are produced by scholars and activists on the ground and come with their own epistemological underpinnings and orientations. Friedner critically examines some of the foundational concepts of the first wave of Deaf Studies, such as "Deaf culture" and "Deaf identity," productively utilizing concepts from outside the field of Deaf Studies (such as from Disability Studies) to unpack some of the assumptions bound up in these terms.

The final chapter in this section, written by Rebecca Sanchez, offers a look at the way in which research informed by "deaf insight" can contribute to approaches and analysis in fields other than Deaf Studies. Sanchez's analysis of Charlie Chaplin's *The Great Dictator* problematizes what for many is an invisible concept—the fetishization of the voice. By bringing a perspective informed by Deaf Studies to a different field, that of the literary analysis of a text seemingly unrelated to deaf people, Sanchez illustrates how new relevancy and legitimacy can be brought to the field of Deaf Studies in the future.

In the second section, "Deaf Ontologies," authors experiment with theoretical frameworks that are based on the ontological experiences of being deaf. This section is not meant to present an exhaustive selection, but rather to illustrate and explore what deaf ontologies look like within various theoretical frames and how deaf ontologies inform deaf scholars' work. In the first chapter of this section, Hannah Lewis and Kirk VanGilder explore what deaf Christian ontologies look like in the context of worship and theology. To do this, they use a dialogic approach, argued to be more grounded in deaf identities and communities, to explore how their personal experiences as deaf theologians working with deaf congregations has influenced their faith and research practice. Continuing the theme established by Sanchez in the previous section, Lewis and VanGilder argue that perspectives rooted in deaf ontologies can provide innovative interpretations of biblical texts and practices of worship that result in a positive valuation of being deaf that flows from being created as such in the image of God.

Analysis of literature with deaf characters offers the framework for Rachel Mazique's chapter, which explores bioethics, eugenics, and the right to life through schema criticism, a new method of social criticism grounded in cognitive science. Mazique's approach is informed by her ontological position as a deaf researcher, and by the perspective of Sign Language Peoples—leading her to identify both "faulty" cognitive schemas and those conducive to "a Deaf bioethics," which seeks to reframe bioethical debates that impact Sign Language Peoples. She offers this type of literary analysis as a strategy for promoting social justice—pointing to the aforementioned tension between rigorous scholarship and advocacy.

Rezenet Moges, in the third chapter of this section, discusses the concepts of intersectionality and the queering of the concept of "Deaf identity." Moges laments the lack of attention paid to LGBTQ sections of deaf communities, offers a critical review of the existing literature in the frame of crip theory, and interviews two queer deaf archivists. Moges also explores how her own identities at the intersection of black, deaf, and lesbian influence her work and life.

The final chapter in this section, by Marieke Kusters, focuses on the intergenerational responsibilities that former and current deaf teachers working in Flemish deaf schools feel toward their deaf pupils. Kusters discusses the ways in which being deaf influences the pedagogical practices of those teachers. The ontological insights gained from their own experiences also motivate the teachers to attempt what Kusters terms "intergenerational correction," or changing the educational system for the better and to benefit their pupils. Kusters explains that she also feels responsibility to contribute to the improvement of deaf education through research.

The third section of the book, "Ethnographic Methodologies," describes the methodologies explored by deaf academics doing ethnographic research, as they pursue approaches that best fit with the experiences of deaf people and deaf communities. Again, this is not meant to be exhaustive description, but rather a starting point for reviewing the innovative research methods used by deaf scholars in recent years. We hope that this section will inform and inspire future research in the field.

The first chapter, written by Dai O'Brien and Annelies Kusters, explores the notion of visucentrism, and how this can inform methods of research and dissemination. The authors describe and evaluate their use of photography and video during research projects. While accepting that visucentric research methods are not always appropriate (e.g., for research with deafblind people they might be less useful), they suggest that these approaches tap into the visual ontologies of deaf people, allowing a deeper connection between researcher and participant, as well as a more accurate representation of deaf peoples' experiences.

Noel O'Connell's chapter is both an exercise in autoethnography, and a presentation of the method as an innovative way of examining the author's own experience as a deaf child in Ireland in the 1970s. He draws on his memories to identify and explore various elements of the deaf experience in this context and suggests that such a research method could be particularly appropriate for deaf people, because it provides a "voice" to deaf academics whose stories traditionally have been silenced by hegemonic narratives attempting to explain away deaf peoples' experiences without regard to their deaf ontologies.

The third chapter in this section, written by Hilde Haualand, discusses how the researchers' own positionality is not only a result of their own experiences and beliefs, but also a result of how they are perceived by others. In her chapter, which outlines Haualand's experiences of conducting research in a multinational context, she explores the implications of "inclusive" practices in research teams and how such practices affected her positionalities during the course of her research project.

The fourth chapter of this section, by Lynn Hou, is based on reflexive metadocumentation as an integral part of ethnographic research of the language and communicative practices of deaf and hearing-signing families in two villages in Mexico. As she produced reflexive metadocumentation of her research progress, she came to terms with how deaf and hearing ontologies shape the interactions among herself, her hearing colleagues, and their research participants, and how these reveal the complexity of their language practices, attitudes, and choices.

The fifth and final chapter in this section is written by Erin Moriarty Harrelson. Moriarty Harrelson discusses how her experience working in Cambodia, in combination with data collected in the United States and on social media, exposed conflict and struggle over representations of deaf communities in various locations. She outlines how differing claims to knowledge, ownership, and power can be brought to light when assumptions of DEAF-SAME are questioned and other levels of privilege are explored.

CONCLUDING REMARKS

This volume explores Deaf Studies as a field that has matured in the sense that it both has a growing body of deaf researchers who make an enormous contribution to scholarship, through employing deaf capital and deaf insight, and a corresponding growth in the breadth of research topics. Given this, the book can suggest ways forward for the field. We hope the present volume will contribute to continuing development and innovation in the field of Deaf Studies, particularly from early-career researchers. In so doing, we are, in fact, engaging in "critical Deaf Studies," a term analogous with critical Disability Studies (Friedner, this volume): a re-evaluation of explanatory paradigms; new terms of engagement in the struggle for social justice; and exploration of the role of positionality, power, and privilege.

This volume only scratches the surface of the exciting new directions that Deaf Studies can take in the future, with many other areas left unexplored. Examples of unexplored or unpublished areas that ultimately did not make it into this book include methodologies of deafblind researchers doing research with deafblind people and the study of the relationships between deaf political associations and deaf academic scholarship. We hope to see further innovation in research methods and methodology to reflect deaf people's visual/tactile experiences of the world, and more experimental approaches to research dissemination. We also hope that a greater number of academics from underrepresented groups will come through in the future and further explore the intersectional identities of deaf people in contemporary society. The future of the field seems bright, with dynamic and exciting research subjects and practices making it into academic discourse.

REFERENCES

Adam, R. (2015). Dissemination and transfer of knowledge to the deaf community. In E. Orfanidou, B. Woll, & G. Morgan (Eds.), *Research methods in sign language studies: A practical guide* (pp. 41–52). Hoboken, NJ: John Wiley & Sons, Inc.

Ahmad, W. I. U., Atkin, K., & Jones, L. (2002). Being deaf and being other things: young Asian people negotiating identities. *Social Science & Medicine,* 55(10), 1757–1769.

Anthias, F. (2012). Transnational mobilities, migration research and intersectionality: Towards a translocational frame. *Nordic Journal of Migration Research,* 2(2), 102–110.

Bahan, B. (1994). Comment on Turner. *Sign Language Studies, 84,* 241–249.

Bahan, B. (2008). Upon the formation of a visual variety of the human race. In H-D. L. Bauman (Ed.), *Open your eyes: Deaf Studies talking* (pp. 83–99). Minneapolis: University of Minnesota Press.

Bahan, B. (2014). Senses and culture: Exploring sensory orientations. In H. Bauman & J. Murray (Eds.), *Deaf Gain: Raising the stakes for human diversity* (pp. 233–254). Minneapolis: University of Minnesota Press.

Baker, C., & Battison, R. (Eds.) (1981). *Sign language and the deaf community.* Silver Spring, MD: National Association of the Deaf.

Baker-Shenk, C., & Kyle, J. G. (1990). Research with deaf people: Issues and conflicts. *Disability & Society,* 5(1), 65–75.

Baker, A., van den Bogaerde, B., Pfau, R., & Schermer, T. (Eds.) (2016). *The Linguistics of Sign Languages. An introduction.* Amsterdam: John Benjamins Publishing Company.

Bakken Jepsen, J., De Clerck, G., Lutalo-Kiingi, S., & McGregor, W.B. (Eds.) (2015). *Sign languages of the world*. Berlin: De Gruyter Mouton.

Barnett, S. (2014). *Being equal: A deafblind community of one* (Unpublished doctoral dissertation). University of Bristol.

Batterbury, S., Ladd, P., & Gulliver, M. (2007). Sign Language Peoples as indigenous minorities: Implications for research and policy. *Environment and Planning, 39*, 2899–2915.

Bauman, H. (2014). DeafSpace: An architecture toward a more livable and sustainable world. In H. Bauman & J. Murray. *Deaf Gain: Raising the stakes for human diversity* (pp. 375–401). Minneapolis: University of Minnesota Press.

Bauman, H.-D. L. (2004). Audism: Exploring the metaphysics of oppression. *Journal of Deaf Studies and Deaf Education, 9*(2), 239–246.

Bauman, H-D. L. (Ed.) (2008). *Open your eyes: Deaf Studies talking*. Minneapolis: University of Minnesota Press.

Bauman, H-D. L. (2008a). Introduction: Listening to Deaf Studies. In H-D. L. Bauman (Ed.), *Open your eyes: Deaf Studies talking* (pp. 1–34). Minneapolis: University of Minnesota Press.

Bauman, H-D. L. (2008b). Postscript: Gallaudet protests of 2006 and the myths of in/exclusion. In H-D. L. Bauman (Ed.), *Open your eyes: Deaf Studies talking* (pp. 327–336). Minneapolis: University of Minnesota Press.

Bauman, H.-D. L., & Murray, J.J. (Eds.) (2014). *Deaf Gain: Raising the stakes for human diversity*. Minneapolis: University of Minnesota Press.

Baynton, D. (1996). *Forbidden signs—American culture and the campaign against sign language*. Chicago: University of Chicago Press.

Baynton, D. (2008). Beyond culture: Deaf studies and the deaf body. In H-D. L. Bauman (Ed.), *Open your eyes: Deaf Studies talking* (pp. 293–313). Minneapolis: University of Minnesota Press.

Bechter, F. (2008). The deaf convert culture and its lessons for deaf theory. In H-D. L. Bauman (Ed.), *Open your eyes: Deaf Studies talking* (pp. 60–82). Minneapolis: University of Minnesota Press.

Bickford, J. A., Lewis, M. P., & Simons, G. F. (2014). Rating the vitality of sign languages. *Journal of Multilingual and Multicultural Development, 36*(5), 513–527.

Bienvenu, M., & Columnos, B. (1986). *An introduction to American deaf culture (videotext)*. Burtonsville, MD: Sign Media.

Bienvenu, M., & Columnos, B. (1989). *Language, community and culture (videotext)*. Durham: University of Durham Deaf Studies Research Unit.

Bienvenu, M. J. (2008). Queer as deaf: Intersections. In H-D. L. Bauman (Ed.), *Open your eyes: Deaf Studies talking*. Minneapolis: University of Minnesota Press.

Bishop, M., & Hicks, S.L. (Eds.) (2009). *Hearing, mother-father deaf: Hearing people in deaf families*. Washington, DC: Gallaudet University Press.

Blankmeyer Burke, T. (2011). *Quest for a deaf child: Ethics and genetics* (Unpublished doctoral dissertation). Albuquerque: University of New Mexico.

Blankmeyer Burke, T., & Nicodemus, B. (2013). Coming out of the hard of hearing closet: Reflections on a shared journey in academia. *Disability Studies Quarterly, 33*(2).

Boland, A. S., Wilson, A. T., & Winiarczyk, R. (2015). Deaf international development practitioners and researchers working effectively in deaf communities.

In M. Friedner & A. Kusters (Eds.), *It's a small world: International deaf spaces and encounters* (pp. 239–248). Washington, DC: Gallaudet University Press.

Breivik, J.-K., Haualand, H., & Solvang, P. (2002). *Rome—a temporary deaf city! Deaflympics 2001.* Stein Rokkan Centre for Social Studies, Bergen University Research Foundation. Report. Available from: www.ub.uib.no/elpub/rokkan/n/n02–02.pdf

Breivik, J.K. (2005) *Deaf identities in the making: Local lives, transnational connections.* Washington, DC: Gallaudet University Press.

Brentari, D. (Ed.) (2010). *Sign languages.* Cambridge: Cambridge University Press.

Brien, D. (1991). Is there a deaf culture? In S. Gregory & G. Hartley (Eds.), *Constructing deafness* (pp. 46–52). London: Pinter Press.

Brueggemann, B. J., & Burch, S. (Eds.) (2006). *Women and deafness: Double visions.* Washington, DC: Gallaudet University Press.

Brueggemann, B.J., & Moddelmog, D. (2002). Coming-out pedagogy: Risking identity in language and literature classrooms. *Pedagogy, 2,* 311–335.

Bryan, A., & Emery, S. (2014). The case for deaf legal theory through the lens of Deaf Gain. In H.-D. L. Bauman & J. Murray (Eds.), *Deaf Gain: Raising the stakes for human diversity* (pp. 37–62). Minneapolis: University of Minnesota Press.

Brubaker, R., & Cooper, F. (2000). "Beyond 'identity'," *Theory and Society, 29,* 1–47.

Calhoun, C., Sennett, R., & Shapira, H. (2013). Poiesis means making. *Public Culture, 25*(2), 195–200.

Callaway, A. (2000). *Deaf children in China.* Washington, DC: Gallaudet University Press.

Capek, C., Woll, B., MacSweeney, M., Waters, D., & McGuire, P.K. (2010). Superior temporal activation as a function of linguistic knowledge: Insights from deaf native signers who speechread, *Brain & Language, 112,* 129–134.

Cardin, V., Orfanidou, E., Rönnberg, J., Capek, C.M., Rudner, M., & Woll, B. (2013). Dissociating cognitive and sensory neural plasticity in human superior temporal cortex. *Nature Communications, 4,* 1473.

Carmel, S. J., & Monaghan, L. (1991). Studying deaf culture: An introduction to ethnographic work in deaf communities. *Sign Language Studies, 73,* 411–420.

Carmel, S. (1997). *A study of deaf culture in an urban deaf community.* Ann Arbor: University of Michigan.

Centre for Deaf Studies. (2008). Conference welcome and introduction. Deaf Studies Today. Academic Conference. 26 September 2008. University of Bristol.

Christiansen, J., & Barnartt, S. (1995). *Deaf President Now!* Washington, DC: Gallaudet University Press.

Cho, S., Crenshaw, K.W., & McCall, L. (2013). Toward a field of intersectionality studies: Theory, applications, and praxis. *Signs: Journal of Women in Culture and Society, 38*(4), 785–810.

Clark, H. D. (2010). *We are the same but different: Navigating African American and deaf cultural identities* (Unpublished doctoral dissertation). University of Washington, Seattle.

Clark, J. L. (2014). *Where I stand: On the signing community and my DeafBlind experience.* Minneapolis, MN: Handtype Press.

Cohen, L. (1995). *Train go sorry: Inside a deaf world.* New York: Vintage.

Cooper, A. (2015). Signed language sovereignties in Viet Nam: Deaf community responses to ASL-based tourism. In M. Friedner & A. Kusters (Eds.), *It's a small world: International deaf spaces and encounters* (pp. 95–111). Washington, DC: Gallaudet University Press.

Cooper, A. (in press). *Deaf to the marrow: deaf social organizing and active citizenship in Việt Nam.* Washington D.C.: Gallaudet University Press.

Cooper, A.C., & Rashid, K. K. (Eds.) (2015). *Signed languages in Sub-Saharan Africa: Politics, citizenship and shared experiences of difference.* Washington, DC: Gallaudet University Press.

Cooper, A. C., & Nguyễn, T. T. T. (2015). Signed language community-researcher collaboration in Việt Nam: Challenging language ideologies, creating social change. *Journal of Linguistic Anthropology, 25*(2), 105–128.

Conama, J. B. (2010). *Finnish and Irish sign languages: An egalitarian analysis of language policies and their effects* (Unpublished doctoral dissertation). University College Dublin.

Conama, J. B. (2013). Situating the socio-economic position of the Irish Deaf community in the equality framework. *Equality, Diversity and Inclusion: An International Journal, 32*(2), 173–194.

Conrad, R. (1979). *The deaf school child. Language and cognitive function.* London: Harper and Row.

Crenshaw, K. W. (1989). Demarginalizing the intersection of race and sex: A Black feminist critique of antidiscrimination doctrine, feminist theory and antiracist politics, *University of Chicago Legal Forum, 1989,* 139–167.

Crenshaw, K. (2002). Background paper for the expert meeting on the gender-related aspects of race discrimination. *Revista Estudos Feministas, 10*(1), 171–188.

Davis, L. J. (2008). Postdeafness. In H-D. L. Bauman (Ed.), *Open your eyes: Deaf Studies talking* (pp. 314–326). Minneapolis: University of Minnesota Press.

De Clerck, G. A. M. (2010). Deaf epistemologies as a critique and alternative to the practice of science: An anthropological perspective. *American Annals of the Deaf, 154*(5), 435–446.

De Clerck, G. (2011). Fostering deaf people's empowerment: the Cameroonian deaf community and epistemological equity. *Third World Quarterly, 32*(8), 1419–1435.

De Clerck, G. A.M., & Paul, P.P. (2015). *Sign language, sustainable development, and equal opportunities.* Gent: Academia Press.

De Meulder, M. (2007). *Giving back: Deaf professionals and the deaf community* (Unpublished master's thesis). University of Bristol, Centre for Deaf Studies.

De Meulder, M. (2014). The UNCRPD and Sign Language Peoples. In A. Pabsch (Ed.), *UNCRPD Implementation in Europe—A Deaf Perspective. Article 29: Participation in Political and Public Life* (pp. 12–28). Brussels: European Union of the Deaf.

De Meulder, M. (2015). A barking dog that never bites?: The British Sign Language (Scotland) Bill. *Sign Language Studies, 15*(4), 446–472.

De Meulder, M. (2016). Promotion in times of endangerment: the Sign Language Act in Finland. *Language Policy.* Advance online publication. doi: 10.1007/s10993-016-9403-5

De Meulder, M., & Murray, J.J. (in press). *Buttering their bread on both sides? The recognition of sign languages and the aspirations of deaf communities. Language Problems & Language Planning.*

Dikyuva, H., Escobedo Delgado, C.E., Panda, S., & Zeshan, U. (2012). Working with village sign language communities: Deaf fieldwork researchers in professional dialogue. In U. Zeshan & C. de Vos (Eds.), *Sign languages in village communities: Anthropological and linguistic insights* (pp. 313–344). Berlin: De Gruyter Mouton.

Dunn, L. M. (1998). The deaf community in the 21st century: A Black deaf perspective. In *Deaf Studies V: Toward 2000—Unity and diversity. Conference proceedings* (pp. 122–128). Washington, DC: College for Continuing Education, Gallaudet University.

Dunn, L. (2008). The burden of racism and audism. In H-D. Bauman (Ed.), *Open your eyes: Deaf Studies talking* (pp. 235–250). Minneapolis: University of Minnesota Press.

Eckert, R. C. (2010). Toward a theory of deaf ethnos: Deafnicity. *Journal of Deaf Studies and Deaf Education, 15*(4), 317–333.

Edwards, T. (2015). Bridging the gap between DeafBlind minds: Interactional and social foundations of intention attribution in the Seattle DeafBlind community. *Frontiers in Psychology, 6,* Art.1497.

Edwards, C., & Harold, G. (2014). DeafSpace and the principles of universal design. *Disability and Rehabilitation, 36*(16), 1350–1359.

Emery, S. D. (2006). *Citizenship and the deaf community.* University of Central Lancashire.

Emery, S. D. (2009). In space no one can see you waving your hands: Making citizenship meaningful to Deaf worlds. *Citizenship Studies, 13*(1), 31–44.

Emery, S. D. (2011). *Citizenship and the deaf community.* Nijmegen: Ishara Press.

Emery, S. D., & Ladd, P. (forthcoming). *Sleepwalking into Eugenics: Genetic interventions and disabled people.*

Emmorey, K. (2002). *Language, cognition, and the brain: Insights from sign language research.* Mahwah, NJ: Lawrence Erlbaum Associates.

Erting, C., Johnson, R., Smith, D., & Snider, B. (Eds) (1994). *The Deaf Way—Perspectives from the International Conference on Deaf Culture, 1989.* Washington, DC: Gallaudet University Press.

Fernandes, J. K., & Myers, S. S. (2010). Inclusive deaf studies: Barriers and pathways. *Journal of Deaf Studies and Deaf Education, 15*(1), 17–29.

Fischer, R., & Lane, H. (Eds.). (1993). *Looking back: A reader on the histories of Deaf communities and their sign languages.* Hamburg: Signum.

Friedner, M. (2014). The church of deaf sociality: Deaf church-going practices and "sign bread and butter" in Bangalore, India. *Anthropology and Education Quarterly, 45*(1), 39–53.

Friedner, M., & Helmreich, S. (2012). Sound studies meets deaf studies. *The Senses and Society, 7*(1), 72–86.

Friedner, M. (2015). *Valuing deaf worlds in urban India.* New Brunswick, NJ: Rutgers University Press.

Friedner, M., & Kusters, A. (Eds.) (2015). *It's a small world: International deaf spaces and encounters.* Washington, DC: Gallaudet University Press.

Friedner, M. (2016). Understanding and Not-Understanding: What do epistemologies and ontologies do in deaf worlds? *Sign Language Studies, 16*(2), 184-203.

Fries, S. (2013). Taube Frauen: Das „zweite Geschlecht" in der (Gehörlosen-) Gemeinschaft? *Lebensdinge,* 34–47.

Fries, S. (2015). *Violence against deaf women in Germany: Collecting and analysing sensitive data.* Paper presented at the 7th International Deaf Academics and Researchers Conference. February 5–7, 2015, Leuven, Belgium.

Foster, S., & Kinuthia, W. (2003). Deaf persons of Asian American, Hispanic American, and African American backgrounds: A study of intraindividual diversity and identity. *Journal of Deaf Studies and Deaf Education, 8*(3), 271–290.

García, O., & Wei, L. (2014). *Translanguaging: Language, bilingualism and education.* New York, NY: Palgrave Macmillan.

García-Fernández, C. M. (2014). Deaf-Latina/Latino critical theory in education: The lived experiences and multiple intersecting identities of deaf-Latina/o high school students (Unpublished doctoral dissertation). The University of Texas at Austin.

Gertz, G., & Boudreault, P. (Eds.) (2016). *The SAGE Deaf Studies encyclopedia.* Thousand Oaks, CA: Sage Publishing.

Goodstein, H. (2006). *The Deaf Way II reader: Perspectives from the Second International Conference on Deaf Culture.* Washington, DC: Gallaudet University Press.

Green, E. M. (2014a). *The nature of signs: Nepal's deaf society, local sign and the production of communicative sociality* (Unpublished doctoral dissertation). University of California, Berkeley.

Green, E. M. (2014b). Building the tower of Babel: International Sign, linguistic commensuration, and moral orientation. *Language in Society, 43,* 1–21.

Green, E. M. (2015). One language, or maybe two: Direct communication, understanding, and informal interpreting in international deaf encounters. In M. Friedner & A. Kusters (Eds.), *It's a small world: International deaf spaces and encounters* (pp. 70–82). Washington, DC: Gallaudet University Press.

Gregory, S., & Hartley, G. (Eds.) (1991). *Constructing deafness.* London: Pinter Press.

Gulliver, M. (2005). *The Deafscape: Landscape and heritage of the Deaf world.* Paper presented at the Institute of British Geographers, Royal Geographical Society Annual Conference, London, September 2, 2005.

Gulliver, M. (2009). *DEAF space, a history: The production of DEAF spaces: Emergent, autonomous, located and disabled in 18th and 19th-century France.* (Unpublished doctoral dissertation). University of Bristol, Centre for Deaf Studies.

Gulliver, M., & Kitzel, M.B. (2016). Deaf geographies. In G. Gertz & P. Boudreault (Eds.), *The SAGE Deaf Studies encyclopedia* (pp. 451–453). Thousand Oaks, CA: Sage Publishing.

Harris, R. (2009). Seizing academic power: Creating deaf counternarratives with commentary. https://www.youtube.com/watch?v=C3Ae20lXJ1I

Harris, R.L., Holmes, H.M., & Mertens, D.M. (2009). Research ethics in sign language communities. *Sign Language Studies, 9*(2), 104–131.

Haualand, H. (2001). *I endringens tegn: diskurser i døvebevegelsen* (Unpublished master's thesis). University of Oslo.

Haualand, H. (2012). *Interpreting ideals and relaying rights—A comparative study of video interpreting services in Norway, Sweden and the United States* (Unpublished doctoral dissertation). University of Oslo.

Haualand, H. M., Ferrara L. N., & Ringso, T. (2016). *Translanguaging in interpreted signed language communication—an exploratory study.* Paper presented at Translanguaging and Repertoires across Signed and Spoken Languages: Insights from Linguistic Ethnographies in (Super)Diverse Contexts, Max Planck Institute for the Study of Ethnic and Religious Diversity. June 20–21, 2016, Göttingen, Sweden.

Hauschildt, S. (2010). *An exploration of identity and status issues as perceived by hearing children of deaf parents* (Unpublished master's thesis). University of Bristol.

Hauser, P. C., Finch, K. L., & Hauser, A.B. (Eds.) (2008). *Deaf professionals and designated interpreters: A new paradigm.* Washington, DC: Gallaudet University Press.

Hauser, P. C., O'Hearn, A., & McKee, M. (2010). Deaf epistemology: Deafhood and deafness. *American Annals of the Deaf, 154*(5), 486–492.

Hauser, P. (2013). *Deaf academics need deaf mentors.* Paper presented at the 6th International Deaf Academics and Researchers Conference, July 18–20, 2013, Lisbon.

Heap, M. (2003). *Crossing social boundaries and dispersing social identity: Tracing Deaf Networks from Cape Town* (Unpublished doctoral dissertation). Stellenbosch University, South Africa.

Higgins, P. (1980). *Outsiders in a hearing world.* Newbury Park, CA: Sage.

Hill, J. C. (2012). *Language attitudes in the American deaf community.* Washington, DC: Gallaudet University Press.

Hochgesang, J. (2015). Ethics of researching signed languages: The case of Kenyan Sign Language (KSL). In A.C. Cooper & K.K. Rashid (Eds.), *Signed Languages in Sub-Saharan Africa: Politics, citizenship and shared experiences of difference* (pp. 11–30). Washington, DC: Gallaudet University Press.

Hoffmann-Dilloway, E. (2011). Writing the smile: Language ideologies in, and through, sign language scripts. *Language & Communication, 31,* 345–355.

Hoffmann-Dilloway, E. (2016). *Signing and belonging in Nepal.* Washington, DC: Gallaudet University Press.

Hoffmeister, R., & Harvey, M. (1996). Is there a psychology of the hearing? In N.S. Glickman & M.A. Harvey (Eds.), *Culturally affirmative psychotherapy with deaf persons.* New York: Routledge.

Holcomb, T. (2013). *Introduction to American deaf culture.* New York: Oxford University Press.

Humphries, T. (1975). *Audism: The Making of a Word.* Unpublished paper.

Humphries, T. (2008). Talking culture and culture talking. In H-D. L. Bauman (Ed.), *Open your eyes: Deaf Studies talking* (pp. 35–41). Minneapolis: University of Minnesota Press.

Humphries, T., Kushalnagar, P., Mathur, G., Napoli, D. J., Padden, C., Rathmann, C., & Smith, S. R. (2012). Language acquisition for deaf children: Reducing the harms of zero tolerance to the use of alternative approaches. *Harm Reduction Journal, 9*(1), 16.

Humphries, T., Kushalnagar, R., Mathur, G., Napoli, D. J., Padden, C., Rathmann, C., & Smith, S. R. (2013). The right to language. *Journal of Law, Medicine and Ethics, 41*(4), 872–884.

Humphries, T., Kushalnagar, P., Mathur, G., Napoli, D. J., Padden, C., Rathmann, C., & Smith, S. R. (2015). Language choices for deaf infants: Advice for parents regarding sign languages. *Clinical Pediatrics, 55*(6), 513–517.

İlkbaşaran, D. (2015). Social media practices of deaf youth in Turkey: Emerging mobilities and language choice. In M. Friedner & A. Kusters (Eds.), *It's a small world: International deaf spaces and encounters* (pp. 112–126). Washington, DC: Gallaudet University Press.

James, M., & Woll, B. (2004). Black Deaf or Deaf Black? Being Black and Deaf in Britain. In A. Pavlenko & A. Blackledge (Eds.), *Negotiation of identities in multilingual contexts.* Clevedon: Multilingual Matters.

Jankowski, K.A. (1997). *Deaf empowerment: Emergence, struggle and rhetoric.* Washington, DC: Gallaudet University Press.

Johnson, R.E., & Erting, C. (1989). Ethnicity and socialization in a classroom for deaf children. In C. Lucas & C. Valli (Eds.), *Sociolinguistics of the deaf community* (pp. 41–83). San Diego, CA: Academic Press.

Johnston, T. (1994). Comment on Turner. *Sign Language Studies, 83*(1), 133–138.

Jokinen, M. (2001). The Sign Language Person—A term to describe us and our future more clearly? In L. Leeson (Ed.), *Looking forward: EUD in the 3rd millennium—the Deaf citizen in the 21st century. Proceedings of a conference to celebrate 15 years of the European Union of the Deaf* (pp. 50–63). Gloucestershire: Douglas McLean Publishing.

Jones, L., & Pullen, G. (1992). Cultural differences: Deaf and hearing researchers working together. *Disability, Handicap and Society, 7*(2), 189–196.

Kannapell, B. (1982). Inside the deaf community. *Deaf American, 34*(4), 21–27.

Kisch, S. (2007). Disablement, gender and deafhood among the Negev Arab-Bedouin. *Disability Studies Quarterly, 27*(4).

Kisch, S. (2008). "Deaf discourse": The social construction of deafness in a Bedouin community. *Medical Anthropology, 27*(3), 283–313.

Kitzel, M.B. (2014). *Chasing ancestors: searching for the roots of American Sign Language in the Kentish Weald, 1620–1851* (Unpublished doctoral dissertation). University of Sussex.

Knoors, H., & Marschark, M. (2014). *Teaching deaf learners. Psychological and developmental foundations.* Oxford: Oxford University Press.

Kochhar-Lindgren, K. (2006). *Hearing difference: The third ear in experimental, deaf, and multicultural theater.* Washington, DC: Gallaudet University Press.

Krausneker, V. (2000). Sign languages and the minority language policy of the European Union. In M. Metzger (Ed.), *Bilingualism & identity in deaf communities, Vol. 6* (pp. 142–158). Washington, DC: Gallaudet University Press.

Krausneker, V. (2009). On the legal status of sign languages: A commented compilation of resources. *Current Issues in Language Planning, 10*(3), 351–354.

Krausneker, V. (2015). Ideologies and attitudes towards sign languages: An approximation. *Sign Language Studies, 15*(4), 411–431.

Kushalnagar, P., Mathur, G., Moreland, C. J., Napoli, D. J., Osterling, W., Padden, C., & Rathmann, C. (2010). Infants and children with hearing loss need early language access. *The Journal of Clinical Ethics, 21*(2), 143–154.

Kusters, A. (2010a). Deaf utopias? Reviewing the sociocultural literature on the world's "Martha's Vineyard Situations." *Journal of Deaf Studies and Deaf Education, 15*(1), 3–16.

Kusters, A. (2010b). Deaf on the lifeline of Mumbai. *Sign Language Studies, 10*(1), 36–68.

Kusters, A. (2012). Being a deaf white anthropologist in Adamorobe: Some ethical and methodological issues. In U. Zeshan & C. de Vos (Eds.), *Sign languages in village communities: Anthropological and linguistic insights* (pp. 27–52). Berlin: De Gruyter Mouton.

Kusters, A. (2014). Language ideologies in the shared signing community of Adamorobe. *Language in Society*, (43), 139–158.

Kusters, A. (2015). *Deaf space in Adamorobe: An ethnographic study in a village in Ghana.* Washington, DC: Gallaudet University Press.

Kusters, A., & De Meulder, M. (2013). Understanding deafhood: In search of its meanings. *American Annals of the Deaf, 157*(5), 428–438.

Kusters, A., De Meulder, M., Friedner, M., & Emery, S. (2015). On "diversity" and "inclusion": Exploring paradigms for achieving Sign Language Peoples' rights. (MMG Working Paper 15–02). http://www.mmg.mpg.de/publications/working-papers/2015/wp-15-02/. Accessed January 28, 2016.

Kusters, A. (forthcoming). Gesture-based customer interactions: Mumbaikars' multimodal and metrolingual strategies. *Translation and Translanguaging in Multilingual Contexts.*

Kusters, A. (2017). When transport becomes a destination: Deaf spaces and networks on the Mumbai trains. *Journal of Cultural Geography.*

Kyle, J., & Allsop, L. (1982). *Deaf People and the community: Final report to the Nuffield Foundation.* Bristol: Centre for Deaf Studies Press.

Ladd, P. (1992). Deaf cultural studies. In M. Garretson (Ed.), *Viewpoints on deafness* (pp. 83-88). Silver Spring, MD: NAD Press.

Ladd, P. (1994). Comment on Turner. *Sign Language Studies, 1085*(1), 329–336.

Ladd, P. (2002). Time to locate the big picture? In A. Baker, B. van den Bogaerde, & O. Crasborn (Eds.), *Cross-linguistic perspectives in sign language research. Selected papers from TISLR 2000* (pp. 3–14). Hamburg: Signum Press.

Ladd, P. (2003). *Understanding deaf culture: In search of deafhood.* Clevedon: Multilingual Matters.

Ladd, P., & Gonçalves, J.C. (2012). A final frontier? How deaf cultures and deaf pedagogies can revolutionize deaf education. In L. Leeson and M. Vermeerbergen (Eds.), *Working with the deaf community: Deaf education, mental health & interpreting.* Dublin: Interesource Group Ireland Limited.

Ladd, P. (forthcoming) Seeing through new eyes—Deafhood pedagogies and the unrecognised curriculum.

Lane, H. L. (1976). *The wild boy of Aveyron: A history of the education of retarded, deaf and hearing children.* Cambridge, MA: Harvard University Press.

Lane, H. L. (1984a). *The deaf experience: Classics in language and education.* Cambridge, MA: Harvard University Press.

Lane, H. L. (1984b). *When the mind hears: A history of the deaf.* New York: Random House.

Lane, H. L. (1992). *The mask of benevolence: Disabling the deaf community.* New York: Alfred Knopf.

Lane, H.L. (2005). Ethnicity, Ethics and the Deaf-World. *Journal of Deaf Studies and Deaf Education, 10*(3), 291–310.

Lane, H., Hoffmeister, R., & Bahan, B. (1996). *A journey into the deaf-world.* San Diego, CA: Dawn Sign Press.

Lane, H., Pillard, R.C., & Hedberg, U. (2011). *People of the eye: Deaf ethnicity and ancestry.* Oxford: Oxford University Press.

Leigh, I. (2009). *A lens on deaf identities.* Oxford: Oxford University Press.

Lewis, H. (2007). *Deaf liberation theology.* Aldershot, England: Ashgate Pub.

Luczak, R. (1993). *Eyes of desire: A gay and lesbian reader.* Boston: Alyson Publications.

Luczak, R. (2007). *Eyes of desire 2: A deaf GLBT reader.* Minneapolis, MN: Handtype Press.

Lutalo-Kiingi, S., & De Clerck, G.A.M. (2015). Perspectives on the sign language factor in Sub-Saharan Africa: Challenges of sustainability. In G.A.M. De Clerck & P.V. Paul (Eds.), *Sign language, sustainable development, and equal opportunities* (pp. 29–64). Gent: Academia Press.

Lutalo-Kiingi, S., & De Clerck, G. (forthcoming). *Developing sustainably? The Ugandan deaf community looking back and forward.* Kampala, Uganda: Fountain Publishers.

MacDougall, J. P. (2012). *Being deaf in a Yucatec Maya community: Communication and identity negotiation* (Unpublished doctoral dissertation). McGill University, Montreal.

Maher, J. (1996). *Seeing language in sign: The work of William C. Stokoe.* Washington DC: Gallaudet University Press.

Malzkuhn, M. L. (2007). *Home customization: Understanding the deaf ways of being* (Unpublished master's thesis). Gallaudet University, Washington, DC.

Marsaja, I G. (2008). *Desa Kolok. A deaf village and its sign language in Bali, Indonesia.* Nijmegen: Ishara Press.

Marschark, M., & Spencer, P.E. (Eds.) (2003). *The Oxford handbook of deaf studies, language, and education* (volume 1; first edition). Oxford: Oxford University Press.

Marschark, M., & Humphries, T. (2009). Deaf studies by any other name? *Journal of Deaf Studies and Deaf Education, 15*(1), 1–2.

Marschark, M., & Spencer, P.E. (Eds.) (2011). *The Oxford handbook of deaf studies, language, and education* (volume 1; second edition). Oxford: Oxford University Press.

Marschark, M., & Spencer, P.E. (Eds.) (2016). *The Oxford handbook of deaf studies in language.* Oxford: Oxford University Press.

Mathews, E. S. (2007). Place, space and identity—Using geography in deaf studies. In *Deaf Studies Today! 2006: Simply Complex (Conference Proceedings)* (pp. 215–226). Oram: Utah Valley University.

McDermid, C. (2009). Two cultures, one programme: Deaf Professors as subaltern? *Deafness and Education International, 11*(4), 221–249.

McKee, M., Schlehofer, D., & Thew, D. (2013). Ethical issues in conducting research with deaf populations. *American Journal of Public Health, 103*(12), 2174–2178.

McKee, R. (2011). Action pending: Four years on from the New Zealand Sign Language Act. *VUW Law Review, 42*(2), 277–298.

McKee, R., & Vale, M. (2014). *The vitality of New Zealand Sign Language project: Report on a survey of the Deaf Community*. Victoria University of Wellington. http://www.victoria.ac.nz/lals/centres-and-institutes/dsru/NZSL-Vitality-Deaf-Community-Survey-Report-Sept-2014-.pdf. Accessed October 27, 2016.

McKee, R., & Manning, V. (2015). Evaluating effects of language recognition on language rights and the vitality of New Zealand Sign Language. *Sign Language Studies, 15*(4), 473–497.

Mindess, A. (2006). *Reading between the signs—Intercultural communication for sign language interpreters*. Yarmouth, ME: Intercultural Press.

Moges, R.T. (2015a). Challenging sign language lineages and geographies: The case of Eritrean, Finnish, and Swedish Sign Languages. In M. Friedner & A. Kusters (Eds.), *It's a Small World: International Deaf Spaces and Encounters* (pp. 83–94). Washington, DC: Gallaudet University Press.

Moges. R.T. (2015b). *"Is the joke on us, deaf anthropologists? Reflections on native anthropology of deaf culture by deaf researchers."* Paper presented at the 7th International Deaf Academics and Researchers Conference, February 5–7, Leuven, Belgium. https://deafacademics2015.wordpress.com/presentations/

Monaghan, L., Schmaling, C., Nakamura, K., & Turner, G.H. (Eds.) (2003). *Many ways to be deaf. International variation in deaf communities*. Washington, DC: Gallaudet University Press.

Morgan, R. (Ed.) (2012). *"DEAF ME NORMAL": Deaf South Africans tell their life stories*. Pretoria: Unisa Press.

Murray, J. (2007). *"One touch of nature makes the whole world kin": The transnational lives of Deaf Americans, 1870–1924* (Unpublished doctoral dissertation). University of Iowa, Iowa City.

Murray, J. J. (2015). Linguistic human rights discourse in deaf community activism. *Sign Language Studies, 15*(4), 379–410.

Myers, S. S., & Fernandes, J. K. (2010). Deaf Studies: A critique of the predominant U.S. theoretical direction. *Journal of Deaf Studies and Deaf Education, 15*(1), 30–49.

Nakamura, K. (2006). *Deaf in Japan. Signing and the politics of identity*. Ithaca, NY: Cornell University Press.

Napier, J., & Rosenstock, R. (2015). *International Sign. Linguistic, usage, and status issues*. Washington, DC: Gallaudet University Press.

Napier, J. (2016). *Linguistic coping strategies of sign language interpreters*. Washington, DC: Gallaudet University Press.

Napier, J., & Leeson, L. (2016). *Sign language in action*. New York, NY: Palgrave Macmillan.

Napoli, D. J., & Mathur, G. (2011). *Deaf around the world: The impact of language*. Oxford: Oxford University Press.

Napoli, D. J. (2014). A magic touch: Deaf Gain and the benefits of tactile sensation. In H. Bauman & J. Murray (Eds.), *Deaf Gain: Raising the stakes for human diversity* (pp. 211–232). Minneapolis: University of Minnesota Press.

Nonaka, A. (2004). The forgotten endangered languages: Lessons on the importance of remembering from Thailand's Ban Khor Sign Language. *Language in Society, 33*, 737–767.

Nonaka, A. M. (2014). (Almost) everyone here spoke Ban Khor Sign Language—Until they started using TSL: Language shift and endangerment of a Thai village sign language. *Language & Communication, 38,* 54–72.

Nyst, V. (2012). Shared sign languages. In R. Pfau, M. Steinbach, & B. Woll (Eds.), *Sign language: An international handbook.* (Handbooks on Language and Communication Science 37) (pp. 552–574). Berlin: Mouton de Gruyter.

O'Brien, D. (2005). What's the sign for "pint"?—An investigation into the validity of two different models to describe Bristol's current Deaf pub culture (Unpublished (master's thesis). University of Bristol.

O'Brien, D., & Emery, S. D. (2014). The role of the intellectual in minority group studies: Reflections on Deaf Studies in social and political contexts. *Qualitative Inquiry, 20*(1), 27–36.

O'Connell, N., & Deegan, J. (2014). "Behind the teacher's back": An ethnographic study of deaf people's schooling experiences in the Republic of Ireland. *Irish Educational Studies, 33*(3), 229–247.

Oliver, M. (1990). *The politics of disablement.* Basingstoke: Macmillan.

Orfanidou, E., Woll, B., & Morgan, G. (Eds.) (2015). *Research methods in Sign Language Studies. A practical guide.* London: Wiley Blackwell.

Padden, C. (1980). The deaf community and the culture of deaf people. In C. Baker & R. Battison (Eds.), *Sign language and the deaf community* (pp. 98–104). Silver Spring, MD: National Association of the Deaf.

Padden, C. (1998). From the cultural to the bicultural: The modern Deaf community. In I. Parasnis (Ed.), *Culture and language diversity and the deaf experience* (pp. 79–98). New York: Cambridge University Press.

Padden, C., & Humphries, T. (1988). *Deaf in America.* Cambridge, MA: Harvard University Press.

Padden, C., & Humphries, T. (2005). *Inside deaf culture.* Cambridge, MA: Harvard University Press.

Palfreyman, N. (forthcoming) Social meanings of linguistic variation in Indonesian Sign Language. *Linguistik online.*

Parasnis, I. (2012). *Cultural and language diversity and the deaf experience.* Cambridge: Cambridge University Press.

Paris, D.G., & Wood, S.K. (Eds.) (2002). *Step into the circle: The heartbeat of American Indian, Alaska Native, and First Nations Deaf Communities.* Salem, OR: AGO Publications.

Paul, P.V., & Moores, D.F. (Eds.) (2012). *Deaf epistemologies: Multiple perspectives on the acquisition of knowledge.* Washington, DC: Gallaudet University Press.

Pfau, R., Steinbach, M., & Woll, B. (Eds.) (2012). *Sign language: An international handbook.* Berlin: De Gruyter Mouton.

Preston, P. (1994). *Mother father deaf: Living between sound and silence.* Cambridge, MA: Harvard University Press.

Quer, J. (2012). Legal pathways to the recognition of sign languages: A comparison of the Catalan and Spanish Sign Language Acts. *Sign Language Studies, 12*(4), 565–582.

Reagan, T. (2006). Language policy and sign languages. In T. Ricento (Ed.), *An introduction to language policy. Theory and method* (pp. 329–345). Oxford: Blackwell Publishing.

Reagan, T. (2011). Ideological barriers to American Sign Language: Unpacking linguistic resistance. *Sign Language Studies, 11*(4), 606–636.

Reffell, H., & McKee, R. (2009). Motives and outcomes of New Zealand Sign Language legislation: A comparative study between New Zealand and Finland. *Current Issues in Language Planning, 10*(3), 272–292.

Reilly, C. B., & Reilly, N. (2005). *The rising of lotus flowers: Self-education by deaf children in Thai boarding schools.* Washington, DC: Gallaudet University Press.

Ruiz-Williams, E., Burke, M., Chong, V.J., & Chainarong, N. (2015). "My deaf is not your deaf": Realizing intersectional realities at Gallaudet University. *It's a small world: International deaf spaces and encounters* (pp. 262–274). Washington, DC: Gallaudet University Press.

Sacks, O. (1989). *Seeing voices.* New York, NY: Vintage Press.

Safar, J. (2014). Village Sign Languages as gefährdete Sprachen: Eine Analyse von Diskursen über Chican Sign Language (Mexiko) (Unpublished master's thesis). University of Hamburg.

Sanchez, R. (2015). *Deafening modernism: Embodied language and visual poetics in American literature.* New York: NYU Press.

Sangalang, J. (2012). *What is privacy in Deaf Space?* (Unpublished master's thesis). Gallaudet University, Washington, DC.

Schein, J. (1989). *At home among strangers.* Washington, DC: Gallaudet University Press.

Schétrit, O. (2016). Approche filmique de la création artistique et des enjeux identitaires des Sourds en France et dans les réseaux transnationaux (Unpublished doctoral dissertation). Ecole des Hautes Études en Sciences Sociales (EHESS), Paris.

Schmaling, C. (2003). A for apple: The impact of Western education and ASL on the deaf community in Kano State, Northern Nigeria. In L. Monaghan, C. Schmaling, K. Nakamura, & Turner, G.H. (Eds.) (2003) *Many ways to be deaf: International variation in deaf communities* (pp. 302–310). Washington, DC: Gallaudet University

Senghas, R. (2016). Sign languages and communicative practices. In N. Bonvillain (Ed.), *The Routledge handbook of linguistic anthropology* (pp. 247–262). New York, NY: Routledge.

Shaw, C. (2015). "We have no need to lock ourselves away": Space, marginality, and the negotiation of deaf identity in late Soviet Moscow. *Slavic Review, 74*(1), 57–78.

Singleton, J.L., Jones, G., & Hanumantha, S. (2012). Deaf friendly research? Toward ethical practice in research involving deaf participants. *Deaf Studies Digital Journal 3.* Available from: http://dsdj.gallaudet.edu/index.php?issue=4&section_id=2&entry_id=123

Singleton, J.L., Jones, G., & Hanumantha, S. (2014). Toward ethical research practice with deaf participants. *Journal of Empirical Research on Human Research Ethics, 9*(3), 59–66.

Singleton, J. L., Martin, A. J., & Morgan, G. (2015). Ethics, deaf-friendly research, and good practice when studying sign languages. In E. Orfanidou, B. Woll, & G. Morgan (Eds.), *Research methods in sign language studies. A practical guide* (pp. 7–20). London: Wiley Blackwell.

Stapleton, L. D. (2014). *The unexpected talented tenth: Black d/Deaf students thriving within the margins* (Unpublished doctoral d). Ames, IA: Iowa State University.

Stapleton, L. D. (2015). The disabled academy: The experiences of deaf faculty at predominantly hearing institutions. *Thought & Action: The NEA Higher Education Journal,* Winter 2015, pp. 55–69.

Stokoe, W. (1960). Sign language structure: An outline of the visual communication systems of the American deaf. In *Studies in Linguistics: Occasional Papers* (No. 8). Buffalo, NY: Department of Anthropology and Linguistics, University of Buffalo.

Stokoe, W. C., Casterline, D.C., & Croneberg, C. (1965). *A dictionary of American Sign Language on linguistic principles.* Washington, DC: Gallaudet University Press.

Sutherland, H., & Rogers, K.D. (2014). The hidden gain: A new lens of research with d/Deaf children and adults. In H.-D. L. Bauman & J. Murray (Eds.), *Deaf Gain: Raising the stakes for human diversity* (pp. 269–282). Minneapolis: University of Minnesota Press.

Sutherland, H., & Young, A. (2014). Research with deaf children and not on them: A Study of Method and Process. *Children & Society, 28*(5), 366–379.

Sutton-Spence, R., & West, D. (2011). Negotiating the Legacy of Hearingness. *Qualitative Inquiry, 17*(5), 422–432.

Swanwick, R. (2015). Scaffolding Learning through Classroom Talk: The Role of Translanguaging. In M. Marschark & P. E. Spencer (Eds.), *The Oxford Handbook of Deaf Studies in Language Research, Policy and Practice* (pp. 45–61). Oxford: Oxford University Press.

Taylor, G., & Bishop, J. (Eds.) (1991). *Being Deaf: The Experience of Deafness.* London: Continuum

Tervoort, B. (1953). *Structurele analyse van visueel taalgebruik binnen een groep dove kinderen [Structural analysis of visual language use within a group of deaf children].* Amsterdam: Noord-Hollandsche Uitgeverij.

Timmermans, N. (2005). *A comparative analysis of the status of sign languages in Europe.* Strasbourg: Council of Europe.

Trowler, P. R., & Turner, G. H. (2002). Exploring the hermeneutic foundations of university life: Deaf academics in a hybrid "community of practice." *Higher Education, 43,* 227–256.

Turner, G. H. (1994). How is deaf culture? Another perspective on a fundamental concept. *Sign Language Studies, 83*(1), 103–126.

Turner, G. H. (2007). The Deaf Studies Project: More questions than answers. *Deaf Worlds, 23*(2&3), 1–16.

Valentine, G., & Skelton, T. (2008) Changing spaces: the role of the internet in shaping Deaf geographies. *Social & Cultural Geography, 9,* 469–486.

Van Cleve, J. V., & Baker-Shenk, C. (Eds.). (1987). *Gallaudet encyclopedia of deaf people and deafness. (Vol. 1–3).* New York: McGraw-Hill Professional.

Van Cleve, J. V., & Crouch, B. (1992). *A place of their own: Creating the deaf community in America.* Washington, DC: Gallaudet University Press.

Van Herreweghe, M., De Meulder, M., & Vermeerbergen, M. (2015). From Erasure to Recognition (and Back Again?): The Case of Flemish Sign Language. In M. Marschark & P. E. Spencer (Eds.), *The Oxford Handbook of Deaf Studies in Language Research, Policy and Practice* (pp. 45–61). Oxford: Oxford University Press.

VanGilder, K. (2012). *Making Sadza with Deaf Zimbabwean Women: A Missiological Reorientation of Practical Theological Method*. Göttingen: Vandenhoeck & Ruprecht.

VanGilder, K. (2015). Exploring the Contours of Deaf-Same: Kinship Bonds and Mutuality in United Methodist Short-Term Missions. In M. Friedner & A. Kusters (Eds.), *It's a small world: International deaf spaces and encounters* (pp. 140–150). Washington, DC: Gallaudet University Press.

Walby, S., Armstrong, J., & Strid, S. (2012). Intersectionality: Multiple Inequalities in Social Theory. *Sociology, 46*(2), 224–240

Wilcox, S. (Ed.). (1989). *American deaf culture: An anthology.* Silver Spring, MD: Linstock Press.

Wilson, A. T., & Winiarczyk, R. E. (2014). Mixed Methods Research Strategies With Deaf People: Linguistic and Cultural Challenges Addressed. *Journal of Mixed Methods Research, 8*(3), 266–277.

Woodcock, K., Rohan, M. J., & Campbell, L. (2007). Equitable representation of deaf people in mainstream academia: Why not? *Higher Education, 53,* 359–379.

Woodward, J. (1975) *How you gonna get to heaven if you can't talk with Jesus: The educational establishment vs. the Deaf community.* Paper presented at the Annual Meeting of the Society for Applied Anthropology, Amsterdam.

Woodward, J. & Horejes, T. (2016). deaf/Deaf: Origins and Usage. *The SAGE Deaf Studies encyclopedia.* Sage Publishing.

Wrigley, O. (1996). *The Politics of Deafness.* Washington DC: Gallaudet University Press.

Young, A. M., & Ackerman, J. (2001). Reflections on Validity and Epistemology in a Study of Working Relations Between Deaf and Hearing Professionals. *Qualitative Health Research, 11*(2), 179–189.

Young, A., & Temple, B. (2014). Approaches to Social Research: the Case of Deaf Studies. Oxford University Press.

Zehnter, J. (2014). I was a stranger and you took me in: Om religiøse og institutionelle dimensioner ved et rehabiliteringsprojekt for hjemløse kvinder i New York City Unpublished master's thesis). University of Copenhagen.

Zeshan, U. (2015). "Making meaning"—Communication between sign language users without a shared language. *Cognitive Linguistics, 26*(2), 211–260.

SECTION I

Developments and Directions in Deaf Studies

2

Deaf-led Deaf Studies: Using Kaupapa Māori Principles to Guide the Development of Deaf Research Practices

Dai O'Brien

The field of Deaf Studies has been established for around 40 years, existing in various university departments and centers around the world, including at Gallaudet University in the United States, the Centre for Deaf Studies at the University of Bristol, England, and the Victoria University of Wellington, New Zealand, to name but three. The discipline established roots in the linguistic study of sign languages, thanks to early groundbreaking work (Tervoort 1953, Stokoe 1960, 1965), before starting to widen in scope to include more political, social, and cultural aspects of the deaf experience of life (Lane 1989, 1999; Padden & Humphries 1988, Turner 2007). The field is now very much interdisciplinary, with the range of current work ably reflected in this volume, from human geography to anthropology, and from theology to linguistics. There is a risk that given the vast range of approaches and theoretical backgrounds each discipline brings to the field, they might not make happy bedfellows. For example, the more quantitative elements of some linguistic or educational approaches may not sit easy with the more avowedly qualitative approaches of anthropological methods. This is a risk in such a small field, because this diversity of approaches and epistemologies could cause a lack of unity or fragmentation, but it also could be considered a strength, providing the field with a wide variety of methodologies and theories with which to engage.

It should be noted that for the purposes of this chapter, the term Deaf Studies is used to refer to all research performed on or with signing (visual or tactile) deaf communities and individuals who identify with those communities, whether the researchers performing the research would consider themselves to be acting in the field of Deaf Studies or not. Research conducted in the field of anthropology, for example, when the focus of the research is signing deaf individuals or communities, would be subsumed under the label of Deaf Studies. Similarly, research conducted using the theories of human geography, or linguistics, or indeed, any study in which the main focus is the cultures, communities, and signed languages of deaf communities is considered, for the purposes of this chapter, Deaf Studies. This is a deliberately provocative stance with which some academics, deaf and hearing, may disagree; but it is taken in an attempt to draw attention to the impact that such work has on representing deaf people in the academy. I accept that others have different definitions of what should be included under the label of Deaf Studies (Fernandes & Myers 2010; see also discussion in the introduction to this volume), but the definition of Deaf Studies used in this chapter is an attempt to "impose on [the field] common principles of vision and division, and thus a unique vision of its identity and an identical vision of its unity" (Bourdieu 1991:224). Using signed languages as the principle of "vision and division" is a way of allowing focus on the concept of Deaf Studies, the reasons for which I hope will become clear as the chapter progresses.

I also accept that for some readers, the use of "community" in this chapter will be problematic. The increased individualization and recognition of individuals in the late modern/postmodern turn problematizes the notion of community (Eagleton 1992, but see also Delanty 2003). Recent scholarship in Deaf Studies also problematizes the notion of a deaf community (again, see the introduction to this volume for more discussion of the problematization of the term "deaf community"). In this chapter, however, I am exercising a certain level of strategic essentialism (Kusters & De Meulder 2013, Ladd 2003) to emphasize the fact that many signing deaf people do, indeed, feel part of a "deaf community." They are part of a sociolinguistic minority group linked by their shared experiences, biology, and community loyalties.

The values of deaf people and deaf communities, those of information sharing, prioritizing visual and tactile-sense languages over spoken or written forms, and collectivism and solidarity with deaf communities (Ladd 2003, Mindess 1999) are often at odds with the values of the academy, where the focus is often on individual progression, publishing journal articles in English-language print journals, preparing for the REF (Research Excellence Framework) assessment (in the United Kingdom), and maintaining a high turnover of research projects without necessarily feeding the findings back to the communities from which the data were gathered (Head 2011). Many deaf academics feel an overriding or equally strong loyalty to the deaf communities with whom they work or in which they live, rather than to the academy (De Meulder 2007, Trowler & Turner 2002). As a consequence, they feel that dissemination of research to deaf communities in sign language, along with consultation with deaf people in research decisions should take priority over, or is equally important to, hegemonic academic values.

Community loyalties also often are shown by being active in various deaf associations, deaf club committees, and other positions of responsibility, which again, can conflict with academic loyalties or commitments. Although it could be argued that this is a false dichotomy and that an academic could, in fact, do both, in practical terms this is rarely the case. Each of these duties takes time, energy, and resources, and as a matter of pragmatism, a deaf academic must choose between the two value sets, or spend vast quantities of time and energy negotiating difficult pathways between the two. In this sense, those deaf academics who navigate these sometimes conflicting priorities could be described as organic intellectuals, academics who have come from within a particular community or social group (Gramsci 1971) and whose loyalties lie with those communities.

Of course, not all deaf academics feel this direct loyalty or connection to specific deaf communities. They may, for example, deliberately or incidentally isolate themselves from other deaf people, or they may work at a remove with deaf people in other countries or communities. Those who do not feel this sense of duty to deaf communities could be termed traditional academics (Gramsci 1971) and could be said to "fit" better into the values of the academy. The potential for tension between the values of organic deaf academics and the academy can result in conflicts between deaf academics who take a more radical, political stance, such as prioritizing dissemination to deaf communities in sign over written dissemination in publications or insisting on deaf leadership of research projects in the field and in the academic structures in which they work, structures which may mandate the status quo (O'Brien & Emery 2014).

In the past, Deaf Studies academics, to define and frame the field, have borrowed approaches and theories from disciplines as diverse as disability studies, feminist and women's studies, Black studies, and queer studies (see Bauman 2008, Brueggemann 2010, and Friedner 2010 for examples of this multidisciplinary engagement and also see Ladd 2003). These borrowings usually are justified on the grounds of shared experiences of oppression or exclusion. Deaf ontologies, however, are not only the result of discrimination due to an inability to hear, but also due to the preferential focus given to visual and tactile experiences, languages, and ways of understanding the world. This means that the rather simplistic comparisons with the discrimination and oppression explored in the disciplines mentioned earlier has limited potential. Not only this, but such comparisons also erase the specific experiences of people used as comparison groups, which could be interpreted as inflicting epistemic violence on these groups. This is not to say that deaf academics and Deaf Studies have nothing to learn from these other disciplines, but that simplistic comparison of experience or uncritical appropriation of theory and approach is not productive. Instead, it can be more useful to look at the ethical and practical frameworks used in these fields and consider whether they can act as guides to developing specific deaf-centric approaches.

How can we develop a framework that is rooted in the values and beliefs of deaf people and deaf communities? How could this framework shift the focus of Deaf Studies away from that of traditional academics rooted in the hegemony of the academic environment, the academic priorities and languages of the hearing academia? Some suggestions have been made in the Deaf Studies literature already (see, for example, Harris et al. 2009, Singleton et al. 2015, Singleton et al. 2014) for "deaf friendly" research ethics, but these have come from within existing hegemonic academic norms, or are relatively uncritical adaptations of existing ethical frameworks, rather than being primarily founded on deaf cultural values. Singleton et al.'s work (2015, 2014) relied on focus groups conducted with staff and students from within Gallaudet University. The fact that all of the participants in this research were staff, students, or researchers at an institution of higher education would suggest that there could be bias in favor of academic values and practices rather than values and practices of nonacademic deaf communities. Harris et al. (2009) suggest that "Investigators should acknowledge that Sign Language community members have the right to have those things that they value to be fully considered in all interactions" (116). Although this is a laudable aim, it remains a suggestion ("*should*") and is written from the perspective of the academic, rather than the community. A model, or guide, for refocusing these ethical frameworks so that they are rooted in the values and beliefs of deaf people and communities could be found in Kaupapa Māori theory.

In this chapter, I suggest that following the example of the Kaupapa Māori[1] research framework would offer more coherency and power of advocacy to the field, in comparison with the less well-connected patchwork of frameworks currently employed. The Kaupapa Māori framework is based on the ontologies and epistemologies of the Māori people of New Zealand. Although Kaupapa Māori frameworks borrow from other academic theories and methodologies, such as critical theory and action research, this framework has been developed by the Māori community, for the Māori community. It was developed in response to pressures on Māori communities and Māori researchers by the hegemonic white European (Pakeha) approach taken by the academy in New Zealand and the challenges that this approach caused for the Māori community. The Kaupapa Māori framework is rooted in the

---

[1] In some references, the word "Kaupapa" in Kaupapa Māori is capitalized, in others it is not. It seems to me that, on balance, it is capitalized more often than not, so it is capitalized in this chapter.

Māori community, in the history, experiences, and beliefs of the Māori people. This approach has created a research framework, which, while not prescriptive in nature, nonetheless outlines key guiding principles for conducting ethical research, research that is acceptable to and supported by the community, and that is rooted in Māori ontologies.

This chapter does not suggest lifting the Kaupapa Māori approach wholesale, but rather suggests using it as an inspiration for developing our own approaches and ethical frameworks in Deaf Studies research; approaches that truly are rooted in the ontologies and epistemologies of deaf people and communities. Findings from a workshop held in the United Kingdom to discuss the creation of such a deaf-led Deaf Studies framework are presented, with a discussion of the initial principles that arose from the dialogue among deaf academics, researchers, and professionals in the workshop. The implications for such a framework also are discussed, along with the possibilities that the adoption of such a framework suggest for the Kaupapa Māori-influenced approaches in Deaf Studies.

KAUPAPA MĀORI THEORY AND RESEARCH

The Māori community in New Zealand is, in many ways, in a similar position to deaf communities in the United Kingdom and other countries. It is a sociolinguistic minority community, with its own language, *te reo* Māori (often shortened, as here, to te reo), community, and culture, which has for many years undergone sustained pressure to integrate into the Pakeha majority (May 2012). In New Zealand academia, the fate and treatment of the Māori community has been similar to that of deaf communities. Māori have been treated as deficient populations in research associated with education and social care, in which the blame for lack of achievement or ill health is placed firmly on their shoulders due to lack of application in school or employment, lack of inherent intelligence, biological inferiority, or other perceived factors (Mahuika 2011). Māori academics also were expected to accept Pakeha hegemony in the academic field, accepting hegemonic practices such as the primacy of the English language and colonialists' history over the indigenous language histories of Māori people and the exclusion of Māori values and the priorities of their communities (Bishop et al. 2003). Māori culture and language were excluded from and devalued in the public sphere through emphasis on the English language and Pakeha values, resulting in declining numbers in te reo speakers and lack of awareness of the Māori culture, until the 1980s, when a social revolution occurred in the way in which Māori thought about themselves.

In 1971, a report published by Richard Benton suggested that te reo was in decline, and by 1974, only 15% of young Māori under the age of 15 were able to speak te reo. Of those who were fluent, more than 38% were over the age of 45 (Te Rito 2008). Te reo was not being passed on from generation to generation due to various cultural pressures, including mainstream education policies. This brought with it additional feelings of shame and the belief that it was no longer a living language, and, therefore, of no use in the modern world (Spolsky 2003). According to the Māori academic, Graham Hingangaroa Smith, this shocked parts of the Māori community into action, and they set up "language nests," te reo-medium childcare groups (Te Kōhanga Reo), which later developed into government recognized and funded te reo-medium schools (kura kaupapa Māori) at both primary and secondary educational levels, which are now developing into tertiary education (Smith 2003). This activist mentality also impacted on Māori academics at the time. Academic research linked to Māori communities then was dominated by medical, historical, and educational research that was informed by Pakeha ontologies and cultural expectations (for a criticism of the similar discourses applied to deaf communities, see Branson & Miller 2002). There was no consideration of the Māori way of being or knowing. For example, medical interventions often ignored the importance of *whanau,* or family, in treatment and support of the patient or affected individual. Following Māori cultural values, whanau are much more likely to play an important role in supporting affected individuals than their equivalents in Pakeha communities (Te Pou 2010). Pakeha academics were presenting themselves as experts in Māori culture, but their research was felt by Maōri people to be unrepresentative of their lives (Mahuika 2011) (for a similar criticism of hearing academics in Deaf Studies, see Baker-Shenk & Kyle 1990). Not only did they feel this way, but the findings of the research were not being fed back into the Māori community. The community was not seeing the benefits of the research based upon its knowledge, its language, and its culture, which had been turned into so many publications gathering dust on academic bookshelves (Walker, Eketone & Gibbs 2006).

Graham Hingangaroa Smith's (1997) PhD dissertation, which reframed the educational and schooling practices of Māori communities as Kaupapa Māori, became the turning point for many Māori researchers. "Kaupapa" can be simplistically translated into English as a policy, initiative, or scheme. Smith's work was the first attempt to frame a research approach rooted in the values of the Māori community from which he came. Smith, and subsequent researchers in the field, established a number of different principles by which Kaupapa Māori research must be conducted in order for it to be acceptable to the Māori community. These principles are not intended as prescriptive, that is, they do not specify that research must utilize a certain method or specific mode of analysis; instead, they provide an overarching philosophy that can guide the intentions and motivations behind the research (Pihama 2001, Lee 2005).

Although some Māori academics hold that it is unproductive to attempt to define Kaupapa Māori research in this way, for the interests of clarity, I will summarize the outline of five principles of Kaupapa Māori research suggested by Walker, Eketone, and Gibbs (2006). There are other summaries of principles written by different Māori academics (see, for example, Hill & May 2013, Kerr et al. 2010, Bishop et al. 2003, and, of course, Smith 1997), but most summaries agree with these basic tenets.

1. *Tino rangatiratanga*—the principle of self-determination. This is "about a Māori-centred agenda where the issues and needs of Māori are the focus and outcomes of research" (Walker, Eketone & Gibbs 2006). One of the advantages of this principle is that "when Māori make decisions for themselves, the 'buy in' and commitment by Māori participants to making the ideas work is more certain and assured" (Smith 2003).

2. Social justice. This principle aims to redress power imbalances and bring about "positive outcomes" for Māori people (Mane 2009). Researchers who utilize the Kaupapa Māori framework believe that Kaupapa Māori research should "enhance the quality of life for Māori" (Walker, Eketone & Gibbs 2006) and ensure that the research they do makes a positive contribution to the Māori community.

3. The Māori worldview. Under this principle, " 'to be Māori' is taken for granted: there is little need to justify one's identity" (Smith 2003). This not only has a legitimating effect on the views of Māori, it also prioritizes the epistemologies and ontologies of the Māori community, such as the importance of respecting others and making contact face-to-face, rather than remaining anonymous through gatekeepers or technologies such as e-mail or telephones (Jones et al. 2010). In the case of Kaupapa Māori research, one implication of this principle is that respecting the Māori worldview has "profound effects on how we see and utilise methodologies and fundamentally shape[s] our relationships to knowledge and practice" (Kerr et al. 2010). It thus plays an essential role in the design and running of research.

4. *Te reo*. This principle of Kaupapa Māori research "asserts Māori language... as integral to its practice" (Mane 2009). The implication of this is that te reo is central to the practice and understanding of the Kaupapa Māori framework. "Te Reo Māori is the only language that can access, conceptualise and internalise in spiritual terms this body of knowledge. From this, we take it that Māori language and Kaupapa Māori knowledge are inextricably bound. One is the means to the other" (International

Research Institute [IRI] 2000). Te reo is, therefore, used as the language of instruction at all levels of te reo-medium education, including at tertiary level. Given the fact that fluency in te reo is not universal in the Māori community, however, this principle is sometimes interpreted as the imperativeness of the "survival and revival of Māori language" (Pihama et al. 2004). For many Māori researchers engaging in Kaupapa Māori research, this means that they include te reo in publications. This could either be in the form of a ritual greeting at the beginning of the publication (Pihama et al. 2004, for example), or te reo is used throughout alongside English (Pihama 2001). Some documents are written in te reo, with a translation into English made available (Department of Internal Affairs 2008).

5. *Whanau*. This principle refers to family, but also includes the idea of "connectedness between Māori" (Walker, Eketone & Gibbs 2006). This is very important, because it not only leads to a shared vision of research, but also respects Māori traditions of knowledge sharing, which in the case of Kaupapa Māori research, includes the results of research projects and community structure (Jones et al. 2010).

These principles combine to produce a research framework rooted in the values and beliefs of the Māori community.

KAUPAPA MĀORI AS A GUIDE FOR DEAF STUDIES

Kaupapa Māori as a research framework is more than just a theory; it is a praxis, that is, "*reflection* and *action* directed at structures to be transformed" (Freire 1996). It is a guide to not only performing research, but to performing research in such a way that challenges the hegemony, the established way of doing things, that has resulted in so much misrepresentation of the Māori community by academia. It is also a direct challenge to postcolonial and "de-colonization" theory, which, according to Smith (2003), places too much emphasis on the colonizers, returning them to the center. Instead, Kaupapa Māori theory places "what it is that we want, what is that we are about and to 'imagine' our future (sic)" (Smith 2003), recentering the focus on the Māori community and its own aims, needs, and aspirations.

For Deaf Studies, a similar recentering must take place. Recent publications have opened a debate about the relations between deaf and hearing academics (Sutton-Spence & West 2011, O'Brien & Emery 2014, Young & Temple 2014, and this volume). Although many hearing academics have made, and continue to make, immensely valuable contributions to the field of Deaf Studies, it is time for deaf academics and deaf communities to consider, as Smith (2003) put it, "what it is that we want, what is that we are about and to 'imagine' our future (sic)." Ladd (2003) has posited that Deaf Studies has long been on the defensive, that it has focused on defending the concepts of deaf culture and community and the value of sign languages. Instead, Kaupapa Māori research challenges us to ignore these "politics of distraction" that keep us on the back foot, and instead focus on "freeing the mind from the grip of dominant hegemony" (Smith 2003).

Of course, in order to do this, it is very important to establish what the values and principles of deaf communities actually are. It should be noted here that I use the plural form of deaf communities. Much like Māori people (Mahuika 2011), deaf people cannot be reduced to a single monolithic concept of "deaf culture" (see Friedner & Kusters 2015, and Friedner in this volume, for further discussion of this, including the principle of DEAF-SAME). Within each (inter)national deaf community, however, or within each local deaf community (depending on the scale on which a particular research project is being held), principles can be agreed upon. The way in which Kaupapa Māori represents the beliefs of the Māori community has been explained as follows,

> Tuakana Nepe (1991:15) . . . states that Kaupapa Māori is the "conceptualisation of Māori knowledge" that has been developed through oral tradition. This is the process by which the Māori mind "receives, internalises, differentiates, and formulates ideas and knowledge exclusively through Te Reo Māori." ... Kaupapa Māori knowledge has its origins in a metaphysical base that is distinctly Māori. As Nepe states, this influences the way Māori people think, understand, interact and interpret the world. (IRI 2000)

A deaf version of this representation of beliefs could be the American concept DEAF-WAY, or the UK version DEAF-HIS [sic] (Ladd, 2003). These glosses attempt to render in English a concept that is expressed easily in sign language. That is, the principle that there are specific ways for deaf people to think about, to experience, and to know the world. In other words, deaf ontologies that are based upon deaf experience of what it is to be deaf.

Little work has been done, however, that attempts to get to the root of what this deaf ontology could be, as opposed to the decades invested in negotiating the Kaupapa Māori framework. Earlier waves of Deaf Studies have tended to be descriptive, rather than exploring what lies at the heart or the root of these beliefs and experiences. But it is important to note, again, that we cannot uncritically adopt Kaupapa Māori principles in Deaf Studies. There are several important differences between Māori and Deaf communities: One such difference is that Māori communities are geographically rooted and located, their traditions are passed vertically from generation to generation within family groups, whereas deaf communities have been described as diaspora communities without a homeland (Emery 2015, Lane 2005), and their traditions are passed mainly horizontally among generations, with very few family groups.

Ladd's Deafhood principle suggests one potential path toward exploring the possibility of a rootedness in community values similar to that of the Kaupapa Māori framework. Deafhood has been described as an exploratory concept, a way for deaf people "to explain to themselves and each other their own existence in the world" (Ladd 2003), but it also has been described by Ladd as a "consciousness-raising strategy" aimed at community regeneration (Kusters & De Meulder 2013) and a way of offering "a chance for a community to find out what it might *become* once the weight of oppression is lifted" (Ladd 2003 [emphasis in original]). Furthermore, by foregrounding the ontological aspects of Deafhood, those aspects that examine the questions of being and becoming (Kusters & De Meulder 2013), the concept of Deafhood could form a starting point for the search for foundations for a deaf-led research framework along the lines of Kaupapa Māori research. By trying to find what it is that the community might become, by deciding which deaf traditions the community must keep and which are a damaging result of colonialism, Deafhood can lead us to the formulation of deaf-led principles that can guide Deaf Studies research in a way that truly reflects deaf ways of being.

Once again, it is worth emphasizing here that by "Deaf Studies" I mean all research that is performed with or on (visual or tactile) signing deaf people, regardless of the theoretical, methodological, or structural background to the study. This reflects the changing nature of the field of Deaf Studies, in that many deaf (and hearing) academics no longer work in dedicated Deaf Studies units or departments, but find themselves embedded in the wider academy. This means that there is more need than ever for a coherent set of guidelines or principles for these academics and researchers to follow, given that they are working in isolated positions where they might not have institutional backing to perform research rooted in the values of deaf communities.

FIRST STEPS

To begin to explore the possibility of utilizing the Kaupapa Māori framework as an inspiration for creating a deaf-led Deaf Studies research framework, I organized and led a one-day workshop in the United Kingdom in 2014. There were seven participants in this workshop, all of whom had experience in working in academia in the United Kingdom, and all of whom strongly self-identified as members of various deaf communities in the country. This experience ranged from working as research assistants and teachers to being lead academics on university courses. Following an initial briefing about the history and principles of the Kaupapa Māori research framework (similar to what was outlined earlier in this chapter), the rest of the day was given over to discussing what could be the founding principles for a similar framework for research with deaf people. To describe what we were discussing, participants in the workshop ended up using a term in British Sign Language, which can be loosely translated as the "deaf research framework." For convenience, I continue to use this term here.

Four preliminary principles were suggested as a result of this workshop. These are summarized here.

1. *The primacy of sign languages*
2. *Self-determination*
3. *Identity preservation*
4. *Community development*

The Primacy of Sign Language

All of the participants in the workshop believed that although sign languages are a central part of deaf life, they are not valued by hegemonic academia. Some of the participants had struggled with working in academia, where they were almost language exiles, and where involvement in their workplace, even in Deaf Studies departments, was limited due to the primacy placed on English rather than sign languages. The importance of using sign languages as the medium of Deaf Studies work went to the heart of much of the discussion in the workshop about various aspects of research. As the language of choice in Deaf Studies departments and research units, sign languages were suggested as the most natural and politically correct choice. As languages in which to conduct research with deaf people and communities, for participant recruitment and informed consent, for research activities, and for subsequent dissemination of findings, again, sign languages were suggested as the most natural language choice. One example of prioritizing sign languages in this way would be the Deaf Academics conferences, in which research findings are shared in International Sign. Another would be Kusters's (2012) practice of gaining informed consent from deaf research participants in sign language, rather than with written consent forms. Both of these examples have their problems. The Deaf Academics conference, by its nature, can exclude hearing academics, non-Western academics subject to the prohibitive cost of travel and visa issues, and those who are not fluent in International Sign. Informed consent statements in sign, rather than in writing, can be in direct conflict with the requirements of research ethics boards. Of course, this principle was understood to bring the deaf research framework into direct conflict with the Anglophone academic world, in which the written English language is fetishized as the language of publication and consent. All participants strongly felt, however, that in order to redress this balance and bring the focus back to deaf community values, primacy must, in principle, be given to sign languages. This is one example of the transformative potential of such a framework or praxis.

Self-determination

Self-determination, in this context, is meant to refer to deaf control of Deaf Studies, with deaf people making the important decisions about how the field is run, how research funding is distributed, and how research is conducted and disseminated. Much like the Māori community in response to Benton's (1971) report, the deaf participants in the workshop felt that there must be "a shift away from waiting for things to be done to them, to doing things for themselves" (Smith 2003). All participants felt that it was important for deaf academics, and deaf communities as a whole, to accept responsibility for the situation of Deaf Studies and challenge the hegemony of hearing-led, medicalized, and linguistic research in favor of research that is valued by deaf communities and gives back tangible benefits to deaf people, with direct impact on policies or practices that have negative effects on their lives (see Emery 2008, and Emery & Ladd ND, Deafhood and Genetics at www.deafhoodgenetics.com, for examples of deaf-led research led by specific deaf community interests). The participants felt that the nature of some linguistic research, which focuses on cataloguing and describing languages, offers little of direct value for those deaf people who consider themselves part of a deaf community. Rather, participants felt that linguistic research should prioritize work that focuses on education of deaf children in sign language, language development and promotion, and development of teaching resources.

It was recognized that some deaf academics may find this a particularly challenging principle. Many deaf academics have, due to the lack of a strong presence of deaf people in the academy, and a lack of academic habitus and capital of their own (O'Brien & Emery 2014), relied at least in part on the patronage of hearing academics. This could take the form of supervision of their PhD studies and subsequent support from hearing supervisors, working on hearing-led research projects, or relying on the advocacy of hearing colleagues rather than self-advocacy in the fight for self-determination and autonomy. Such reliance does not deny the hugely valuable contributions of hearing academics to Deaf Studies, or deny hearing academics and allies a place in the future of Deaf Studies, but does demand a fundamental renegotiation of the ways in which deaf and hearing academics work together (see Jones & Pullen 1992 for an account of deaf-hearing relations in academic research). Participants in the workshop did not feel that it was impossible for hearing people to make a contribution to the field.

If the principles of the deaf research framework were followed, hearing academics could make valuable contributions to the field of Deaf Studies, in much the same way as Pakeha researchers could follow the Kaupapa Māori framework (Smith 1999, Hill & May 2013). Indeed, in much the same way as not every Māori researcher will be able to conduct Kaupapa Māori research (Lee 2005), not every deaf person would be able to conduct research following the deaf research framework; for example, those who do not have a deep knowledge of sign language or a commitment to deaf communities and cultures.

Identity Preservation

This principle was linked to preservation of deaf identities on both an individual and collective level. "Deaf identities" in this context meant being role models as signing deaf persons and upholding the values of their deaf communities, such as the primacy of sign languages, loyalty to community members, and so on. This concept is one of the founding concepts of the field of Deaf Studies (see introduction chapter, this volume, for more discussion). It was felt that the pressure to conform to the hegemonic behaviors, beliefs, and attitudes of the academy could lead deaf academics to become "more hearing", to forego signing in favor of trying to communicate through spoken languages, to take on individualist academic behaviors that would clash with the collective nature of deaf communities. Participants felt that it was important for deaf academics to preserve their deaf identities in these circumstances, to act as role models for deaf people who might wish to become involved in academia, and to act as cultural models for others who may not understand the values of deaf cultures and communities. This does not just mean using sign languages, it also means exhibiting a commitment to promoting and supporting other deaf people, such as by acting as mentors or advocates for them in higher education. A deaf research framework would have such a positive deaf identity as its core and would work to preserve and develop this identity. On a professional level, deaf academics would, therefore, have a responsibility to represent, promote, and develop a deaf academic identity, in other words, to prove that it is possible to be a successful academic as a signing deaf person.

Community Development

This principle was very much linked to Principle One, the centrality of sign languages, and Principle Three, the preservation of deaf identities. It stated that all research conducted under a deaf research framework should contribute in some way to the development of deaf communities. This contribution could be through supporting language rights, improving educational provision for deaf people, and so on. A key element of this was that deaf people and deaf communities should be consulted about the content and direction of research. This consultation could take the form of an initial discussion with the community involved, or representatives of that community, to consider what their priorities from the research would be. The researcher then would create and conduct research projects in partnership with these community representatives to ensure that the needs and priorities of the community remained an integral part of the project, and that the outcomes of the research directly contributed to strengthening and supporting the deaf community. Such projects could be seen as a form of action research. One such example would be the Our Space meetings set up by John Walker in Brighton, in the United Kingdom,[2] in which community members were invited to share their knowledge, experience, and skills with one another, based on the "communities of practice" approach (Wenger 1999).[3]

Of course, rather than suggesting that this workshop led us to any answers or principles that we can agree on as foundational for a deaf research framework, we must admit that the workshop could be seen as raising more questions than answers. Significantly, although all the participants considered themselves members of the UK deaf community, they all were, or had been, practicing academics. There were no participants in the workshop who were not involved in academia in some way, so the perspectives of the nonacademic sector were absent. This is a definite weakness in the initial findings of this workshop. The workshop was meant, however, as merely the beginning of a process of exploring the implications of a research framework. The involvement of nonacademic deaf people is a definite priority for the future.

This discussion also highlighted the question of how to police such a framework? Inevitably, any process that is community-based and rooted in activism would have to be self-policed. This could take the form of published guidelines (written and signed), much like those published by various professional bodies, such the British Sociological Association, or the American Anthropological Association (both of which are available on the respective association websites). Some

---

[2] http://www.sussexdeafhistory.org.uk/category_id__37.aspx

[3] Interestingly, a reviewer of this chapter questioned whether a theoretical volume such as this one, exploring deaf ontologies, would fall foul of this principle. Of course, without reference to a discussion group of deaf people to thoroughly explore this issue, a firm answer cannot be given. My own feeling is, though, that this volume, being written and edited solely by deaf people, exploring issues that are inextricably linked to the experience of being deaf, and placing primacy on work done by deaf academics, meets three of the four principles suggested. The only one it does not meet, that of the primacy of sign languages, is a result of the compromises one must currently make in academia—prioritizing English publication over sign.

participants believed that it eventually would be necessary or desirable to set up some kind of deaf-led deaf academic body or network, which would not only approve research that followed the deaf research framework and provide guidance to prospective researchers on how to conduct such research, but also eventually be able to award research funding itself. The priorities of this body in awarding research funding would follow the principles outlined earlier in this chapter. A major element in the assessment of applications for funding would, therefore, be the project's potential contribution to deaf communities, not merely its contribution to the academy. However, the practicalities of setting up this body and gaining control of research funding allocation remain to be discussed.

GOING FORWARD

I suggest that rather than answering all these questions, our workshop on a potential deaf research framework opened up negotiation about, and revealed, many barriers that deaf academics and deaf communities face in engaging effectively and constructively with the academy. These barriers could prevent this deaf research framework from being developed, disseminated, and utilized across the academy. However, the nature of the change being suggested here, that of challenging the hegemony of the academy, of making changes in the way in which a whole field of academic study should be run, opens up debate about the very nature of academic pursuit. What is considered to be "academic" varies immensely among different fields. For example, the quantitative nature of physics, chemistry, and other "hard sciences" as opposed to the qualitative nature of fine art or drama. Why, then, should Deaf Studies not have a different approach to academia? Why should it not have its own unique frameworks and rules to determine what is of worth within the field?

This pilot work took place in the United Kingdom. It is important to note here that I am not advocating a global essentialism of the deaf experience. Understanding, appreciation, and valuing of variation at a local, national, and international level would be an essential foundation of a deaf research framework. Such a framework must be for all deaf people, and so must be diverse and recognize the diversity within and among deaf communities (IRI 2000). Some principles could be considered universal; for example, the biologically rooted affinity for communication through the visual and tactile mode of sign language. This is only the first step to exploring the possibility and the potential of a deaf research framework, and it will require much more investigation, discussion, and negotiation by many other deaf academics and deaf people before it can become a reality.

CONCLUSION

Kaupapa Māori research took a long time to become established in the Māori community. Indeed, it remains "unknown territory for a significant part of the Māori population" (Mane 2009). Through decades of hard work and negotiation, however, it has become an accepted approach utilized by many different services and researchers in New Zealand—in health care, social care, education, and other settings (IRI 2000). In many different ways, Māori principles now influence the way in which the New Zealand Government work with Māori people. These principles are rooted in the Māori culture and community and ensure that Māori people are engaged with and benefit from the services on offer (IRI 2002). These principles also are informing Deaf Studies practices in New Zealand (Smiler & McKee 2007) by providing a framework through which to explore the dual heritage of deaf Māori. Although some sections of the Māori community may not yet know or understand the reasons for taking Kaupapa Māori approaches, as a research framework, as a theory, and as praxis, it is delivering tangible benefits for the Māori communities of New Zealand.

As already mentioned, Kaupapa Māori research is not prescriptive in the sense that it imposes particular research methods or disciplinary rules. Instead, it is about ensuring that the philosophy behind the research is in tune with the philosophy of the Māori community. It is suggested that a deaf research framework would provide similar scaffolding approaches for deaf communities. Engaging with such a research framework would not preclude any particular research areas so long as appropriate consultation and inclusion of deaf stakeholders was incorporated into project design. Similarly, it would not preclude any particular research methods, although it would promote engagement with methods most suitable for working with deaf people. These could include methods that prioritize visual and tactile experiences or expression, that include collective data collection such as focus groups and group interviews as well as individual interviews, and that prioritize signed forms of consent and dissemination over written forms. Such an engagement with a deaf research framework also would demand that research provide a tangible benefit for the deaf communities from which the research data was gathered.

By rooting their research framework and praxis in the epistemologies and ontologies of the Māori community in New Zealand, Māori academics have ensured that the feelings, beliefs, and priorities of the Māori community are reflected in the work that they do (see Beaton et al. 2015, Rata et al. 2012, for examples). Their struggle to achieve this has been long and hard, but the movement started from a situation of colonialism, academic underachievement, and exclusion from the academy (Jane 2001). Deaf academics start from very much the same position, with the Deaf Academics organization (DeafAcademics.org) having only 400 members worldwide (not all of whom are deaf, or, indeed, work in academia) (O'Brien & Emery 2014) and deaf children being failed in school at every level (see, for example, Marschark, Lang & Albertini 2002, Lang 2002). Deaf people "cannot afford to 'wait' to be invited into research academies" (Lee 2005), but must try to formulate ways in which deaf people and communities can be included in research activities as equals. As Smith has written, "we can't do any worse than the current system is doing—there is only one way to go—upward" (Smith 2003).

REFERENCES

Baker-Shenk, C., & Kyle, J. G. (1990). Research with deaf people: Issues and conflicts. *Disability & Society, 5,* 65–75.

Bauman, H.-D. L. (2008). *Open your eyes: Deaf studies talking.* Minneapolis: University of Minnesota Press.

Beaton, A., Smith, B., Toki, V., Southey, K., & Hudson, M. (2015). Engaging Māori in biobanking and genetic research: Legal, ethical, and policy challenges. *The International Indigenous Policy Journal, 6*(3). Retrieved from http://ir.lib.uwo.ca/iipj/vol6/iss3/1.

Bourdieu, P. (1991). *Language and symbolic power.* Cambridge: Polity Press.

Branson, J., & Miller, D. (2002). *Damned for their difference: The cultural construction of deaf people as disabled.* Washington, DC: Gallaudet University Press.

Brueggemann, B.J. (2010). The tango, or, what Deaf studies and disability studies do-do. In S. Burch & A. Kafer. (Eds.), *Deaf and disability studies: Interdisciplinary perspectives* (pp.245–265). Washington, DC: Gallaudet University Press.

Bishop, R., Berryman, M., Tiakiwai, S., & Richardson, C. (2003). *Te Kōtahitanga: The experiences of Year 9 and 10 Māori students in mainstream classrooms.* Wellington: New Zealand Ministry of Education.

De Meulder, M. (2007). GIVING BACK. Deaf professionals and the Deaf community. Unpublished MSc dissertation, University of Bristol.

Delanty, G. (2003). *Community.* London: Routledge.

Department of Internal Affairs. (2008). Official version of te aho matua o ngā kura kaupapa Māori: and an explanation in English. *New Zealand Gazette, 32,* 733–746.

Eagleton, T. (1992). *The illusions of postmodernism.* Oxford: Blackwell.

Emery, S.D. (2015). A deaf diaspora? Imagining deaf worlds across and beyond nations. In M. Friedner & A. Kusters. (Eds.), *It's a small world: International deaf spaces and encounters.* Washington, DC: Gallaudet University Press.

Emery, S. D. (2008). *The mental health needs of deaf Black minority ethnic people.* Greater Glasgow and Clyde National Health Service Board Mental Health Partnership.

Emery, S. D., & Ladd, P. (ND). Deafhood and Genetics. Retrieved from http://deafhoodgenetics.com/index.php/welcome.

Fernandes, J.K., & Myers, S.S. (2010). Inclusive Deaf Studies: Barriers and pathways. *Journal of Deaf Studies and Deaf Education, 15*(1), 17–29.

Freire, P. (1996). *Pedagogy of the oppressed.* London: Penguin Books.

Friedner, M. (2010). Biopower, biosociality and community formation: How biopower is constitutive of the Deaf community. *Sign Language Studies, 10*(3), 336–347.

Gramsci, A. (1971). *Selections from the prison notebooks*. Geneva: International Publishers.

Harris, R., Holmes, H. M., & Mertens, D. M. (2009). Research ethics in sign language communities. *Sign Language Studies, 9*(2), 104–131.

Head, S. (2011). The grim threat to British universities. *The New York Review of Books, 58*(1). Retrieved from http://www.nybooks.com/articles/archives/2011/jan/13/grim-threat-british-universities/.

Hill, R., & May, S. (2013). Non-indigenous researchers in indigenous language education: Ethical implications. *International Journal of the Sociology of Language, 219*, 47–65.

International Research Institute for Māori and Indigenous Education. (2000). *Māori research development: Kaupapa Māori principles and practices, a literature review*. International Research Institute for Māori and Indigenous Education (IRI): University of Auckland.

International Research Institute for Māori and Indigenous Education. (2002). *Iwi and Māori provider success: a research report of interviews with successful Iwi and Māori providers and government agencies*. International Research Institute for Māori and Indigenous Education (IRI): University of Auckland.

Jane, S. (2001). *Māori participation in higher education. Tainui graduates from the University of Waikato, 1992 to 1997* (Unpublished doctoral dissertation). University of Waikato.

Jones, L., & Pullen, G. (1992). Cultural differences: Deaf and hearing researchers working together. *Disability, Handicap & Society, 7*, 189–196.

Jones, B., Ingham, T., Davies, C., & Cram, F. (2010). Whānau Tuatahi: Māori community partnership research using a Kaupapa Māori methodology. *MAI Review 3*. Retrieved from http://www.review.mai.ac.nz/index.php/MR/issue/view/17.

Kerr, S., Penney, L., Moewaka Barnes, H., & McCreanor, T. (2010). Kaupapa Māori Action Research to improve heart disease services in Aotearoa, New Zealand. *Ethnicity & Health, 15*(1), 15–31.

Kusters, A. (2012). Being a deaf white anthropologist in Adamorobe: Some ethical and methodological issues. In U. Zeshan & C. de Vos (Eds.), *Sign languages in village communities: Anthropological and linguistic insights*. Berlin: Mouton de Gruyter.

Kusters, A., & De Meulder, M. (2013). Understanding Deafhood: In search of its meanings. *American Annals of the Deaf, 158*(5), 428–438.

Ladd, P. (2003). *Understanding deaf culture: In search of deafhood*. Clevedon: Multilingual Matters.

Lane, H. (2005). Ethnicity, ethics and the Deaf-World. *Journal of Deaf Studies and Deaf Education, 10*(3), 291–310.

Lane, H. (1999). *The mask of benevolence: Disabling the deaf community* (2nd ed.). San Diego, CA: Dawn Sign Press.

Lane, H. (1989). *When the mind hears: A history of the Deaf*. New York: Vintage Books.

Lang, H. G. (2002). Higher education for deaf students: Research priorities in the new millennium. *Journal of Deaf Studies and Deaf Education, 7*, 267–280.

Lee, J. (2005). *Māori cultural regeneration: Pūrākau as pedagogy*. Paper presented at "Indigenous (Māori) pedagogies: Towards community and cultural regeneration." Centre for Research in Lifelong Learning International Conference, Stirling, Scotland. Retrieved from http://www.kaupapamaori.com/assets/crll_final.pdf.

Mahuika, N. (2011). "Closing the gaps": From postcolonialism to Kaupapa Māori and beyond. *New Zealand Journal of History, 45*(1), 15–32.

Mane, J. (2009). Kaupapa Māori: A community approach. *MAI Review, 3*. Retrieved from http://www.review.mai.ac.nz/index.php/MR/issue/view/17.

Marschark, M., Lang, H.G., & Albertini, J.A. (2002). *Educating Deaf students: From research to practice*. Oxford: Oxford University Press.

May, S. (2012). *Language and minority rights. Ethnicity, nationalism and the politics of language* (2nd ed.). London: Routledge.

Mindess, A. (1999). *Reading between the signs: Intercultural communication for sign language interpreters*. Yarmouth: Intercultural Press.

O'Brien, D., & Emery, S.D. (2014). The role of the intellectual in minority group studies: Reflections on Deaf Studies in social and political contexts. *Qualitative Inquiry, 20*(1), 27–36.

Padden, C., & Humphries, T. (1988). *Deaf in America: Voices from a culture*. Cambridge, MA: Harvard University Press.

Pihama, L. (2001). *Tihei mauri ora Honouring our voices: Mana wahine as kaupapa Māori theoretical framework* (Unpublished doctoral dissertation). The University of Auckland.

Pihama, L., Smith, K., Taki, M., & Lee, J. (2004). *A literature review on Kaupapa Māori and Māori education pedagogy*. The International Research Institute for Māori and Indigenous Education. Auckland, New Zealand: University of Auckland.

Rata, A., Hutchings, J., & Liu, J.H. (2012). The Waka Hourua Research Framework: A dynamic approach to research with urban Māori communities. *The Australian Community Psychologist, 24*(1), 64–75.

Singleton, J.L, Martin, A.J., & Morgan, G. (2015). Ethics, deaf-friendly research, and good practice when studying sign languages. In E. Orfanidou, B. Woll & G. Morgan (Eds.), *Research methods in sign language studies: A practical guide* (pp. 7–20). Hoboken, NJ: Wiley-Blackwell.

Singleton, J.L., Jones, G., & Hanumantha, S. (2014). Toward ethical research practice with deaf participants. *Journal of Empirical Research on Human Research Ethics, 9*(59), 59–66.

Smiler, K., & McKee, R. L. (2007). Perceptions of Māori Deaf Identity in New Zealand. *Journal of Deaf Studies and Deaf Education, 12*(1), 93–111.

Smith, G. (2003). *Indigenous Struggle for the Transformation of Education and Schooling*. Keynote Address to Alaskan Federation and Natives (AFN) Convention. Anchorage, Alaska. Dates for Conference October 23, 2003.

Smith, G. (1997). *The development of kaupapa Māori: Theory and praxis* (Unpublished doctoral dissertation). University of Auckland.

Smith, L. T. (1999). *Decolonizing methodologies: Research and indigenous peoples*. New York: Palgrave.

Spolsky, B. (2003). Reassessing Māori regeneration. *Language in Society, 32*, 553–578.

Stokoe, W. C. (1960). Sign language structure: An outline of the visual communication systems of the American Deaf. *Studies in Linguistics: Occasional Papers, 8.* Buffalo, NY: Department. of Anthropology and Linguistics, University of Buffalo.

Stokoe, W. C., Casterline D.C., & Croneberg, C.G. (1965). *A dictionary of American sign languages on linguistic principles.* Washington, DC: Gallaudet College Press.

Tervoort, B. T. M. (1953). *Structurele analyse van visueel taalgebruik binnen een groep dove kinderen.* Amsterdam: N.V. Noord-Hollandsche.

Trowler, P. R., & Turner, G. H. (2002). Exploring the hermeneutic foundation of university life: Deaf academics in a hybrid "community of practice." *Higher Education, 43,* 227–256.

Turner, G. H. (2007). The Deaf Studies project: More questions than answers. *Deaf Worlds, 23*(2&3), 1–26.

Te Rito, J.S. (2008). Struggles for the Māori language: He whawhai mo te reo Māori. *MAI Review, 2.* Retrieved from http://www.review.mai.ac.nz/index.php/MR/issue/view/10.

Walker, S., Eketone, A., & Gibbs, A. (2006). An exploration of Kaupapa Māori research, its principles, processes and applications. *International Journal of Social Research Methodology, 9,* 331–334.

Wenger, E. (1999). *Communities of practice: Learning, meaning and identity.* Cambridge: Cambridge University Press.

Sutton-Spence, R., & West, D. (2011). Negotiating the legacy of hearingness. *Qualitative Inquiry, 17,* 422–432.

Young, A., & Temple, B. (2014). *Approaches to social research: The case of Deaf Studies.* Oxford: Oxford University Press.

3

Academic and Community Interactions in the Formation of Deaf Studies in the United States

Joseph J. Murray

The idea of Deaf Studies in the United States sprang from and remained closely tied to a long tradition of deaf community activism during its formative years. The first person to publicly broach the idea of Deaf Studies was the Executive Director of the U.S. National Association of the Deaf, Frederick Schreiber, who explicitly called for an activist field of study in 1971: "If deaf people are to get ahead in our time, they must have a better image of themselves and their capabilities. They need concrete examples of what deaf people have already done so that they can project for themselves a brighter future. If we can have Black studies, Jewish studies, why not Deaf studies?" (as quoted in Bauman, 2008). Schreiber's call was a vision of an academic field with a close connection to the lived experiences of deaf people. He drew upon existing academic fields as a means of validating the existence of deaf people as an American minority. Schreiber also saw a tight connection between academic practice and individual empowerment, leading in turn to group empowerment.

The academic discipline of Deaf Studies emerged at universities in the United States and the United Kingdom. Bristol University, in the United Kingdom, received a research grant in 1978 that eventually led to an independent Deaf Studies Trust in 1984, then the creation of the Centre for Deaf Studies in 1986 (Kyle J., personal communication, February 24, 2016). In the United States, a deaf studies degree program was founded at Boston University in 1981, followed by California State University at Northridge (CSUN) in 1983. Bristol established a diploma course in 1985 with formal Bsc and MSc programs in Deaf Studies following in 1999 (History of CDS, 2013). Gallaudet University opened a Deaf Studies undergraduate program in 1994, followed by a master's program in 2002. Today, a number of courses and programs with the name Deaf Studies exist in the United States and other locations around the world (primarily in Europe). Degree programs exist at

Humboldt University in Berlin, Utrecht University in the Netherlands, at the University of Central Lancashire in the United Kingdom, and the University College of London, among others, with the latter program having a master's degree with a deaf studies component. At some colleges in the United States, most notably Utah Valley University and CSUN, undergraduate majors in Deaf Studies number in the hundreds. Many of these programs are designed to teach American Sign Language (henceforth ASL) to second language learners, provide sign language interpreter training, or train teachers in the field of Deaf Education. The number of programs that focus on Deaf Studies as a cultural studies field is smaller, with fewer than 10 institutions in the United States with BA programs as of this writing. With the closure of Bristol University's Centre for Deaf Studies degree programs after the 2012–2013 academic year due to funding cuts, Gallaudet University currently has the only remaining MA/Msc in Deaf Studies as a cultural studies field (Bauman & Murray 2016). But these programs cannot be credited with originating the field of deaf studies. For this, we must turn to the rediscovery of sign languages beginning two decades earlier.

This chapter looks at the beginning of the field of Deaf Studies in the United States. The efforts of the first generation of scholars in ASL and Deaf Studies were dedicated to translating deaf people's lived experiences to wider society. An important part of this was the selection and presentation of aspects of these lives that showed deaf people as members of a cultural and linguistic minority. Deaf Studies scholar Tom Humphries calls these actions, undertaken by academics and deaf community members, "talking culture," or presenting cultural "artifacts" of being Deaf for wider public consumption (Humphries 2008). I look at the development and reception of the idea of ASL as a language and its use in a university setting—Gallaudet University— as an example of the complex interaction between academic practice and community activism that took place in the early decades of Deaf Studies. This interaction shows the key role that deaf ontologies played in the formation of the field of Deaf Studies, and in the subsequent shift in public perceptions of deaf people and ASL. This chapter relies on published work, supplemented by interviews and personal conversations with key historical actors. These interviews were conducted by a team at Gallaudet University and were done in 2015 in preparation for a celebration of the 50th anniversary of the publication of the first dictionary of ASL that presented the language according to linguistic principles.[1]

---

[1] The interview team was led by Marvin Miller, with faculty advisor Arlene B. Kelly. I am grateful to them for granting me access to these interviews.

THE ROLE OF AMERICAN SIGN LANGUAGE RESEARCH
IN CREATING DEAF STUDIES

The modern era of linguistic research in ASL grammar began in the 1960s, when a hearing English professor at Gallaudet, William Stokoe, published *A Dictionary of American Sign Language on Linguistic Principles* with two deaf coauthors, Dorothy Casterline and Carl Croneberg (Stokoe, Casterline & Croneberg 1965). The Linguistics Research Laboratory (LRL), established at Gallaudet University in 1971 from a National Science Foundation grant, was an important point of entry for many deaf and hearing researchers into the field (Armstrong 2000). The Salk Institute's Biological Studies' Laboratory for Cognitive Neuroscience in La Jolla, California was another location where deaf ASL users participated in research about ASL. Battison (2016) points to a research program established by Harlan Lane in 1975 at Northeastern University in Boston, Massachusetts as making up the third important research cluster on ASL in these early years. Lane hired two deaf people, Marie Jean Philip and Ella Mae Lentz, as ASL instructors and both would become important figures in the study of ASL. This era was a fertile time for new discoveries in sign language linguistics, with many of the participants in this research, both deaf and hearing, recalling "personal epiphanies" when encountering the study of ASL as a language (Emmorey & Lane 2000). These participants found their previous understanding of "signing" (without naming "signing" as a language) being replaced by a discourse of linguistic distinctiveness and of ASL as the language of a defined community— the American deaf community (Emmorey & Lane 2000).

Throughout this chapter, I use the words "rediscovery" and "reemergence" in relation to the historical moment generally considered to have begun with the release of *A Dictionary of American Sign Language on Linguistic Principles.* This was not the first such moment in deaf history. With "reemergence" I seek to highlight the long and shifting history of public perceptions of sign languages, which have existed for several centuries in a wide variety of societies around the world. Deaf people have long sought recognition for their sign languages as languages worthy of use in daily life and in education (for an early example of deaf writing in this vein see Desloges 1779). Sophia Rosenfeld (2001) notes the prominence of sign language in the early years of the French Revolution. Douglas Baynton (2002) uncovers, in "The Curious Death of Sign Language Studies in the Nineteenth Century," an earlier tradition of research on sign language by educators of deaf people. This tradition disappeared with the 20th-century dominance of oralist narratives, which precedes the history in this chapter. These were two of the many cultural moments in history in which sign languages gained the attention of the wider societies in which they existed. In addition to promoting sign languages, deaf communities have long sought autonomy via group identity. They claimed recognition of themselves as a group of people with "interests peculiar to ourselves, which can be taken care of by ourselves," a sentiment expressed by deaf American Theodore Froelich (1880:39) at an Ohio convention establishing the world's first national association of deaf people. The 1960s mark the most recent reemergence of sign languages in academic study and in public life, and this chapter places this moment in the context of late-20th-century U.S. society.

The rediscovery of ASL in the 1960s set off an era of sustained academic intervention in the deaf community, radically reshaping perceptions of deaf people and sign language from a pathological view to one of deaf people as constituting a cultural and linguistic minority in American life. Although research in ASL was instrumental in the formation of a *cultural* understanding of deaf people, the idea of deaf people constituting a distinct group of people within larger society preceded and influenced the rediscovery of ASL (Stokoe 1960; see also Sok 2012). As seen by the Schreiber quote in the first paragraph of this chapter, members of the American deaf community were increasingly influenced by the spirit of the civil rights movement of the 1960s and 1970s, with a renewed focus on new ideas to combat oralist educational philosophies and an increasingly assertive self-definition of themselves as a minority (Jankowski 1997). Definitions of deaf people as constituting a minority in U.S. society also emerged among psychologists and social scientists in these decades (Sok 2012). In 1956, sociologist Anders Lunde wrote that a view of a deaf person as "an individual adrift in a hearing society" was inaccurate, with many deaf people members of a "well-integrated group" of others like themselves (Lunde 1956 as reprinted in Stokoe 1960:12 [2005 reprint]). These early attempts at understanding deaf people outside of pathological frameworks as described by Stokoe (1960) only catalyzed into a larger movement with the rediscovery of ASL. The conditions for a shift from pathological to cultural views could not rely on academic investigation alone. It was the interaction of deaf and hearing individuals involved in the creation of a new field of academic research, working alongside the desires of deaf people for change, which created the conditions necessary for the emergence of a cultural minority view of deaf people.

The impact of the rediscovery of ASL as a language sparked a change in deaf community and public perceptions. Signing was no longer simply a verb—something that people did. It became a noun—something with a proper name and a key position in the conceptual framework of deaf people as a cultural minority. This change is shown in the material produced for ASL learners. Lottie Riekoff's *Talk to the Deaf*, first published in 1963, assured its readers "the sign language, being a language of natural grammar and pantomime can be easily learned," but successful signers needed to sign with movements "free and graceful rather than stiff or angular." (Riekoff, 1963, vii–viii). By way of contrast, the 1980 textbook, *A Basic Course in American Sign Language*, listed "Sentences with Predicate Adjectives," "Directional and Non-Directional Verbs," and "Using Two Third Person Pronouns" (Humphries et al. 1980:v) among the 22 lessons students were to learn as they studied "the native language of thousands of Deaf people who have Deaf parents." The textbook went on to emphasize, "For them, it is not only a first language but also carries with it the culture of generations of Deaf people in America" (Humphries et al. 1980:1). The link between language and culture was an integral part of the rediscovery of ASL, and one that spawned the conceptual framework upon which the field of Deaf Studies was founded.

THE LINGUISTICS RESEARCH LABORATORY: CREATING SPACE FOR CULTURAL DISCOURSES

The Linguistics Research Laboratory (LRL) at Gallaudet University was an important space for the development of this new discourse of cultural and linguistic distinctiveness. Although Gallaudet College (as it was then known) was not hostile to "signing," it was still a space heavily dominated by the patriarchal status quo in deaf education and pathological views of deaf people were as prevalent there as they were elsewhere in the United States. Deaf and hearing researchers involved in the LRL during its operation from 1971 to 1984 portrayed the LRL as a space apart from the rest of Gallaudet, as "the one light" on a campus otherwise hostile to nonpathological views of deaf people (C. Baker-Shenk, personal communication, December 1, 2015). The removal of the LRL to a building on the periphery of the campus was an attempt by the administration to marginalize the laboratory, but, as one participant put it, this ended up being the "worst, ie: best" thing the administration could have done, because it gave the laboratory the "ability to grow in our own space" free from constant political battles (Dennis Cokely, personal communication, December 1, 2015).

Participants remember the LRL as a space where people actively sought to create social change. Several participants recall the laboratory as a space for "social justice work" with "research not for the sake of research itself but for what it meant for deaf children, deaf people and others" (Cokely, video interview, December 18, 2015). Carol Padden, reminiscing on the early years of the laboratory, recalled a feeling among LRL participants that they were "a special group of people" who were doing things the rest of the campus could not understand. Although they could not have predicted the results of their work, they did feel that "we were doing something right" (Padden, C. videotaped interview, December 18, 2015). This mission was reflected not only in

the feeling of outsider status, but also in community-building activities, such as regular Friday afternoon gatherings, with research discussion taking place alongside the literal breaking of bread baked by (and
quaffing of beer brewed by) Stokoe.

This space involved both deaf and hearing people moving toward
new ways of working with one another. Interviewed participants
remembered the LRL as a space in which, for many, deaf and hearing
people were able to have sustained conversations with one another for
the first time, exploring new ways of being deaf and hearing together.
Benjamin Bahan recalls attending the Friday sessions as an undergraduate student and feeling that "my opinion, my view mattered" even
though he was in a room filled with hearing PhDs (Bahan, personal
communication, December 1, 2015). MJ Bienvenu, deaf, and Charlotte
Baker-Shenk, hearing, recall the forging of an "ally" relationship during their work together at the LRL (Baker-Shenk & Bienvenu, personal
communication, December 1, 2015[2]). Dennis Cokely saw the daily
interactions at the Lab as one in which cultural consciousness emerged
through everyday interaction, with the placement of hearing co-
workers desks so that its persons' backs were to the wall as an opportunity to learn about "deaf eyes" and "deaf ways of seeing" (Cokely,
personal communication, December 1, 2015).

For Deaf participants, the LRL was a space in which they found a new
way of understanding themselves as a cultural and linguistic minority. Ella Mae Lentz remembers Carol Padden bringing her into the LRL
and introducing her to the idea that her signs made up a language.
Although she previously had adhered to more English-like signing,
and only used ASL in a mocking manner as a form of linguistic slum-
ming, the exposure to ASL linguistics made her re-evaluate her language use (Lentz, E.M. videotaped interview, December 18, 2015). MJ
Bienvenu recalls her years at the LRL as a time of intense learning and
processing of new ideas about ASL, learning which spilled over to her
personal life. Bienvenu would interrupt friends in mid-conversation to
marvel how their use of raised eyebrows validated emergent research
that showed this was a part of ASL grammar (Bienvenu, personal communication, December 1, 2015), an epinany echoed by others at the time
(Lentz, E.M. videotaped interview, December 18, 2015). For hearing
researchers such as Baker-Shenk and Cokely, learning ASL by sustained

---

[2] The December 1, 2016 conversations took place during a free-ranging discussion among a
group of faculty, students, and visitors at the Department of ASL and Deaf Studies at Gallaudet
University. The following individuals from the period studied were present: Benjamin
Bahan, Charlotte Baker-Schenk, MJ Bienvenu, Dennis Cokely, Barbara LeMaster, and Barbara
Kannapell. When comments refer to a conversation or agreement between two participants, the
comments are referenced with both names.

personal interaction with deaf people, in and out of the lab, was a trans-formative experience (Baker-Schenk & Cokely, personal communication, December 1, 2015).

In addition to being a place for personal epiphany, the LRL was a space in which formative concepts in the field emerged. The LRL allowed deaf researchers and participants to imagine new ways of being deaf, as opposed to the pathological discourses prevalent at Gallaudet and in larger American society. The individuals mentioned in the previous paragraphs all went on to publish widely cited works (in both print and video), which discussed the idea of deaf people as having a culture, the characteristics of this culture, and how deaf and hearing people could negotiate cultural differences. The personal experiences and activities of the members of the LRL inspired the emergence of important ideas in the field of Deaf Studies.

This was an important moment in moving awareness of ASL as a language from the field of linguistics into the larger deaf community. Previously, as Padden and Humphries recount, Stokoe's dictionary spurred negative reactions from deaf people at Gallaudet. A deaf professor, Gilbert Eastman, recollected thinking "How dare a hearing person write such a dictionary of deaf people's language? How dare he represent his [Eastman's] language in this bizarre form—a collection of nonsensical symbols, squiggles, and invented vocabulary?" (Padden & Humphries 1988). Eastman writes of the time, "some people, including deaf people were deaf to our true Sign Language . . .. American Sign Language." (Eastman 1980:25). Lentz recalls being met with perplexity when she started signing in ASL, with her friends asking her why she was aligning herself with "uneducated" deaf people (Lentz, video interview, December 18, 2015). The LRL created a space for nonpathological ways of being deaf and it trained a group of deaf people who could carry these ideas out to the larger U.S. deaf community.

This claim to authority based on personal experiences as native signers was a key component of early ASL awareness. It was one encouraged by hearing linguists as an attempt to promote the authority of deaf people's lived experiences alongside academic discourses (Bienvenu & Baker-Schenk, personal communication, December 1, 2015). Although the initial focus of linguists was on deaf people from deaf families, this focus on personal experiences opened up opportunities for other deaf people to claim authority alongside academics. Deaf American storyteller Eric Malzkuhn, presenting at the First International Symposium on Sign Language Research in Stockholm, Sweden in 1979, opened his presentation by remarking, "I'm not sure exactly WHY I was selected, since I am, assuredly, no linguist." Malzkuhn presented himself as taking a "pragmatic" approach to his work with artistic representation in ASL, saying he "was primarily interested in communication." (Malzkuhn 1980:235). Malzkuhn was one of the mid-20th-century ASL storytellers, a forerunner of canonical figures who came later, such as Clayton Valli, Ella Mae Lentz, and Dorothy Miles (Humphries 2008). Gilbert Eastman, at the same conference, framed his presentation as a look at "my personal experience in sign language research" (Eastman 1980:121), being careful to explain, "I am neither a linguist, nor a sociologist, nor a psychologist, nor an anthropologist, nor a person in a scientific field." Eastman was a professor of theater and "a native user of American Sign Language." Even deaf sociolinguist Barbara Kannapell, in a paper on bilingual teaching materials at the same conference, verified her claims through "informal research on the actual usage of these ASL signs by deaf people," framing her conclusions through the lens of being both "a deaf person and a sociolinguist." (Kannapell 1980:198). These quotes show how deaf people saw their personal experience carry authority in the field of sign language research.

The rediscovery of ASL led to a shift in power relations in the deaf community in the United States. Linguists prioritized native users of the language and linguists decided early on that this meant deaf people from deaf families. Ben Bahan recalls Ursula Bellugi of the Salk Institute intentionally selecting deaf people from deaf families as research informants, excusing those from hearing families. Noting the informants were paid, and their knowledge thus assigned economic value, Bahan reflects on the underlying message given to deaf people from hearing families: "You have no value." This was a significant change from earlier decades, when membership in deaf families was seen as hereditarily problematic and even a source of shame (Malzkuhn 2016, Ennis 2015, Humphries 2008). The issue, Bahan correctly noted, was that the link between language and community status had changed (Bahan, personal communication, 2015a). Whereas professionals in the "field of deafness" considered hard-of-hearing and English-dominant deaf people to be ideal exemplars of their work (Ladd 2003, Lane 1993), linguists upended this hierarchy, one also reflected to some degree in the U.S. deaf community (Padden & Humphries 1988). The designation of a narrow group of mostly white middle-class ASL signers as native informants overlooked the diversity of ASL, including Black ASL, and has proved to be overly restrictive (Myers & Fernandes 2010). Nonetheless, it created new power relations in the deaf community.

The creation of a corpus of deaf researchers in ASL opened a space for community debate on alternative ways of understanding deaf people and sign language. Bienvenu recalls going to dinner with her deaf sister and a deaf friend and having her sister turn to her and say, "OK, now explain ASL to her." This was the moment, Bienvenu recalled, when she realized she was part of a larger community movement (personal communication, December 1, 2015). In 1972, students at Gallaudet founded an "Ameslan" club (an early acronym for American Sign Language), which wrote articles in the student newspaper in English using ASL grammar (Eastman 1980), a public assertion of deaf people as ASL users. This was especially noteworthy considering the status attributed to written English proficiency among Gallaudet students, as earlier described by Lentz. The introduction to a 1977 publication, *American Sign Language: Fact and Fancy,* published by Gallaudet's Public Service Programs, stated the publication's purpose was for readers to "learn about American Sign Language, and be excited by the infinitely challenging and creative possibilities that engage us when we use any language at all" (DiPietro, in Markowitz, 1977, unpaged). The goal of the publication was not only to dispel myths about ASL, but also to encourage pride in the use of the language.

This shift from "sign language" or "signing" to "ASL" continued to be contested long into the 1990s, reflecting what Padden and Humphries call "the anxiety of culture," (Padden & Humphries 2009). The (U.S.) National Association of the Deaf's annual *Deaf American Monograph* series, edited by Merv Garrettson, was one of the few discursive spaces in English available for deaf people to write about the struggles over culture and language within the U.S. deaf community. The 1990 *Monograph* had several articles dealing with a provocative question of the time: How did deaf people define ASL? Larry Stewart, opened his article by noting (as other contributors did) that he was not a linguist, and he asked for a consensus in which "we open our arms to any and all forms of sign communication that are used by deaf people" (Stewart 1990:123). Harvey Goodstein wrote, "a couple of my deaf colleagues jokingly remarked they had to face an 'identity crisis' each time they were asked as to which sign language they were using: ASL, PSE (a taboo?), Sign English, a combination thereof or what? How we miss the good old days when we all could communicate in sign without thinking twice as to which sign system was being used at the moment." (Goodstein 1990:49). PSE (Pidgin Signed English) was an invented sign system based on English. Leo Jacobs, writing in the same volume, suggested "ASL . . . should be treated in a very generic way," (53) echoing Goodstein's contention that everything from " 'clubroom signs' to "ASL in English word order" could be considered under an "all-inclusive" version of ASL. Goodstein specifically refers to linguistic research on sign languages, as well as to the advent of sign systems such as SEE (Seeing Essential English), as overturning what he and other contributors to the volume saw as a benevolent era in which signing was simply done, not queried.

But the reality was that linguistic research in ASL had empowered a movement that sought to distinguish and promote ASL as distinct from the Signed English systems established in earlier decades. The academic authority granted to ASL and the development of a discourse to describe alternative ways of being deaf enabled challenges to existing practices in the field of deaf education. The Total Communication philosophy of the 1970s was developed as "a liberal approach to the use of both oral and manual means of communication with deaf people" (Evans 1982:1). Described by proponents as a philosophy and not a particular method, it was ostensibly grounded in the needs of deaf learners for whichever communication method worked best for that learner. Deaf leaders of the time supported this approach, seeing it as a way to reintroduce sign language in deaf education. But with the introduction of ASL, Total Communication was now seen as a halfway measure. The use of invented manual systems intended to represent English, such as Seeing Essential English (Anthony 1977) or Pidgin Signed English (Gustason et al. 1972) also was contested. Clayton Valli and Ceil Lucas, a deaf–hearing team researching contact signing in the U.S. deaf community wanted to ensure that their research could not be misinterpreted as advocacy for the use of this form of signing in deaf education (TBC News 1994). ASL researchers presented linguistic evidence that such artificial systems were not languages and deaf children should learn via a natural language, which was ASL (Johnson et al. 1989).

The legitimation of ASL spawned the bilingual/bicultural movement advocating this form of education for deaf children. Clayton Valli opened his article in the 1990 *Monograph* with a long list of linguistic and sociolinguistic research on ASL/English bilingualism, leveraging research from this field to argue for the presence of ASL in deaf education classrooms (Valli 1990). Valli called for the use of ASL in the classroom, particularly at Gallaudet (Valli 1990:129). The use of the term "sign communication," Valli wrote, was a cover for the "taboo" of using ASL, and noted, "we Deaf people, and especially Deaf children, are suffering" from the refusal to use ASL in the classroom (Valli 1990:131). The term "sign communication" was being used in this period to refer to any kind of signing, including signing that adhered closely to English word order. Valli and others rejected this term as a cover for refusal to use ASL, with Valli writing "discussion of ASL is frowned upon" among faculty members at Gallaudet (Valli 2013:129). In the same issue of the *Monograph*, Barbara Kannapell wrote of the controversy referred to by Goodstein, and criticized him for what she saw as an attempt to confuse the distinction between ASL and English as separate languages. Kannapell defined the debate over ASL at Gallaudet as "between deaf advocates of ASL and English as two separate languages and deaf people who want a combination of both languages without acknowledging fully that ASL is a language." (Kannapell 1990:67). This alliance between academic research and deaf community goals was a prominent part of the field of Deaf Studies and ASL linguistics in its early days.

The conversations from the LRL and other academic spaces migrated to other fields and to larger public spaces, through conferences and video and print publications. The understanding of deaf people as a cultural and linguistic minority spurred the establishment of courses in ASL. Businesses emerged that saw a market in this new consciousness, selling "artifacts of culture" (Humphries 2008) to deaf and hearing audiences. A number of ASL textbooks were released in this period, with one, *A Basic Course in American Sign Language*, selling a quarter of a million copies (LeMaster 2001). Patrick Graybill, Ken Glickman, and others traveled the country offering performances in and about ASL to deaf and hearing audiences. Publishing houses such as TJ Publishers, Dawn Sign Press, and Sign Media Incorporated (SMI) were incorporated in the 1970s and 1980s. Upon the closure of the LRL in 1984, Dennis Cokely expanded SMI into a full-time venture the next year as a way to continue its work on ASL in another venue, seeing the videos his company produced as "an opportunity for accomplished deaf people to show their talent" (personal communication, December 1, 2015). SMI has produced 350 videos to date. The products from these companies were among the "artifacts of culture" Humphries (2008) discusses and included videotaped ASL performances, videos about deaf culture, and ASL translations, including a multivolume ASL synopsis (Cokely et al. 1993) of Harlan Lane's 537-page magnum opus on deaf history, *When the Mind Hears* (1984). The Bicultural Center (TBC) was one of the most prominent of a number of businesses (mostly run by sole proprietors) that provided workshops on ASL and Deaf Culture. TBC, SMI, Dawn Sign Press, and other businesses seemed to be sustainable financial enterprises, indicating a growing market for ASL and deaf culture in the 1980s and 1990s, with the latter two still in operation today.

This outpouring of work was spurred by a feeling that real changes were taking place in deaf people's lives as a result of this new orientation to ASL and deaf culture. John Vickrey Van Cleve, a hearing historian who was a pioneering scholar in U.S. Deaf History, writes that scholars at Gallaudet felt the 1980s offered "a unique opportunity to nudge the world in a positive direction" for deaf people (Van Cleve 2016:14). MJ Bienvenu, Marie Philip, Jack Gannon, Harlan Lane, and others led workshops and produced videotapes that presented deaf people's history and culture to the community and to wider society. Clayton Valli, Ella Mae Lentz, Dorothy Miles (in the United Kingdom), Benjamin Bahan, Nathie Marbury, and Sam Supalla developed poems, stories, and other literature in ASL, often working with the publishing companies mentioned earlier (see Supalla, S. J., and Bahan, B. J. [2000], Valli 1995, Lentz 1995, Marbury 1994, among others). Carolyn McCaskill, Glenn Anderson, and Lindsay Dunn constantly sought to expand the field's boundaries to include the perspectives of deaf people of color. Conferences were key sites for the transmission of ideas in ASL among scholars, professionals in ASL and sign language teaching, and deaf community members, with a series of Deaf Studies conferences at various locations around the country in the 1990s (hosted by

Gallaudet University's College of Continuing Education) that provided spaces for the exploration of this new field by academics and community members. All these spaces brought academic understandings of ASL and deaf culture to both the wider deaf community and, via ASL classes, to society at large.

THE CULTURAL TURN

An early and important step in the establishment of the field of Deaf Studies was the definition of deaf people as having a culture. Humphries writes that establishment of the field required deaf people to "assemble the material of our world that is unique to us," (Humphries 2008:37) in order to present alternative ways of understanding deaf people outside of pathological frameworks. This material was assembled and presented via the concept of "deaf culture." Carol Padden's 1980 article, "The Deaf Community and the Culture of Deaf People," set the theoretical parameters for the early decades of Deaf Studies, and her two books with Tom Humphries (1988 and 2005) are still standard textbooks in university classrooms across the United States, providing students with their first introduction to deaf people. Padden's 1980 article drew a distinction between the concepts of community and culture and proposed a definition of deaf culture grounded in experientially based discourses. Padden adopted a definition of community that included both deaf people and hearing people who "actively support the goals of the community and work with Deaf people to achieve them" (Padden 1980:92). This distinction between community and culture was tied to a larger question: How do we understand deaf people as a cultural group if they exist alongside hearing people? The cultural turn had to account for a constant interaction between deaf and hearing people in everyday life and yet account for the existence of what was termed a separate deaf culture. Padden's solution was to split community and culture, to allow for hearing people, especially signing hearing people, to be a part of deaf lives, while still preserving a sphere of distinctiveness for deaf people called "deaf culture."

Padden defined culture as "a set of learned behaviors of a group of people who have their own language, values, rules for behavior, and traditions" (Padden 1980:92). The article then discusses "some identifying characteristics of the American deaf culture," such as the value deaf people accorded to sign language and the emphasis on social interaction with other deaf people. Padden's evidence for her definition of deaf culture were "first based on intuition—my own understanding of how I grew up as a child of Deaf parents and how I interact with other Deaf people" (Padden 1980:95), as well as on literature published by Deaf people. This focus on the experientially based narratives of deaf people can be seen as a continuation of the prioritization of native informants and personal experience described earlier in the discussion of the early years of ASL linguistics. Padden's work has advanced considerably in nuance and sophistication from the ideas presented in this initial article, but it remains important because it set the terms for much work in Deaf Studies over the next decade, and beyond.

The influence of Padden's focus on "identifying characteristics" cannot be overstated, both in academic work and in its influence in shaping deaf community discourse on the concept of deaf culture. Deaf community members and academics (deaf and hearing) set out to "talk culture" and "produce these examples of our difference" (Humphries 2008:37). The videotape series *American Deaf Culture* (Bienvenu & Colonomos 1985) showcased self-identified culturally deaf people, often from deaf families or with long periods of matriculation at schools for deaf people, giving examples of "identifying characteristics" of deaf culture. Each video in the series had a title closely paralleling aspects of culture identified in Padden's 1980 article: Language and Traditions, Values, Rules of Social Interaction, Group Norms, and Identity (Bienvenu Colonomos 1985). One example of a characteristic of deaf culture reproduced across several works is the norm of introducing oneself with one's name and where one is "from," with the from being the deaf residential school from which the deaf person presumably matriculated (Philip 1997). Works such as Sherman Wilcox's *American Deaf Culture: An Anthology* (Wilcox 1989) compiled writings by deaf and hearing people on deaf ways of living in the world. Susan Rutherford's "Funny in Deaf, Not in Hearing" (1989) explored differences in deaf and hearing jokes, based not only on language play but also on different life experiences. Marie Jean Philip, an early and important theorist of Deaf Culture, in an ASL lecture translated into English and published in 1997, outlined a litany of cultural behaviors of culturally deaf people, which distinguished them not only from hearing people but also from non-culturally deaf people, defined as those who did not grow up using ASL (Philip 1997). This "invisible line that separates Deaf and hearing cultures" required hearing interpreters to know various cultural rules, such as how to resolve arguments (the person with whom the problem originated needed to apologize first) and the role of reciprocity in maintaining cultural connections (Philip 1997:58–59). The aim of this body of work was to confirm this new conceptual framework of deaf culture.

The project of promoting a cultural view of deaf people was, as several participants in a 1994 forum in *Sign Language Studies* noted, an explicitly political project. Trevor Johnston defined the project as one in which "deaf activists and theorists are not only defining but also creating and developing Deaf culture" (Johnston 1994:134–135). Graham Turner, whose article initiated the forum, was careful to frame his inquiry as a means of improving the concept of deaf culture and thus allowing the "strength of our political impact [to be] enhanced" (Turner

1994:108). The project was political because it attacked entrenched medical ideologies that had heretofore controlled representations of deaf people to larger society. Lane (1992) describes how this initial resistance to deaf culture among educators, psychologists, audiologists, and other professionals who worked with deaf people was a struggle over who had the power to define what it meant to be deaf. The story of this resistance against deaf culture will not be told here, but suffice it to say that the concept of culture proved effective in challenging, but not displacing, earlier pathological views of deaf people. It is also important to note that a newer wave of work in Deaf Studies (discussed by the editors in the Introduction to this volume) has challenged the cultural model as the most appropriate one to use when understanding deaf lives (Baynton 2008, Davis 2008).

The use of the concept of deaf culture emerged alongside earlier terms used by deaf people to describe their lives. Benjamin Bahan, drawing on his "experience growing up with Deaf people and conversations with five Deaf friends who also grew up with Deaf people" (Bahan 1994:241), observes that terms in ASL such as DEAF WORLD or DEAF WAY were common in the deaf community but were not (yet) adopted by academics. DEAF WORLD referred to a "group of people" and a sense of commonality, emphasized by the term DEAF-SAME-ME (243). According to this group of six deaf people, the concept of DEAF WORLD was "formed out of a need for sameness rather than the need to create an 'us-versus-them' dichotomy" among deaf people (244). The concept of DEAF WORLD, Bahan wrote, was one that emphasized the experience of being deaf. The DEAF WORLD was one in which deaf latecomers to the community and to using ASL were welcomed, provided they adopted the right attitude to other deaf people. Concepts in ASL such as DEAF WORLD and DEAF WAY or DEAF TYPICAL were signs that forecast a uniquely deaf way of being to other insiders. The term DEAF CULTURE was more what Humphries (2008) has called a "coming to voice," a term that was oriented toward representing deaf people to others. But a representation to others invariably takes on its own life.

The introduction of the concept of "deaf culture" created new power relations within the deaf community. Bahan observed that "there are people in the Deaf World who have used the definition of Deaf Culture proposed by others to create stratification inside the Deaf World" (Bahan 1994:245). Among deaf people, these terms could be translated into ASL in ways that highlighted a different understanding of themselves. The sign DEAF could be qualified with a BIG D and SMALL D, glossing the Deaf/deaf distinction adopted in written literature in Deaf Studies. So deaf people could tell others (and be told) in ASL exactly how Deaf they really were. Bahan notes the phrase YOU NOT DEAF CULTURE foregrounded "a new boundary in the Deaf World." This was used to delineate who were and who were not members of the deaf community and influenced the rise of a companion phrase: YOU NOT DEAF WORLD. Such stratification, Bahan writes, did not exist before the introduction of the concept of deaf culture (Bahan 1994:245–246).

The use of deaf culture veered toward the prescriptive when used to judge a person's cultural competencies. Although Bahan notes these phrases are ostensibly negative, he also saw them as having "value in raising consciousness among Deaf people about their world" (Bahan 1994:246). That is, although definitions of culture could be used as a checklist for deaf people to evaluate themselves, this evaluation was an important part of deaf people's emergence from medical/pathological definitions that had been imposed on them earlier.

The cultural turn brought about new concepts that reshaped how deaf people perceived themselves and their relationship to hearing people and larger society. The term deaf culture displaced, but did not wholly replace, earlier terms such as DEAF WORLD in that they received more attention from scholars and thus gained more cultural authority among deaf people themselves. The idea of deaf people constituting a cultural minority could be easily understood by other academics and by larger society, corresponding as it did to ongoing discourses in the late 20th century on minority group identities. The idea of deaf culture privileged those who exhibited behaviors corresponding to definitions and descriptions of deaf culture advanced in the field of Deaf Studies. These descriptions also became prescriptions, used as the impetus for community-wide conversations and confrontations aimed at shifting individual deaf community members' self-perceptions. The emergence of the field of Deaf Studies, growing out of an alliance between sign language linguists and deaf people, had a profound effect on the 20th century U.S. deaf community.

DEAF STUDIES TODAY

This rough map of the early years reveals a number of blank spaces. We know William Stokoe's thoughts and experiences through his writings and a biography (Maher 1996), but what of his deaf research assistants, Dorothy Casterline and Carl Cronenberg, and the other deaf researchers and research assistants at the linguistics laboratories in Washington, DC and California? What ideologies and motivations drove the creation of the early sign language textbooks such as *A Basic Course in Sign Language*, the *American Sign Language Green Books*, and the *Signing Naturally* series? How large was the market for ASL and Deaf Culture in Deaf Studies' early years? Not coincidentally, the bilingual–bicultural movement in U.S. deaf education emerged at this time and the history of this movement, still ongoing, is largely unexplored.

What we do know is that the final two decades of the 20th century saw academics and activists, both deaf and hearing, laying the groundwork for an unprecedented shift in the ways deaf people were viewed. This shift emerged in the ways deaf people understood themselves and it also encompassed a concerted effort to create a shift in larger public perceptions of deaf people. It involved a partnership between academics and deaf community members that ultimately sought to promote new perceptions of deaf people. Linguistics and sociolinguistics were a prominent part of the field of deaf studies for much of its history. Even today the most common academic training of full-time tenure-track faculty in Deaf Studies programs in the five most prominent university settings in the United States (Gallaudet, National Technical Institute for the Deaf at the Rochester Institute of Technology, California State University, Northridge, Utah Valley University, Boston University) is in linguistics or sociolinguistics (this pattern is to be found mostly among full professors, with the lower academic ranks showing more disciplinary diversity). Deaf researchers began their training in linguistic research laboratories, which served as incubators for the first generation of scholars and teachers of Deaf Studies. These fields were seen, by practitioners and by deaf community members, as lending support to the project to reintroduce ASL to deaf education, in changing individual and community self-perceptions, and as enhancing the status of deaf people in society at large.

Some preliminary conclusions can be drawn from an initial look at the literature from the early days of Deaf Studies. In addition to the aforementioned tensions between medical and cultural models, within the community over new ways of representing deaf lives, and between various understandings of ASL, there are several unexplored tensions for scholars studying this era. One is the tension between written and signed language. The story of the cultural turn is easy to find in the print materials of the era, of which there is an abundance. The videotapes distributed by publishing companies consist largely of storytelling or performances with only a few textbooks that aim to explain culture (see, for example, Marbury 1994, 1996, Bienvenu 1989). As we saw earlier, much of the work done by deaf people in explaining ASL and deaf culture to one another was done in ASL, both in personal encounters and at workshops and conferences around the country. Not only is there no overview of this output, we do not even know which of these conferences may have been videotaped or where these videotapes might be. This is especially problematic in light of the shift in video recording technologies to digital formats and the resulting loss of older video playback technologies. What this means is that there is a real danger that the story of the cultural turn, an era of promotion and recognition of a signing community, will be told largely based on written sources. Related to this is the privileging of academic over community narratives. Tensions between these narratives emerge at certain points in the literature, most notably with the concept of "deaf culture," versus DEAF WORLD as noted earlier in Bahan (1994).

A final tension should be an inherent part of any field of cultural study: the inherited traditions of academic disciplines, the relentless pressure for market-oriented degree programs, which makes up today's university environment, and curricular practices that seek to accommodate both. Curricula are reflections of current knowledge, but they are also ideological artifacts that seek to define the field of study. The rapid expansion of ASL instruction in colleges and universities across the United States has prompted the establishment of classes or programs in Deaf Studies. Many of these programs appear to be located in the existing academic structure, which means being in (Deaf) Education, Audiology, or Foreign Language Departments. These disciplinary spaces shape course offerings in Deaf Studies, textbooks produced to meet this market, and thereby the contours of the field. This is a trend Humphries also has noted in the realm of deaf art and literature, and he raises concerns about the viability of art produced to meet a market dominated largely by hearing second-language learners (Humphries 2008:39). Paddy Ladd has warned of the colonialization of Deaf Studies by the ideologies of existing disciplines, particularly in education and audiology (Ladd 2003). The expansion of ASL teaching also has created a large number of jobs related to culture and ASL teaching. It is unclear how many of these jobs are taken by deaf people—anecdotal observation indicates the cultural turn has provided quite a few teaching jobs for hearing people who learned ASL in adulthood, taking us further away from ASL and Deaf Studies initial idealization of deaf people as native bearers of cultural and linguistic knowledge. Parallel to these events, we see the rapid growth of video blogs and social media networks, which have enabled a wider array of cultural productions (especially in ASL) than previously possible. What impact do these cultural productions have on the academic field of Deaf Studies?

CONCLUSION

This chapter surveys the earliest years of Deaf Studies as an academic field, touching on the turn to conceptions of deaf people as a cultural community and some of the "anxieties of culture" this turn inspired. The scholarship in Deaf Studies discussed in this chapter has become considerably more complex since the 1980s and 1990s and should not be read as representative of current thought in the field. This chapter shows that deaf ontologies were a foundational part of the field of Deaf Studies, with deaf experiences influencing the formation and dissemination of a cultural perspective on deaf people. Although some deaf community responses veered to the prescriptive, even this prescriptive discourse is evidence of a search for experiences rooted in deaf lives. The story of Deaf Studies in its earliest years is still not fully told, but we can see "talking culture" was spurred by hearing academics and deaf people inside and outside of academe, drawing on academic ideas and authority, but shaped by deaf experiences. The cultural turn is the story of academic and community activism working on a successful project to shift public perceptions of deaf people and sign language.

The past few decades have, indeed, seen a change in the way deaf people and sign languages are perceived by the larger U.S. society. Denigrated as a "primitive" gestural system for much of the 20th century, ASL is now the third most widely taught "foreign" language in U.S. colleges and universities, with slightly over 100,000 people taking ASL classes every year (Goldberg et al. 2015). The increasing presence of deaf people and sign language in the mainstream media (Murray 2015) lends social respectability to the idea of a deaf community and deaf people as cultural beings. This had led to a remarkable transformation of ASL's status and showcases ways in which deaf people's lives and standing in wider society have changed since the emergence of the field of Deaf Studies. This shift ranges from mundane (but important) daily interactions between deaf and hearing people to new laws that reshape how deaf people receive services and accommodations. Deaf people could stop apologizing for not understanding waiters in restaurants and, instead, demand the restaurant staff either use ASL or provide them with a pen and paper for communication. Video relay services, authorized by the U.S. government in 2000, offer ASL-based telephone calls where cross-cultural interaction receives federal reimbursement on a minute-by-minute basis (Brunson 2011, Haualand, this volume). The cultural turn sparked a fertile period of self-empowerment and self-awareness in the U.S. deaf community, indubitably changing many lives for the better.

The cultural turn was definitive, but also in ways that Deaf Studies would do well to examine anew. The focus on the personal experiences of a deliberately limited set of people—native users of ASL from deaf families—had at least two serious problems. First, concepts grounded in the beliefs and experiences of (broadly middle-class) white deaf people from deaf families, most of whom attended deaf schools in the 1960s and embarked on their careers in the 1970s and 1980s, cannot be said to be representative of the experiences of all deaf people in the United States. The class, race, and language experiences of deaf people are so much more variegated than those of this particular group of people. The historically specific context of this generation, who grew up during a time when many deaf people attended residential schools, and social clubs for deaf people were popular meeting spaces, needs to be taken into account. This is something the field has acknowledged (Wrigley

1996, Bauman 2008, Myers & Fernandes 2010) and is addressing, as seen by the contributions to this volume (such as Moges's chapter).

The second limitation is the uncritical use of personal experience narratives as an evidentiary base for critical deaf theory. The use of the personal experiences of deaf people as the basis of academic theory was an emancipatory strategy in the early years of Deaf Studies. It allowed deaf people to claim value in their lives and create spaces outside of the control of existing pathological ideologies. Nonetheless, this was a strategy of strategic essentialism (as noted in Ladd 2003) and one with limitations beyond those addressed earlier. Although one solution may be to present the personal experiences of a wider variety of deaf people, we cannot simply continue to "produce these examples of our difference" and show even more "artifacts of ourselves" (Humphries 2008) without also placing these narratives into wider academic conversations. Narratives of personal experience privilege studies *within*. Humphries asks us to move from asking "how are we different to how are we being" (Humphries 2008:41). This means re-examining the role and uses such narratives can play in Deaf Studies (see O'Connell, this volume). The Editors' Introduction (this volume) outlines multiple directions now being taken by scholars who are moving the field in new thematic and theoretical directions.

As a cultural studies field, Deaf Studies emerged within an emancipatory context in which deaf and hearing people worked together to respond to the needs of late-20th-century deaf communities. Although this chapter focuses on the U.S. case, similar trajectories have been noted in other countries. Research on sign languages created new and empowering ways for deaf and hearing people to relate to one another, to understand the deaf community, and to make an impact on deaf lives, particularly in promoting cultural views of deaf people (see, among others, Ahlgren 1980, Brennan & Hayhurst 1980, Hansen 1980, Mally 1993, Gras 2008). The 20th-century development of sign language research in the United Kingdom began in the 1970s, directly influenced by Stokoe's work (Brennan & Hayhurst 1980:235). The recognition of British Sign Language as a language brought about "a renewal at various levels within and around the deaf community" (Brennan & Hayhurst 1980:236). In Sweden, Brita Bergman initiated linguistic research on sign language in 1976 with two deaf researchers, Lars Åke Wikström and Lars Wallin (Ahlgren 1980), the latter of whom, in 1994, became one of the first deaf Europeans to receive a PhD in linguistics. In Denmark, the decade of the 1970s saw a change in attitudes toward Danish Sign Language among deaf people and hearing professionals who worked with deaf people. Early research in Dansk Tegnsprog (DTS) [Danish Sign Language] received "stimulus" from Stokoe and the LRL, with a leading Danish researcher visiting the LRL several times during that decade (Hansen 1980:248). This change could be seen in a shift from teaching DTS in Danish word order to pedagogy that emphasized DTS as an independent language of the deaf community (Hansen 1980). Gertrud Mally's story of her evolution as a German sign language (DGS) teacher from 1977 onward shows the micropolitics of deaf–hearing interactions in introducing sign language to deaf education and other fields as DGS slowly became recognized over the next decade (Mally 1993). A 1985 Hamburg congress on sign language exposed the author to the fact of sign language research in these countries and to the idea that DGS was "a fully developed linguistic system…equal next to spoken and written German" (Mally 1993:189). In these and other countries, an understanding of one's sign language as a legitimate language promoted new conceptualizations of deaf people, which were used to counter earlier pathological models of deafness.

Talking culture in the first decades of Deaf Studies allowed aspects of deaf lives—which were called deaf culture—to talk and to be listened to. A new century brings new contexts. Scholarship is emerging in response to issues such as support for sign languages (De Meulder 2015, McKee & Manning 2015) or biological and genetic ideologies that fail to see the value of deaf lives (Bauman & Murray 2014, Mazique, this volume), among other issues demanding attention. Deaf people have managed to survive in myriad societies across human history as signing communities within speaking societies. How? Deaf Studies' response to this and other questions will be rooted in deaf people's lives, lives lived in a wide range of ways across a dizzying array of social, temporal, and cultural spaces. To do justice to this diversity, Deaf Studies also should work within this shifting landscape of mobile and strategic social positionings, going beyond talking culture to find the many ways in which deaf lives are lived in a continuous conversation with the world.

REFERENCES

Ahlgren, I. (1980). The sign language group in Stockholm. In I. Ahlgren & B. Bergman (Eds.), *Papers from the First International Symposium on Sign Language Research* (pp. 3–7). Leksand, Sweden: Swedish National Association of the Deaf.

Anthony, D. A., & Shawver, A. (1977). *The seeing essential English manual.* Davenport, IA: National Foundation for the Advancement of Communication for the Deaf.

Armstrong, D.A. (2000). William C. Stokoe, Jr, Founder of Sign Language Linguistics: 1919–2000. Published May 4, 2000. Retrieved from http://gupress.gallaudet.edu/stokoe.html

Bahan, B. (1994). Comment on Turner. *Sign Language Studies, 84*, 241–249.

Bahan, B. (2015a). Personal communication. March 10, 2015.

Bahan, B. (2015b). Personal communication. December 1, 2015.

Baker-Shenk, C. (2015). Personal communication. December 1, 2015.

Battison, R. (2016). Sign language research: Pre-1980. In G. Gertz & P. Boudreault (Eds.), *Sage encyclopedia of Deaf Studies* (pp. 842–847). Los Angeles: Sage Press.

Bauman, H-D. L. (2008). Introduction: Listening to Deaf Studies. In H-D.L. Bauman (Ed.), *Open your eyes: Deaf studies talking* (pp. 1–32). Minneapolis: University of Minnesota Press.

Bauman, H-D. L., & Murray, J.J. (2016). Deaf Studies. In G. Gertz & P. Boudreault (Eds.), *Sage encyclopedia of Deaf Studies* (pp. 273–276). Los Angeles: Sage Press.

Baynton, D. (2002). The curious death of sign language studies in the nineteenth century. In W.C. Stokoe, D. F. Armstrong, M.A. Karchmer, & C.J.V. Van (Eds.), *The study of signed languages: Essays in honor of William C. Stokoe* (pp. 13–34). Washington, DC: Gallaudet University Press.

Baynton, D. (2008). Beyond culture: Deaf Studies and the Deaf Body. In H-D. L. Bauman (Ed.), *Open your eyes: Deaf Studies talking* (pp. 293–313). Minneapolis: University of Minnesota Press.

Davis, L. J. (2008). Postdeafness. In H-D. L. Bauman (Ed.), *Open your eyes: Deaf Studies talking* (pp. 314–326). Minneapolis: University of Minnesota Press.

Bauman, H.-D. L., & Murray, J. J. (Eds.) (2014). *Deaf Gain: Raising the stakes for human diversity*. Minneapolis: University of Minnesota Press.

Bienvenu, M. J., Colonomos, B., & Sign Media, Inc. (1985). *An introduction to American deaf culture*. Silver Spring, MD: Sign Media.

Bienvenu, M.J. (1989). *Deaf Culture autobiographies on video*. Sign Enhancers, Inc. [producer].

Bienvenu, M.J. (2015). Personal communication. December 1, 2015.

Brennan, M., & Hayhurst, A. B. (1980). The renaissance of British Sign Language. In C.L. Baker & R. Battison (Eds.), *Sign language and the deaf community: Essays in honor of William C. Stokoe* (pp. 233–244). Silver Spring, MD: National Association of the Deaf.

Brunson, J. L. (2011). *Video relay service interpreters: Intricacies of sign language access*. Washington, DC: Gallaudet University Press.

Cokely, D., Graybill, P., Weinstock, J., Norman, F., Eastman, G. C., Clerc, L., Lane, H. L., . . . Sign Media, Inc. (1993). *When the mind hears*. Burtonsville, MD: Sign Media.

Cokely, D. (2015a). Personal communication. December 1, 2015.

Cokely, D. (2015b). Videotaped interview. December 18, 2015. Interviewed as part of M. Miller & A.B. Kelly [producers], *DASL 50th Anniversary*. Washington, DC: Gallaudet University Department of ASL and Deaf Studies.

Desloges, P. (1779). *Observations d'un Sourd et Muèt, sur un cours élémentaire d'éducation des sourds et muets*; publié en 1779 par M. L'abbé Deschamps, Chapelain de l'Eglise d'Orléans. Paris: B. Morin.

De Meulder, M. (2015). A barking dog that never bites? The British Sign Language (Scotland) Bill. *Sign Language Studies, 15*(4), 446–472.

Eastman, G. (1980). From student to professional: A personal chronicle of Sign Language. In W.C. Stokoe, C.L. Baker-Shenk & R. Battison. *Sign language and the deaf community: Essays in honor of William C. Stokoe* (pp. 9–32). Silver Spring, MD: National Association of the Deaf.

Emmorey, K., & Lane, H. (2000). *The signs of language revisited: An anthology to honor Ursula Bellugi and Edward Klima*. Mahwah, NJ: Lawrence Erlbaum Associates, Inc.

Ennis, W. T. (2015). *Hereditarian ideas and eugenic ideals at the National Deaf–Mute College* (Unpublished doctoral dissertation). University of Iowa.

Evans, L. (1982). *Total communication: Structure and strategy*. Washington, DC: Gallaudet College Press.

Fernandes, J. K., & Myers, S. S. (2010). Inclusive Deaf Studies: Barriers and pathways. *Journal of Deaf Studies and Deaf Education, 15*(1), 17–29.

"A history of CDS: the heritage that will be lost with its closure." (2013). http://www.savedeafstudies.org.uk/?p=480 Posted June 27, 2013. Accessed February 10, 2016.

Froelich, T. (1880). The importance of association among mutes for mutual improvement. In *Proceedings of the National Convention of Deaf-Mutes* (p.39). New York: New York Institution for the Deaf and Dumb.

Goldberg, D., Looney, D., & Lusin, N. (2015). Enrollment in languages other than English in United States institutions of higher education. Fall 2013. New York: Modern Language Association. Internet resource.

Goodstein, H. (1990). American Sign Language. In M. Garretson (Ed.), *Eyes, hands, voices: Communication issues among deaf people (A Deaf American Monograph), 40 (1,2,3,4)* (pp. 47–49). Silver Spring, MD: National Association of the Deaf.

Gras, V. (2008). Can signed language be planned? Implications for interpretation in Spain. In C. Plaza-Pust & E. Morales Lopez (Eds.), *Sign bilingualism: Language development, interaction, and maintenance in sign language contact situations* (pp. 165–194). Amsterdam: John Benjamins Publishing Company.

Gustason, G., Pfetzing, D., Zawolkow, E., & Norris, C. B. (1972). *Signing exact English*. Los Alamitos, CA: Modern Signs Press.

Hansen, B. (1980). Research on Danish Sign Language and its impact on the deaf community. In C.L. Baker & R. Battison (Eds.), *Sign language and the deaf community: Essays in Honor of William C. Stokoe* (pp. 245–263). Silver Spring, MD: National Association of the Deaf.

A history of CDS: The heritage that will be lost with closure. (2013). Published June 27, 2013. Retrieved from http://www.savedeafstudies.org.uk/?p=480

Humphries, T., Padden, C., & O'Rourke, T. J. (1980). *A basic course in American Sign Language*. Silver Spring, MD: T.J. Publishers.

Humphries, T. (2008). Scientific explanation and other performance acts in the reorganization of the DEAF. In K.A. Lindgren, D. DeLuca, & D. J. Napoli (Eds.), *Signs and voices: Deaf culture, identity, language, and arts*. Washington, DC: Gallaudet University Press.

Jankowski, K.A. (1997). *Deaf empowerment: Emergence, struggle, and rhetoric*. Washington, DC: Gallaudet University Press.

Johnson, R. E., Liddell, S. K., & Erting, C. J. (1989). *Unlocking the curriculum: Principles for achieving access in deaf education*. Washington, DC: Gallaudet University Press.

Johnston, T. (1994). Comment on Turner. *Sign Language Studies, 83*(1), 133–138.

Kannapell, B. (1980). A Preliminary Report on Developing Bilingual Teaching Materials To Teach Deaf Students. In I. Ahlgren & B. Bergman (Eds.), *Papers from the First International Symposium on Sign Language Research* (pp. 189–205). Leksand, Sweden: Swedish National Association of the Deaf.

Kannapell, B. (1990). Personal Reflections. Current Issues on Language and Communication Among Deaf People. In M. Garretson (Ed.), *Eyes, hands,*

voices: Communication issues among deaf people (A Deaf American Monograph),
40 (1,2,3,4) (pp. 65–69). Silver Spring, MD: National Association of the Deaf.

Kyle, J. (2016). Personal communication with M. De Meulder. February 24, 2016.

Ladd, P. (2003). *Understanding Deaf culture: In search of Deafhood.* Clevedon: Multilingual Matters.

Lane, H. (1992). *The mask of benevolence.* San Diego, CA: DawnSignPress.

LeMaster, B. (2001). *Anthropological linguistics and deaf language policies in the US and Ireland.* Available at http://ccat.sas.upenn.edu/plc/SLA/lemaster.html Accessed February 10, 2016.

Lentz, E. M. (1995). *The treasure: Poems by Ella Mae Lentz.* In Motion Press.

Lentz, E. M. (2015). Videotaped interview. December 18. 2015. Interviewed as part of M. Miller & A.B. Kelly. [producers], "DASL 50th Anniversary." Washington, DC: Gallaudet University Department of ASL and Deaf Studies.

Maher, J. (1996). *Seeing language in sign: The work of William C.* Stokoe. Washington, DC: Gallaudet University Press.

Mally, G. (1993). The long road to self-confidence of the deaf in Germany. In R. Fischer & H.L. Lane (Eds.), *Looking back: A reader on the history of deaf communities and their sign languages* (pp. 177–198). Hamburg, Germany: Signum Press.

Malzkuhn, E. (1980). Nonverbal Utterances. In I. Ahlgren & B. Bergman (Eds.), *Papers from the First International Symposium on Sign Language Research* (pp. 235–245). Leksand, Sweden: Swedish National Association of the Deaf.

Malzkuhn, M. (2016). "Compromising for Agency: The Role of the NAD during the American Eugenics Movement, 1880–1940." In B. Greenwald & J.J. Murray (Eds.), *In our hands: Essays in deaf history, 1780–1970* (pp. 171–192). Washington, DC: Gallaudet University Press.

McKee, R., & Manning, V. (2015). Effects of language planning and policy on language rights and the vitality of New Zealand Sign Language. *Sign Language Studies, 15*(4), 473–497.

Marbury, N. (1994). *Deaf culture lecture: Cultural differences.* Salem, OR: Sign Enhancers, Inc.

Marbury, N. (1996). *Deaf culture: Shared wisdom for families.* Sign Enhancers, Inc. [producers].

Markowitz, H. (1977). *American Sign Language: Fact and Fancy.* Washington, DC: Gallaudet University Public Service Programs.

Murray, J. J. (2015). Linguistic human rights discourse in deaf community activism. *Sign Language Studies, 15*(4), 379–410.

Padden, C., & Humphries, T. (1988). *Deaf in America: Voices from a culture.* Cambridge, MA: Harvard University Press.

Padden, C., & Humphries, T. (2005). *Inside deaf culture.* Cambridge, MA: Harvard University Press.

Padden, C. (2015). Personal communication. December 1, 2015.

Padden, C. (2015). Videotaped interview. December 18. 2015. Interviewed as part of M. Miller & A.B. Kelly [producers], "DASL 50th Anniversary." Washington, DC: Gallaudet University Department of ASL and Deaf Studies.

Philip, M. (1997). Deaf culture and interpreter training curricula. (Unpublished manuscript).

Reikoff, L. (1963). *Talk to the deaf.* Springfield, MO: Gospel Publishing House.

Rosenfeld, S. A. (2001). *A revolution in language: The problem of signs in late eighteenth-century France.* Stanford, CA: Stanford University Press.

Rutherford, S.D. Funny in Deaf—Not in Hearing. In Wilcox, S. (Ed.) (1989). *American deaf culture: An anthology* (pp. 65–81). Silver Spring, MD: Linstok Press.

Sign Media Incorporated. "About sign media." Retrieved from http://signmedia.com/info/smi.htm

Stewart, L. (1990). Sign Language: Some Thoughts of a Deaf American. In M. Garretson (Ed.), *Eyes, hands, voices: Communication issues among deaf people (A Deaf American Monograph), 40 (1,2,3,4)* (pp. 117–124). Silver Spring, MD: National Association of the Deaf.

Sok, S. (2012). *An investigation into the formation of deaf culture concept in Deaf Studies* (Unpublished master's thesis). Gallaudet University, Washington, DC.

Stokoe, W. (1960/2005). Sign language structure: An outline of the visual communication systems of the American deaf. Reprinted in *Journal of Deaf Studies and Deaf Education, 10*, 4–35.

Stokoe, W. C., Casterline, D. C., & Croneberg, C. G. (1965). *A dictionary of American Sign Language on linguistic principles.*Silver Spring, MD: Linstock Press.

Supalla, S. J., & Bahan, B. J. (2000). *Bird of a different feather: &, For a decent living.* San Diego, CA: DawnSignPress.

Turner. G. (1994). How Is Deaf Culture?: Towards a Revised Notion of a Fundamental Concept. *Sign Language Studies, 83*(1), 103–126.

Valli, C. (1990). A taboo exposed: Using ASL in the classroom. In M. Garretson (Ed.), *Eyes, hands, voices: Communication issues among deaf people (A Deaf American Monograph), 40* (1,2,3,4) (pp. 129–131). Silver Spring, MD: National Association of the Deaf.

Valli, C., & Ceil, L. (1994). Deaf and hearing teams. *TBC News* 68 (May/June), 8–9.

Valli, C. (1995). *ASL poetry: Selected works of Clayton Valli.* San Diego, CA: Dawn Pictures.

Van Cleve, J. V. (Fall 2016). *A Place of Their Own* in History. *Sign Language Studies, 17*(1), 12–24.

Wilcox, S. (Ed.) (1989). *American deaf culture: An anthology.* Silver Spring, MD: Linstok Press.

Wrigley, O. (1996). *The politics of deafness.* Washington, DC: Gallaudet University Press.

4

The Emergence of a Deaf Academic Professional Class during the British Deaf Resurgence

Maartje De Meulder

This chapter is based on research I carried out in 2006, looking at the role of deaf academic professionals in a research and teaching institute located in a mainstream university in the United Kingdom, and their relationship with the British deaf community (De Meulder 2007). More specifically, the chapter focuses on those deaf professionals who work in an academic setting (as lecturers, researchers, research assistants, and/or in the academic administration) and how they relate with and to the deaf community, as well as their individual work settings. Consequently, in this chapter, I use the term "deaf academic professionals" to describe them.

This chapter has to be seen and read as a historical chapter, both in terms of when the research was carried out (a decade ago) and in terms of the period that is the main focus of the research, a period that Ladd (2003) calls the "Deaf Resurgence." This was a period of change taking place across Western Europe and the United States in the 1970s and 1980s. According to Ladd (2003), it was characterized by five features: (1) the recognition by linguists of sign languages as bona fide languages; (2) the return of sign languages to deaf education and the wider public domain; (3) the growth of sign language television; (4) the recognition of the concepts of "Deaf history" and "Deaf culture"; and (5) the founding of Deaf Studies (similar processes in the United States from the 1960s onward are described in Murray, this volume). It was a period of reinvigoration and revival after a long period of oralism.[1]

Since the research was carried out, we have come a long way: The number of deaf professionals in the United Kingdom has steadily increased, with deaf professionals working in educational settings, the mental health sector, the care professions, as ordained ministers, in youth work, language instruction, advocacy, and the academy. This

---

[1] Oralism was the dominant educational ideology in deaf education for much of the 20th century. It prioritised the instruction of spoken language over the use of sign language.

chapter focuses on this last setting. Here, the situation has changed drastically, too, compared with 10 years ago: An increasing number of deaf people in the United Kingdom are pursuing and achieving master's and doctoral degrees,[2] and some of them go on to work in academic environments.[3]

Ladd (2003) calls the professional class that emerged during the Deaf Resurgence the "subaltern-elite." Further on in this chapter, I expand on the origins and meaning of this term. Ladd states there is a need for research into "the experiences of the new subaltern-elite; how becoming professional affects cultural dynamics and the strategies involved" (Ladd 2003:450). Indeed, due to the behaviors and values often observed in deaf communities, such as the importance placed on collectivism, information sharing, and reciprocity (Mindess 2000, Ladd 2003, Philip 1993), extra pressures were and still are visited on this group of professionals. They are expected to give back to their local and/or national communities and often become trapped in a situation where they have to adapt to "hearing" norms and values in their training and workplace and face huge difficulties concerning attitudes toward them (hearing-centered values, ignorance of their skills, tokenism, and unequal power balances, to name but a few). At the same time, they want to remain strongly involved in the deaf community. These are issues already seen in other minority groups, such as the Black community (Landry 1987, Blackwell 1975) and indigenous groups (Tuhiwai Smith 2012).

This chapter is structured as follows: After I have introduced the subaltern concept, I move on to a literature review on the main topics of this research. I then talk about the methodology for this research, after which I present and analyze the results of interviews I carried out with four deaf subaltern-elite academic professionals. The chapter concludes with a discussion regarding the situation of the current generation of deaf scholars.

THE "CLASS"-BASED CONCEPT AND THE SUBALTERN CONCEPT

Ladd (1998) was the first author to distinguish different groups within the British deaf community, because he found this lack of distinction to be one of the main weaknesses in Deaf Studies cultural analysis[4]:

---

[2] Based on my observations, as of 2016 there are at least 10 deaf people who obtained PhDs in the UK after 2010, and at least six deaf people are currently pursuing a PhD degree. However, the problem in the UK seems to be that while several PhDs have been advertised recently specifically wanting deaf applicants, the supply line of available/qualified/interested young deaf people seems scarce or has dried up.

[3] Here too, the supply line is scarce, especially because of the specific profile of some advertised jobs which are often linked to sign language linguistics, sign language interpreting or sign language teaching.

[4] See also Carmel (1997), Padden and Humphries (2005) and Robinson (2010) for a (historical) analysis of class issues in the American deaf community.

Little or no mention is made of the cultural significance of different groups within Deaf communities—they are all constructed as sharing the same culture in equal measure. Furthermore, although limited mention is made of Deaf families, hard of hearing and mainstreamed Deaf young people and the like, there is almost no mention of the distinctions of class, race, gender, age and sexual orientation (Ladd 2003:260).

Ladd (2003) found that conventional definitions of "class" are a Western construction and cannot automatically be applied to the experience of minority cultures. He thought the term "subaltern" to be more useful for his cultural analysis because it offered a possibility to correct academic bias, given that it enables a demarcation of social distinctions in groups that do not fall into conventional Western class divisions. He uses the term "subaltern" to distinguish between "what we might call 'grass-roots' and 'intellectual' members of minority cultures" (Ladd 2003:19).

"Subaltern" is a term derived from Gramsci (1971) and represented by the work of Guha (1982) and Spivak (1996). It refers to "any group of people denied meaningful access to 'hegemonic' power" (Ladd 2003:81) and "subject to the hegemony of the ruling classes" (Ashcroft et al. 2000:215). It was brought into postcolonial discourse to situate the social position and discourse of "ordinary" people in relation to those of the intelligentsia and comprador groupings (Ladd 2003). In postcolonial theory, the term "comprador" refers to the intelligentsia "whose dependence may be compromised by a reliance on, and identification with, colonial power" (Ashcroft et al. 2000:55). Guha's (1982) work was instrumental in exposing the version of history within postcolonial India written by elite groups, and how subaltern groups had played an important part in resisting the British but had been "written out" of history by elite groups, who controlled the hegemonic discourse.

STATUS AND CLASS DISTINCTIONS DURING ORALIST AND SOCIAL WELFARE COLONIALISM

Ladd (2003) gives an extensive account of "class" differences within the British deaf community during the period of oralist and social welfare colonialism (circa 1900–1960). Up till now, Ladd is the only one who has investigated these issues in the UK deaf community; hence this chapter will rely on his work quite heavily. During this period, the only deaf people who were *not* subaltern were some deaf missioners and welfare workers, a few high-ranking members of the BDDA,[5] and some oralist children of the wealthy. Virtually all the deaf club members worked in

[5] British Deaf and Dumb Association, as it was then called (currently British Deaf Association).

manual trades and had become illiterate (and thus subaltern) in comparison with previous generations. Indeed, under oralism, the removal of sign languages from deaf education left the majority of deaf people with no access to education at all. This led to the missioners of the Church of England, most of whom were hearing, taking nearly absolute hold over the clubs.

Nevertheless, Ladd (2003) identified class dimensions and patterns of resistance related to class. These dimensions did not seem to be based on deaf people's jobs (they were almost all blue-collar workers, i.e., performing manual labor). Neither did it seem to be based on educational level, given that in general, deaf club members were ill-educated. These dimensions also did not seem to be based on hearing status, because according to Ladd (2003) at the time there seemed to be no sign for "HARD OF HEARING" (Ladd 2003). Differences appeared to be based mainly on the class background of the parents of each group and on the attitude toward the missioners, leading to two distinct groups; on the one hand, a Signed English-using group, the "middle class," who, according to Ladd, avoided conflict with the missioners or took an active role by becoming their "favoured group," and on the other hand, a British Sign Language (BSL) using subaltern group, the "working class," who revolted against the missioners and was not afraid to challenge them. The missioners gave the middle class group token positions of power (e.g., on the deaf club committee), but to keep these, group members had to be successful according to the missioners' deafness model. This meant that most of them had some hearing or were deafened after acquiring English, which allowed them to succeed better under the oralist educational ideology. It also meant that they internalized the negative perceptions of BSL from the missioners, looked down on BSL signers, and used SSE (Sign Supported English) themselves. Ladd (2003) calls them "petit bourgeois" or, to stay within the class distinctions, "elite-subalterns." Under oralism, the division between subalterns (with no command of the majority language) and elite-subalterns (with some command of it, if only superficially, by being able to partially hear it, speak it, read it, or write it), was thus reinforced, because those with better hearing had a better chance of acquiring English.

THE EMERGENCE OF A DEAF PROFESSIONAL CLASS: THE "SUBALTERN-ELITE"

By 1980, the power balance between the deaf middle class (the elite-subalterns) and the deaf subalterns began to swing in the latter's direction. Indeed, linguistic research on BSL became increasingly prominent at universities; there were changes in the educational system toward sign bilingual education, and BSL became increasingly visible on television and in public life. Although the first two series of *See Hear*[6] were still delivered in Signed English with voicing, after campaigns to change this in the third series one presenter was permitted to use BSL[7] and BSL was added to the BBC's language teaching series accompanied by a guide signed by Princess Diana (Miles 1988). Princess Diana[8] was instrumental in raising the public profile of BSL and deaf signers, by learning BSL herself, by becoming a patron of the BDA in 1983, and by being present at the launch of the first ever BSL Dictionary in 1992. All these evolutions benefited deaf BSL signers (many of them from deaf families), who were at that time almost all functionally monolingual in BSL (Conrad 1979) and employed in blue-collar jobs. Deaf BSL signers began to occupy professional positions, most of them within deaf-related areas; for example as sign language tutors, research assistants, and mental health aides. Specifically for Deaf Studies research in this period, Turner (2007) mentions the increasing focus of research institutes such as the Centre for Deaf Studies in Bristol and the Deaf Studies Research Unit in Durham on training of deaf people to prepare professionals in all deaf-related areas who, as BSL signers, would be sensitive to deaf issues.

Because deaf subalterns now obtained professional posts and training and began to participate in the deafness discourse, the subaltern concept became problematic. In the 1990s the signs "GRASS-ROOTS" and "GRASS-ROOTS-OUT" emerged, with the latter indicating those who had "uprooted" themselves from the subaltern community. Although these signs illustrated that the British deaf community started to make a distinction between professionals and subalterns, Ladd (2003) states there are reasons to believe that this group of deaf professionals was still essentially subaltern. To reflect this, he decided to continue to use the term "subaltern" to refer to this professional group but add a demarcation, using the term "subaltern-elite"[9] (not to be confused with the "elite-subalterns," the group that was granted privileges during the era of oralist and social welfare colonialism).

Indeed, both the subaltern and the subaltern-elite group still shared BSL as their first language and had a common cultural background based around the deaf school experience. They both experienced oralism and internalized its effects, resulting in, for example, low levels of

---

[6] *See Hear* is a weekly magazine programme for the British deaf community on BBC Two established in 1981, and one of the longest-running UK television series. See Ladd (2007) for a historical overview of the programme.

[7] It was not until 1987 before the whole programme was presented in BSL (Ladd 2007).

[8] To see Princess Diana signing BSL, see https://www.youtube.com/watch?v=yelE5nmK0dg.

[9] Ladd (2003) admits this is a somewhat simplified demarcation and is not unproblematic in the context of, for example, mainstreamed young deaf people and minority groups within the British deaf community.

self-confidence. Both groups shared knowledge of deaf organizations and deaf history and traditions. Although the English skills of the professional group had improved because of their professional demands and training, they still felt uncomfortable with printed and spoken English discourse. The professional group still socialized with the deaf community, albeit in different forms than before, was still committed to maintaining and developing the deaf community (although they had different roles and strategies for doing so—I describe these later in the chapter), and were still treated as "deaf" (i.e., functionally monolingual in BSL) by the hegemonic discourses (Ladd 2003).

COLLECTIVIST VALUES AND "STICKING OUT"

The rise of this deaf professional class was not met with total enthusiasm by the subaltern community, as evidenced by the development of the sign "GRASS-ROOTS-OUT" to indicate how the professionals were perceived as having moved away from their "grass-roots," that is, their deaf club background. Redfern (1995:8) describes the emergence of the professional class as a double-edged sword leading to a weakened status for both the deaf clubs and the deaf professionals.

> [There are] Those who have moved out of the Deaf clubs or who are still in the clubs but in a smaller role, either giving up or reducing their voluntary work [...] They are now finding it difficult to maintain their old friendships. Sometimes it's because the conversation at the Deaf club has become boring for those who are now working professionally. [...] And the people who still enjoy their Deaf clubs find it difficult to relate to their old friends who are now professional workers and are now becoming "workaholics." The consequence is that the Deaf clubs have become weakened because of the loss of their leaders and the leaders have lost their support network.

Ladd (2001) points out six sources of stress for deaf professionals. One of these stress-sources is having to walk a tightrope all the time: deciding when to pass on information to deaf subaltern people and when not to, when to talk about their jobs and when not to, always facing the risk of being accused of "talking smart." Another source of stress is the risk of rejection because of their changed status:

> [...] they walk a tightrope between a search for conversation levels which match their newly awakened vision and thirst for information and knowledge, and finding ways to remain within their local community (Ladd 2001: no page number).

It would appear that many of the deaf professionals who emerged during this period have been the victims of "tall poppy treatment." They were not allowed to "stick out,"[10] and overt and covert actions were set in place to pull them down. This is commonly known as the "crab theory" or "crab antics." As early as 1949 in the United States, Murphy mentioned this issue, although he did not use the term "crab theory":

> There have been many leaders of the deaf who were glad to devote their time and effort toward a better deaf world, and who had no thought of recompense for their work. [. . .] In many cases the deaf try to hinder their leaders. They say things that are untrue about the leader trying to create distrust of him among his followers. This is very discouraging to the leaders and it is fortunate that only a few of them have quit (Murphy, 1949:5).

Moore and Levitan (1993) also describe this behavior:

> Oppressed in blatant and subtle ways from a very early age, Deaf people have traditionally reacted by huddling into something like solidarity: "Let's endure this together; are we all here?" This group loyalty has in turn fostered a rigid conformist mentality. If I'm oppressed by the Hearing culture, and you're oppressed, we can help each other out, but if you do something to rock the boat or break loose from the group, even if it will ultimately benefit me, you've disrupted the order of things and behaved disloyally to your Deaf culture (Moore & Levitan 1993:271–272).

The issue at stake was thus not only jealousy but also the *perception* of disruption and disloyalty. Indeed, Humphrey and Alcorn (2001:29) found that within a collectivist framework status and identity are defined "by one's connection within the group."

DEAF COMMUNITIES AND THE VALUE OF EDUCATION/QUALIFICATIONS

Education and qualifications have been a longstanding controversial issue in deaf communities. In 1980, Higgins (1980:55) mentioned that

> In almost no other marginalized group is so little value attached to the extent of one's education, and seldom is the attainment of educational distinction such a cause for suspicions as to one's loyalty to the community.

This quote needs to be contextualized both in space (the United States) and in time (some 35 years ago). More recent research is needed to establish the value of education and qualifications in present-day deaf communities. Friedner (2015), for example, demonstrates the high value attached

---

[10] The verb "stick out" is derived from a BSL sign that was often used during the interviews for this research.

to education in urban Indian deaf communities. Ladd mentions tensions between Gallaudet graduates and the American deaf community:

> Sectors of the American Deaf community also resent the amount of power and influence its [Gallaudet University's] alumni have had, and their perceived attitudes towards subaltern Deaf [. . .] (Ladd 2003:58).

Gallaudet graduates were accused of having a "snobbish" attitude, of thinking that they were better than others and thus choosing the "individual way." Padden and Humphries (1988) refer to Bragg and Bergman's play, "Tales from a Clubroom," from 1981. In one particular scene, the character Mark Lindsey, a Gallaudet graduate, enters the deaf club. Will Grady, one of the club coordinators, warns Lindsey about his attitude:

> Grady: Say, you use some strange signs.
> Lindsey: What do you mean, strange?
> Grady: You fingerspell big words. "Operate, opretate [sic]." I don't know how to fingerspell it. And you use fancy signs . . . Our signs are good enough for us. I'm older than you, so let me give you some advice. You came here to make some new friends, right? (Lindsey nods.) If you want to be accepted, don't act like a smartass or you won't make any friends.
> (Padden & Humphries 1988:66–67)

Although the literature in this part mostly refers to the United States, it is relevant to the UK situation. Willis (1977),[11] in his ethnographic study of (hearing) working class high school students (or "lads") in a British industrial town, describes a process wherein the "lads" distance themselves from the school culture and requirements and develop their own counterculture. This counterculture is built, among other things, on a working class discourse of privileging practical knowledge, life experience, and "street wisdom" over theoretical knowledge, attributing high value to the group, expressing opposition to academia, and glorifying hard manual labor. The "lads" feel that what the school is trying to offer them, namely, formal knowledge and skills, will not serve them in life and will lead to their rejection by their peers because such things are considered "feminine." By setting themselves up for working class jobs, the lads were merely reproducing their class positions.

Ladd (2003:181) mentions elitist attitudes toward BSL and its users by graduates of the Mary Hare Grammar School.[12] Young et al., in their study of a deaf school and two psychiatric units with a mixed

---

[11] Thanks to Michele Friedner for bringing this study to my attention.
[12] Mary Hary Grammar School is a deaf school in southern England established in the 1940s with spoken English as the (only) language of instruction. Because it mostly selected

Deaf-hearing staff, discussed the "qualifications versus skills-debate." In all three organizations they analyzed, a key issue was "[. . .] the tension between the low occupational status of the majority of deaf staff and their high intrinsic value in delivering an effective service (Young et al. 1998:4). All three organizations were in a situation where they had to cope with the problem of the relationship between the "unqualified" skills and experience of the majority of deaf staff and the "qualified" skills and experience of the majority of hearing staff. Qualified hearing staff could no longer assume that their mere qualifications were enough to do the job, while deaf staff with relevant skills and experience began to question the value of professional qualifications and those who possess them (Young et al. 1998). This "qualifications versus skills" question and the meaning of education and qualifications turned out to be a significant and recurring topic in the interviews discussed in the data portion of the research.

METHODOLOGY

Interviews

The informants for this research were four deaf staff members working within a UK academic research and teaching institute within a mainstream university: Kate, Helen, Neil, and Sue.[13] They were all members of the group of deaf professionals (subaltern-elite) that emerged during the Deaf Resurgence and all came from a deaf school background. The informants all had been active in maintaining and developing their relationships with their local and national deaf community and had reflected on that relationship. They knew each other as colleagues, and also knew from each other they were being interviewed for this research. The functions they had at the time of the research ranged from teaching BSL to carrying out research projects themselves (mostly on BSL), being involved as research assistants, and/or working in university administration. At the time of the research, none of the informants held a postgraduate (master's degree) qualification.

A semistructured interview schedule was used with a prepared list of general questions, but any interesting points brought up by the informants were followed up. All but one staff member were interviewed in the same period in 2006, so it was possible to triangulate thoughts and opinions from one interviewee in an interview with another. All interviews were carried out in British Sign Language and video recorded.

---

hard-of-hearing and deafened children, who were discouraged from seeking contact with the deaf community, Ladd (2003:181) describes it as "a useful instrument for oralist propaganda."

[13] Because of confidentiality issues these are fictional names.

The participants were accustomed to being filmed during interviews and to working with a camera, so this was not a major issue.

Three staff members were interviewed two times, whereby each interview lasted on average one and a half hours. The fourth staff member could only be interviewed for 50 minutes, due to time constraints for both the staff member and me. The data in BSL were then translated to English. In doing so, I tried to stay as close to the BSL meaning as possible. In some instances I chose to use glossing, that is, the nearest equivalent to the sign in printed text.

All informants were offered the option of confidentiality. I gave them this option for two reasons. Firstly, interviews conducted within an academic workplace might obtain nonoptimal answers due to informants' fears about losing their positions, or fears about how their answers might affect their professional relationship with the workplace and/ or colleagues (Santini 2001). Secondly, some of the informants' statements are personal in nature. I thus changed the informants' names and other "give-aways," and removed any features of the data that could reveal their identities. I also chose to not reveal the name of the research and teaching institute, because this would jeopardize informants' anonymity.

Positionality

I came to the research field as a MA student at the University of Bristol. Hailing from Belgium, BSL is not my first sign language, but when I started the interviews for the research I had been living in the United Kingdom for almost a year. I had been using BSL on a daily basis and in different situations; for example, at the Centre for Deaf Studies, at my student home, in the homes of other signing students, and in social situations such as the deaf pub. Although I had insider status being deaf myself, I was a relative outsider in and newcomer to the British deaf community. In addition, my status as a MA student, that is, as someone pursuing a qualification in higher education, made me different from the informants, who at the time did not have this qualification.

HISTORY OF THE INSTITUTE'S RELATIONSHIP WITH THE LOCAL DEAF COMMUNITY

The history and situation of the institute where the four informants were employed at the time, and its relationship with the deaf community based in the same city, had a profound impact on the role of the four informants and their own relationships with the community. All the informants asserted that in the early days of the institute, around the end of the 1970s, strong ties existed with the local deaf community because all deaf staff members employed at that time ("subaltern-elite") came from the local community, in contrast with research units in other locations.[14] Deaf people, often without traditional academic backgrounds, were appointed as members of university staff.

> Through our work, the community became interested, because we travelled back and forth between the university and the community. They knew about our work, but they never thought about us as from the university, "high level," professionals … The same for the three of us [the three deaf research assistants employed at that time], we never thought about ourselves like that. It was just a job; pass on information to them and connect with them. (Kate)

The institute also engaged with the community through courses and research projects. Turner (2007) describes the trend at that time in Britain for Deaf Studies research and theoretical advances to go hand-in-hand with dissemination, and efforts of research institutes to disseminate information in ways accessible to all relevant stakeholders in the public domain. Murray (this volume) found that the early days of the Deaf Studies field in the United States also demonstrated an alliance between academic research and deaf community goals. In the 1980s, the institute set up certificate and noncertificate courses, which offered local deaf people access to the latest thinking on sign language, "deaf community," and "deaf culture." Informants saw these as very useful and beneficial to the relationship with the community because the courses allowed deaf people to come together and share information and insights, which they would then take to the larger community. Neil believed that the institute

> [...] always positively supported the community [...]. They always tried to empower the community through involvement in projects, and also involved the local deaf school. As a result, several deaf people from the local community became students at the Institute, studying for a certificate. Before, they worked in a factory or an office, but after they got a certificate, they went to work in a deaf school or for a deaf organisation.

This illustrates how the institute itself was instrumental in creating a group of deaf professionals through awareness raising and training. All informants believed that around the beginning of the 1990s, the situation began to change. During this period, the institute began to set up interpreting courses, which at the end of the 1990s became a BA course in Deaf Studies (later an MA would be added). In the mid 2000s, new deaf and hearing staff members from outside the local community were recruited, and the focus shifted more toward teaching hearing students. With the advent of the bachelor's and master's degrees,

---

[14] Graham Turner, personal communication, March 8, 2016.

the university raised entrance requirements and gradually fewer deaf students entered the program.

> When the degrees started, it all changed. The deaf community felt they had no access. At that moment, there became a divide between the Institute and the community. (Kate)

Informants also stated that after some time, the local deaf club began to suffer from consultation fatigue (see also Singleton et al. 2015 for the risk of "overtesting") and became less motivated to participate in research because they felt they received nothing back from it. Around the time my research was carried out, the institute was still trying to disseminate information to the local community, but this happened in different ways than before, mainly through DVDs that were sent out to the deaf club without staff members really meeting people. Lack of financial resources also was mentioned as a reason for the divide with the community. Before, the institute had, for example, funded programs to allow deaf families to host hearing students as a way to allow for linguistic and cultural immersion. This funding dried up, and so did the deaf community's involvement. Informants also felt deaf peoples' ethos changed, and they wanted to be paid for their contribution.

> When I was young, I often volunteered, and I was very happy to do that. I did it all my life, and I'm still doing it now. But a lot of people see that differently; they expect to earn money. When the deaf community began to expect to get paid for their contribution, there became a divide. And now, it's very difficult to involve deaf people at all. The ethos changed. [...] (Neil)

The introduction of the undergraduate degrees not only meant that informants had to invest more time in teaching hearing students, but also that hearing students outnumbered deaf students and, according to informants, became "overpowering" in relation to the knowledge and information most deaf people had. They all had strong feelings about this.

> Because we teach hearing people, I feel I can't give back to the deaf community. [...] I'm not comfortable with that. Hearing students achieve a degree, and know more [about sign language and culture] than deaf people themselves! But it is their [deaf] culture, their language! When I have information, I want to give it to deaf people! But we give it to hearing people. That's very frustrating. (Kate)

This also led to informants valuing their volunteer work for the deaf community very much.

> I'm worried about only teaching hearing students, and I think a lot of staff here feel the same. [...] I'm frustrated, because I have a

lot of information, but I give it all to hearing students. That's why I still hold on to my volunteer work. I also still teach [deaf students]. That way, I can encourage deaf people, cultivate their skills ... If I couldn't do that, I wouldn't be happy. (Neil)

All informants referred to their support of the deaf community, either locally or nationally, and the use of their skills for its benefit, as "giving back." For Kate it was something she grew up with:

I have a role there [in the deaf community]. I felt that through my upbringing and I still feel that. I have a *duty* towards the deaf community. I'm not used to say that, but I feel I have it. Nobody tells you that you have it, or that you *must* do something, but I feel ... If I would do nothing, I would feel guilty.

An important aspect of this giving back was that informants knew *to whom* they were giving back.

Maybe they [hearing professionals] give back, too, but to the hearing world in general, to people they don't know, they didn't grow up with. I give back to my community; I grew up there. (Helen)

"Giving back" could happen in various ways. Informants asserted that in the early days of the institute, it happened, for example, through joint research projects and dissemination within the deaf community, that it was "part of the job." Now, however, giving back happened in more individual ways. Helen signed the news on television and felt that this was her way of giving something back. She felt that hearing people see this as a professional job whereas for her it was a way of giving back. This statement was somewhat ambiguous given that she was paid for this work, too. As a deaf interpreter, however, she might feel more connected to the community for whom she is working (Stone 2009). Kate was involved in awareness-raising activities concerning deaf women's health and in the local deaf club, as well as in a national deaf organization. Neil performed his volunteer work in teaching and in his commitments to a national deaf organization. This corresponds with McDermid's (2009) account of the collectivist framework in which deaf staff members in U.S. institutions engaged, that is, their shared value of community involvement and reciprocity.

Neil observed that the university recently became more aware of the importance of academics serving their communities:

Recently, they [the university] said that they would support staff who are involved in supporting their community. They never said that before! So they've started to see it. Maybe we, as staff, should let them know that we want to work for the community one day a week or something.

Ladd (2003) confirms that in collectivist cultures like deaf cultures, "giving back" is linked to what one is doing with the qualifications and status one has achieved through education.

THE PROFESSIONAL STATUS OF THE DEAF STAFF MEMBERS

Kate did not find it easy to cope with her changed professional status. "I feel ... I moved on, while they [subaltern deaf people] are still the same. It hurts so see that."

When she goes to the deaf club, she feels she often has to behave carefully.

> In the deaf club, I'm just Kate, "ROLE-NOTHING," I'm the same as everyone else. I have to, because if I behave differently, they [deaf people] will feel a power divide.

This statement is ambiguous, because Kate does not make clear whether she wants to be treated "the same as everyone else," or behaves like that (although she knows she is not) to conform to others' expectations of her. Sue remarked that how other deaf people react to her professional status depends on the context and that it takes time for people to accept her as a person instead of as a professional only.

> One of the things I like very much is going out to the [...][15] club [in another place]. A lot of deaf people there don't know about my job, so I can just mix with them. There I am just Sue, not university. But at other places, deaf people know who I am. But I think after a while, they become used to it. Also, the older people, they say, "UNIVERSITY CLEVER-CLEVER," but at the same time, they don't really care. It's different from the younger people, my age group, they know about my job.

Still, their professional status meant that deaf people had certain expectations of deaf professionals, and they often are asked for help and advice, sometimes at the expense of their own free time in social situations.

> In my free time, I often went to social events with my wife. But it wasn't really social, because deaf people always had to ask me things or talk to me about work. I told them, "I'm not working now, I need to switch off!" But they really can't see I need to relax. My wife was quite upset about that, told me that I had [a] right to my own time. But when people ask me something, I always try to talk with them; I can't just say "bugger off!" That's not me. I now understand why they felt they had to do that. If you are hearing and you

---

[15] Name withheld for confidentiality reasons.

have questions about the course, you can e-mail, or phone, ask others, or read. But deaf people are not really confident with e-mail, if they read they don't understand it and there are not many people they can ask for help. So they come to me. I need to recognize that but still, it's very difficult. That's part of the reason some of us—I say *some*, because others are still going—went less to social events, because they couldn't cope with those expectations." (Neil)

This corresponds with Kusters et al.'s (this volume) statement that because of the perceived "DEAF-SAME" feelings and the privileged position of deaf professionals, they sometimes experience high expectations of deaf communities and that failure to respond to such requests can result in distrust or disappointment.

DIVIDE BETWEEN THE PROFESSIONAL GROUP AND THE COMMUNITY

Informants often had a hard time meeting both their professional demands and those of the deaf club. Because of their specific skills, there was often a high demand for them to be involved in all kinds of matters related to deaf organizations.

Work at university means a heavy commitment, and that means I'm less involved in the community. Some deaf people are quite upset about that. They say I think I'm better than them, that I avoid them but that's not true! I'm just often very tired, worn out. That's hard. There is a lot of misunderstanding. (Neil)

When they declined demands because of lack of time or energy, they often were accused of selfishness and warned that this would affect the situation at the deaf club.

Some people from the community blame the ones that left (or come less often) because of their professional demands. They feel we "left" the community and blame us for the decline of the deaf club. They say "you created this." (Neil)

Kate, however, felt that this divide between the professional group and the deaf community only partly had to do with demands and time pressure. Although a professional job, indeed, demands a sustained commitment of time and energy, she believed the divide is also due to the professional group not knowing how to relate to their friends and acquaintances in the deaf club anymore, and to the professional group's thirst for "information" they believe is not available in the deaf club.

It's not only about time; it's also about that they [the professionals] don't know what to say. There is a difference between their knowledge and the community's. The professionals don't know what to talk about; they feel the community is only everyday, simple talk. But it *is* possible to talk, they just don't know how, they forgot. They want information, and feel they can't get that information in the deaf club. But if you make time to slow down, to sit and talk, it will happen automatically, it *is* there. But you can't just go and expect all this to happen from the first instance. It needs time. (Kate)

The problem, however, not only had to do with the professional group's attitudes but also with the "subaltern" deaf people themselves, she said.

I'm worried about the deaf club. Hearing people have their own local pub where they can just sit and chat. But increasingly, deaf people say they will only come when there is "something on." If there is nothing on, they don't know what to do and think it is boring. But it's not boring! You have time for conversation. But deaf people don't know how to have a conversation with each other anymore. [...] They work in a hearing environment, can't talk there, most of them can't talk with their family, they sit in front of the television focused on hearing life, but they forgot what a deaf life is, really. (Kate)

This divide between the professional and the subaltern group, Kate said, was caused by an increasingly competitive environment in which deaf professionals had to "compete" against their hearing peers.

I want them all together again, to be connected. We really need that. Because who created this division? Hearing society. [...] Because deaf people feel competition with hearing people, feel they have to strive to as high a level as possible. But they forget the deaf community. (Kate)

Sue had a different view on this. Although she recognized the value of collectivity, she believed it is just a fact that things change, and that it is a good thing to have different groups within the community:

Why should deaf people always stay together, like in a ghetto? Why should you stay in the same group just because you're deaf? [...] Why should I force myself to come to a place when there is another group in a different place where I fit much better because we have the same interests? That's a good thing! Some deaf women are housewives and want to talk with each other about their children. That's fine! That's not a bad thing. I think it's just about accepting things change. The same is true for the club culture, which has become a pub culture. That's life, things change. Text messages influence us, subtitles, ... People stay more at home now. Some people think that's a bad thing, some that's a good thing but again, life just changes. That's it. (Sue)

With "club culture becoming a pub culture," Sue refers to the growing "pub scene" in many UK cities in which young deaf people go to pubs rather than deaf clubs in order to interact and socialize not only with other young deaf people but also with hearing people. For an analysis of this pub scene and interactions that occur there, see O'Brien (2005).

WALKING A TIGHTROPE

A recurring theme in the interviews, also described by Ladd (2003) was that of informants having to walk a tightrope all the time in terms of how to behave, what to say and when. Because of their status, the informants were quickly seen by subaltern deaf people as pedantic or "talking smart."

> I don't start to talk about my work and politics myself. When they [subaltern deaf people] start and bring that up, I'm happy to join, but I don't start myself. (Kate)

Although a normal social scene was not perceived as problematic most of the time, the informants felt this changed when there was politics involved, information had to be given, or decisions made, for example, at the deaf club's annual general meeting (AGM). In this situation, informants felt they became a "professional" for the other deaf people present, and they tried to stay low profile.

> Some deaf people say like "THEIRS-UNIVERSITY." Like at the deaf club AGM, I always try to be low profile and not to stand up to say something. I leave it to the deaf people there. Sometimes when I do stand up, I see some deaf like *(looks disapproving)* "UNIVERSITY-AGAIN." (Helen)

They were also very well aware, however, of their status and ability to exert influence without being perceived as doing so. Even here, the line between when to be involved and not was very thin.

> When I'm involved in a meeting or AGM, I just leave it. It's better not to stand up. But you can play that smart, that's our skill. You can't make them feel like they are under pressure, but you can say something like "why don't you try this, or...". So that they think *they* make the decision, not you. I can't just say "I disagree, you are wrong!" I really can't do that. But there is a dangerous line between where they will say, "why are you not involved, come on!" and where I think, "better not now, you can do this yourselves, don't rely on us." (Neil)

THE "PROFESSIONAL" LABEL AND THE MEANING OF "QUALIFICATIONS"

The "professional" label was something all informants felt strongly about, agreeing it is a "hearing label" highly valued in hearing society but with virtually no significance in the deaf community.

> In the hearing world, it's important to show we are professionals, show them we *can* do things. So that they know deaf people have a high level of achievement. For deaf people it means nothing. If you show it, there will be a high level–low level divide, immediately. I just had the opportunity, they didn't . . . (Kate)

The professional label was seen rather as a leverage that could be used to show hearing people one's worth, something which was not perceived to be necessary and/or socially acceptable among deaf people.

> Sometimes, in the deaf school, I had to tell people explicitly: "I am a lecturer, I have a high-level function. Treat me accordingly." I would never say that in the deaf community. (Helen)

Neil, while very aware of his capacities and skills, realized that "out there" in "the hearing world," these are not recognized as such:

> When I would change jobs, I will need to show my qualifications. Here at the Institute, they all know me, they know my skills, my knowledge. But out there [in the hearing world], I'm worth nothing. That's what I mean with differing perspectives on professionalism in deaf and hearing worlds.

Informants observed that in their professional environment, qualifications were seen as important by hearing but not by deaf staff members.

> Recently, staff here began to put qualifications behind their names, like BA, or MA, or PhD. But it's only hearing staff who do this; deaf staff don't bother. Deaf staff members only do this when they have to confront the hearing world. To let hearing people know: "I have this qualification." But they will not do the same in the deaf world. There is a different way there to profile yourself, and they judge you on different standards and values. (Neil)

This "judgment" is linked to what Neil calls "approval" from the community. Getting this approval means it is OK to "stick out," that is, to achieve professional status. Approval is linked to demonstrating one's loyalty to the community—by showing up regularly—and to one's attitude. This approval does not depend on someone's qualifications, but rather means:

[. . .] the group says: "you have permission." They *give* you approval. It is not linked to your "piece of paper," your qualification. Collective communities have their own approval. (Neil)

This relates to Humphrey and Alcorn's (2001) finding that connections to the group are important for one's status and identity within a collectivist culture.

Ladd (2003) mentions it might be surprising that a respectable social standing does not come naturally to professionals and claims that "[. . .] in Deaf communities, with their strong belief in cultural collectivism, *attitude* is, or can be, all" (58–59).

I'm a professional, but I'm still in the deaf community, I still go to the deaf club. That means that deaf people see I'm still around, and they accept my professional status. But some people stick out and never come back. And if they come, deaf people in the club immediately start to say: "What is he/she here for?" (Helen)

Neil disapproved of the behavior of some of the professional group's members, who, because they now had a qualification, expected to be treated differently.

I'm worried, because some deaf people get qualifications, and from then on, they expect everyone to admire them. When that is not happening, they become bitter. They expect that because they have a degree, a red carpet is being rolled out for them. But that's not happening. Even the opposite is happening: They are rejected, and have no approval from the community. (Neil)

Helen had similar feelings about the group of "new" deaf professionals:

I feel the young professionals don't value that you need approval. They just come and don't think about approval, they don't feel they need that. When I go to the deaf community, I really feel that's my community, I feel happy they approve me and accept me. That really means a lot to me. The community is like home, like a family. But for young people, that's completely different; they have different values, different beliefs. They just come to the deaf club and that's fine, but they know they can go to other places as well. DEAF-INSIDE-VALUE-NOT-THERE.[16]

Still, the issue of qualifications remained very sensitive and ambiguous. Sometimes it was not clear whether informants really thought

---

[16] I used glossing for this part of the quote because it has a rich cultural meaning which is difficult to translate in one English sentence.

qualifications are not important, or that they thought they are important but are difficult to achieve.

> Before, deaf people could say, "Well, I'm deaf, you know," as a sort of excuse. That's not possible anymore. I think that's both positive and negative. Positive because deaf people now can achieve many things but negative because despite that, they still confront many barriers. So where does that leave us? (Neil)

Also, the informants' view on education and qualifications might be informed by their experience with and observations of hearing (qualified) professionals; for example, hearing teachers in the deaf school. Informants observe that (unqualified) deaf teachers are way ahead in competency compared with their qualified hearing peers, which might lead them to question the very value of those qualifications (see also Kusters, this volume):

> Here in the deaf school, the deaf teachers are not qualified. But to be fair, their service and skills are really amazing, often much better than those of the qualified [hearing] teachers. But these deaf teachers are not paid on a professional level; their status is still very low. Some of them just left because they are frustrated. They still confront that glass ceiling because it is very difficult for them to become a qualified teacher. That really disappoints me because they are way ahead in competency and capacity, but they can't get the qualifications! (Neil)

This links to the "qualifications versus skills" debate mentioned by Young et al. (1998). Although Neil jokingly said he has "a degree of life," he also wondered about his need to gain a degree.

> But some deaf people say: "What for'? Why would you do that?" But I know I will have a problem out there without qualifications. [...] Society forces us; they make these qualifications important. I'm like torn between the university community and the deaf community. (Neil)

Talking about the hierarchy of values in deaf and hearing worlds, he said he has a strong deaf perspective, which means, "I value skills, knowledge and experience over qualifications. I respect qualifications, but they are not important to me."

These accounts represent what Ladd (2003) has termed "double binds"; situations that place minority cultural members and their allies in strategic dilemmas resembling "no win" situations. Neil's last quote, in particular, expresses this double bind: pursuing qualifications may lead to him being rejected by some deaf people and be seen as "betraying" the deaf community, while not pursuing them means limiting his own professional opportunities and development.

A "deaf perspective" is described as valuing skills and knowledge over qualifications. This also links with the "double bind" situations; "cultural forms which are rationalized as 'Deaf', yet perpetuate the oppression" (Ladd 2003:418) and result in damage to cultural unity. There is an interesting parallel here with the accounts of the working class "lads" in Willis's (1977) study, whose counterculture is built on a similar discourse of privileging practical knowledge ("a degree of life") over theoretical knowledge and the high value attributed to the group.

THE CURRENT GENERATION OF DEAF SCHOLARS: ARE THEY STILL SUBALTERN?

The research carried out in 2006 had a specific focus: the experiences of deaf academic professionals ("subaltern-elite") who emerged during the Deaf Resurgence, and their relationship with the ("subaltern") deaf community. It is an interesting exercise to review these data in light of the current situation in the United Kingdom. Based on my observations (and in the absence of any official statistics), it seems that postgraduate degrees are not that controversial anymore; indeed, a growing number of deaf students in the United Kingdom have obtained them (including all of the four informants) or are pursuing them. The current generation—as opposed to the one interviewed for this chapter—has had better access to the regular curriculum and/or sign bilingual education and with that, to higher education. Although deaf PhDs remain less numerous, an increasing number of deaf people are obtaining them, too.

It is crucial to realize that although the number of deaf scholars is steadily growing, their influence over the fields in which they work remains small. A very small number are leading research projects or are eligible to apply for research grants as principal investigators. Most work under hearing principal investigators, and their social, cultural, and linguistic capital is often not recognized by the academy (O'Brien & Emery 2014). Also, the power of deaf scholars in relation to hearing scholars is not to be overestimated (for a discussion of this, see, for example, Kusters et al., this volume, O'Brien, this volume, O'Brien & Emery 2014; for a different perspective, see Sutton-Spence & West 2011).

But the *relative* power deaf scholars hold compared with the majority of deaf people is significant, and one can discuss whether Ladd's (2003) subaltern and subaltern-elite categories are still applicable or even relevant. Indeed, Spivak (1990) and others have suggested that once the subaltern can "speak" (in a metaphorical sense),[17] they are no longer

---

17 The concept "speak" might be confusing in a Deaf Studies context. Spivak (1990) clearly meant this in a metaphorical sense, as in "contributing to hegemonic discourses."

subaltern. Ladd (2003) has stated there is interplay between subaltern and elite, which cannot be captured in this limited bipolar perspective, which is why he created the subaltern-elite category. Still, it can be discussed whether the current generation of deaf scholars, for example, the ones involved in writing this volume, can be called "subaltern-elite." Ladd (2003) described his own position as "subaltern-elite" based on self-ascribed "subaltern" characteristics, such as experience of oralism (although in a different way than a monolingual deaf person in sign language), experience of being audiologically deaf in a hearing world, and his socialization with the deaf community. He was aware though that this appellation required vigilance, because of English being his first language, his privileged position as a bilingual, and his lack of a deaf school experience.

In later reflections on this,[18] Ladd expressed doubts about this assessment of himself as "subaltern-elite," describing his position as something of a "historical anomaly" coming as he did from the first generation of individual mainstreaming in the United Kingdom (Ladd 1979). His historical positioning, both in respect to oralism and the subsequent Deaf Resurgence, meant that the position he most resembled was the subaltern-elite category, which was reinforced by a strong commitment to the understanding, support, and advocacy of subaltern views. Nonetheless, his immersion in a monolingual "hearing" world for the first 22 years of his life meant that he missed out on the crucial deaf school experience, and his in-depth cultural familiarity with that hearing world, and his privileged position as a bilingual with English as his first language, meant that the subaltern-elite category was only the most useful grouping for the purposes of Ladd's (2003) research, rather than a definitive positioning.

Ladd's position actually prefigures the current generation of deaf scholars, many of whom went to hearing schools for all or most of their schooling, including the authors of this volume (see Kusters et al., this volume, for further discussion). Taking Ladd's experience as a point of reference, we can compare it to these authors. All of us are to some extent "insider researchers" who conduct research on the cultural, racial, or ethnic group to which we belong (Moges 2015) based on deaf ontologies and employing deaf capital.[19] Ladd (2003:19) claimed that in order to become such an insider researcher, "one must spend years learning to think and feel in ways and methods designed by white, middle-class, able-bodied males within majority society academic structures," which leads to the question of how representative of minority communities

---

[18] Personal communication, Paddy Ladd, March 8, 2016.
[19] See also Haualand, this volume, for a discussion of positionality of deaf researchers.

such a person actually is, and how that affects the nature of his or her research. This is a relevant observation in light of the current generation of deaf scholars. Although we might be subaltern because of our deaf ontologies, our educational background and linguistic competencies make us very different from the previous generation of subaltern-elite who were the subject of this chapter, and this might call into question the very meaning of a deaf ontology. Our having obtained academic degrees means we have gone through traditional academic structures. By not only having access to but increasingly contributing to hegemonic discourses, for example, by publishing in mainstream journals in English or other majority languages and by publishing in volumes such as this, our voice becomes part of and changes these discourses. Additionally, most of the current generation of deaf scholars have a high command of English and/or other written languages, often a high command of one or several sign languages, and most of them are transnationally mobile. Further, the majority are White and middle-class, and there continues to be a huge absence of people of color, disabled deaf scholars, and other minorities (see also Emery 2014, Ruiz et al. 2015). Deaf scholars effectively *do* gain prestige and advantage from their positions and publications—which are barely accessible to those who are not English literate and/or not well-versed in academic jargon. In that sense, deaf scholars are elite not only compared with the majority of deaf people but also compared with many hearing people. It is, therefore, vitally important that deaf scholars (and deaf professionals in other domains) display awareness of this privileged status and remain self-reflective practitioners; otherwise, they risk simply reinforcing hegemonic structures and perceptions of oppression.

However, this volume also demonstrates that many of the current generation of deaf researchers, while having gone through traditional academic structures, use this experience and expertise to challenge those very structures and hegemonic thinking. They are "organic intellectuals," striving "to change the prevailing or dominant perceptions and discourses of Deaf culture and sign language" (O'Brien & Emery 2014:30). In that sense, they are still "giving back"—in myriad ways. For many of them, their positionality, research ethics, and relationships with deaf communities are important issues that influence their work, although the ways in which they give back might be articulated differently than the previous generation, if only because of their educational background and cultural, linguistic, and deaf capital.

WAYS FORWARD

The issue of deaf scholars and their relationship with deaf communities has not decreased in relevance. It is a much-discussed topic, not in the least among deaf scholars themselves. The 1st International Deaf

Academics and Researchers Conference in 2002 included a panel, "Our identities in the Deaf and academic communities. [. . .] What can I as a Deaf researcher contribute to the Deaf community and to the academic community?" The 3rd conference in 2006 had as its main theme, "What do deaf academics mean for the world?"; the 4th conference in 2008, "The role of Deaf Academics in the Pursuit of Social Justice," the main rationale being that "many Deaf academics and researchers have found themselves working in the academia which itself is a cultural institution hence by default, was the mainstay of reproducing inequalities in societies."[20] The 7th conference, in 2015, had several presentations linked to researchers' positionalities and relationships with their communities. In the United Kingdom, three "Bridging the Gap" events have been organized, two in 2014 and one in 2015, which discussed, among other things, community engagement in Deaf Studies research.

With this chapter, I am not aiming to create or reproduce any perceived or false (historical) dichotomies between "the deaf community" and "deaf scholars" or between "deaf scholars" and "the academy," as if loyalty to one necessarily means a "betrayal" of the other, and as if the position of any deaf scholar is stalemated from the start and full of double binds. To do so would not advance the status of deaf communities or the position of deaf scholars themselves. As this volume demonstrates, many deaf scholars *do* value their academic work and output, their publications (whether written and/or signed), and their contribution to the academy. But it also demonstrates that many deaf scholars value their connection with their communities, the impact their work might have on them, and the improvement of deaf lives that may come as a result of it. I agree with O'Brien (this volume) though that in practical terms, this loyalty to both often plays out problematically because of time, energy, and resources. This might be even more so for the current generation of deaf scholars, many of whom are working in an increasingly market-driven academic environment focused on individual progression, publications in English, and availability of funding.

What is needed is a healthy balance, wherein deaf communities learn to appreciate the contribution deaf scholars make (and the choices they sometimes have to make in terms of their community engagement); the academy learns to appreciate and acknowledge the diverse roles deaf scholars play and their commitment to deaf communities; deaf scholars reflect on their role and status and often privileged positions vis-à-vis these communities (both deaf and hearing) of which they are a part and in which they perform research; and Deaf Studies as a field reflects more intensively on its raison d'être and its relationship to the very people it purports to serve.

---

[20] http://www.deafacademics.org/news/article.php?id=70

ACKNOWLEDGMENTS

I would like to thank Hilde Haualand, Hannah Lewis, Annelies Kusters, and Dai O'Brien for their generous and useful comments on earlier drafts of this chapter. Also, a sincere thanks to my four informants for sharing their insights and perspectives, and to Paddy Ladd for sparking my interest in this topic and the many conversations about it.

REFERENCES

Ashcroft, B., Griffiths, G., & Tiffin, H. (2000). *Post-colonial studies. The key concepts.* London & New York: Routledge.

Blackwell, J.E. (1975). *The black community. Diversity and unity.* New York: Dodd, Mead & Company.

Carmel, S. (1997). *A study of deaf culture in an urban deaf community.* Ann Arbor: University of Michigan.

Conrad, R. (1979). *The deaf school child. Language and cognitive function.* London: Harper and Row.

De Meulder, M. (2007). *GIVING BACK. Deaf professionals and the Deaf community* (Unpublished master's thesis). University of Bristol.

Emery, S. (2014). Our newly published article out now: Deaf academics and academia. https://tigerdeafie.wordpress.com/2014/01/23/our-newly-published-article-out-now-deaf-academics-and-academia/. Accessed February 26, 2016.

Friedner, M. (2015). *Valuing deaf worlds in urban India.* New Brunswick, NJ: Rutgers University Press.

Gramsci, A. (1971). *Selections from the prison notebooks.* London: Lawrence and Wishart.

Guha, R. (1982). On some aspects of the historiography of colonial India. In R. Guha (Ed.), *Subaltern Studies I* (pp. 1–8). Delhi: Oxford University Press.

Higgins, P.C. (1980). *Outsiders in a hearing world. A sociology of deafness.* London: Sage Publications.

Humphrey, J.H., & Alcorn, B.J. (2001). *So you want to be an interpreter? An introduction to sign language interpreting* (3rd ed.). Amarillo, TX: H & H Publishing Company.

Ladd, P. (1979). Making plans for Nigel: The erosion of identity by mainstreaming. In G. Montgomery (Ed.), *The integration and disintegration of the deaf in society.* Edinburgh: Scottish Workshop Publications.

Ladd, P. (1998). *In search of Deafhood: Towards an understanding of British Deaf Culture* (Unpublished doctoral dissertation). University of Bristol.

Ladd, P. (2001). *Further explorations in Deaf Sociology.* Resource Materials for Advances in Deaf Studies, University of Bristol.

Ladd, P. (2003). *Understanding Deaf Culture: In search of Deafhood.* Clevedon: Multilingual Matters Ltd.

Ladd, P. (2007). Signs of Change: Sign Language and Televisual Media in the UK. In M. Cormack & N. Hourigan (Eds.), *Minority language media. Concepts, critiques and case studies* (pp. 229–247). Clevedon: Multilingual Matters.

Landry, B. (1987). *The new Black middle class.* Berkeley: University of California Press.

McDermid, C. (2009). Two cultures, one programme: Deaf professors as subaltern? *Deafness and Education International, 11*(4), 221–249.

Miles, D. (1988). *British Sign Language. A beginner's guide.* London: BBC Books.

Mindess, A. (2000). *Reading between the signs. Intercultural communication for Sign Language interpreters.* Yarmouth, ME: Intercultural Press.

Moges, R. (2015). *"Is the Joke on us, Deaf Anthropologist?" Reflections on native anthropology of Deaf culture by Deaf researcher(s).* Presented at the 7th International Deaf Academics and Researchers Conference, Leuven, February 6, 2015.

Moore, M.S., & Levitan, L. (1993). *For hearing people only.* Rochester, NY: MSM Productions, Ltd.

Murphy, F. (1949). Moiphy's column. *Silent Worker, 1*(5), 5.

O'Brien, D. (2005). *What's the sign for "pint"?—An investigation into the validity of two different models to describe Bristol's current Deaf pub culture* (Unpublished master's thesis). University of Bristol.

O'Brien, D., & Emery, S. (2014). The role of the intellectual in minority group studies: Reflections on Deaf Studies in social and political contexts. *Qualitative Inquiry, 20*(1), 27–36.

Padden, C., & Humphries, T. (1988). *Deaf in America. Voices from a culture.* Cambridge, MA: Harvard University Press.

Padden, C., & Humphries, T. (2005). *Inside Deaf Culture.* Cambridge MA: Harvard University Press.

Philip, M. (1993). *Cross-cultural comparisons: American Deaf Culture and American majority culture.* Westminster, CO: Front Range Community College.

Redfern, P. (1995). Deaf professionals: A growing stream. *Deafness, 11*(1), 8–10.

Robinson, T. (2010). "We are of a different class": Ableist rhetoric in Deaf America, 1880–1920. In S. Burch & A. Kafer (Eds.), *Deaf and Disability Studies: Interdisciplinary perspectives* (pp. 5–21). Washington, DC: Gallaudet University Press.

Ruiz-Williams, E., Burke, M., Chong, V.J., & Chainarong, N. (2015). "My deaf is not your deaf": Realizing intersectional realities at Gallaudet University. In A. Kusters & M. Friedner (Eds.), *It's a small world: International deaf spaces and encounters* (pp. 262–274). Washington, DC: Gallaudet University Press.

Santini, J. (2001). *The role models. Multicultural politics at bilingual deaf schools in Britain* (Unpublished master's thesis). University of Bristol.

Singleton, J. L., Martin, A. J., & Morgan, G. (2015). Ethics, deaf-friendly research, and good practice when studying sign languages. In E. Orfanidou, B. Woll, & G. Morgan (Eds.), *Research methods in Sign Language Studies. A practical guide* (pp. 7–20). London: Wiley Blackwell.

Spivak, G. (1990). *The post-colonial critic: Interviews, strategies, dialogues.* S. Harasym, Ed. London: Routledge.

Spivak, G. (1996). *The Spivak reader.* D. Landry & G. Maclean, Eds. London: Routledge.

Stone, C. (2009). *Toward A deaf translation norm.* Washington, DC: Gallaudet University Press.

Sutton-Spence, R., & West, D. (2011). Negotiating the legacy of hearingness. *Qualitative Inquiry, 17*(5), 422–432.

Tuhiwai Smith, L. (2012). *Decolonizing methodologies: research and indigenous peoples* (2nd ed.). London: Zed Books.

Turner, G. H. (2007). The Deaf Studies Project: More questions than answers. *Deaf Worlds, 23*(2–3), 1–26.

Willis, P. E. (1977). *Learning to labor: How working class kids get working class jobs.* Farnborough: Saxon House.

Young, A., Ackerman, J., & Kyle, J. (1998). *Looking on. Deaf people and the organisation of services.* University of Bristol: The Policy Press.

5

Doing Deaf Studies in the Global South

Michele Friedner

INTRODUCTION: DOING WHAT AND WHERE?

In this essay, I will not provide a pedagogical or prescriptive account of how to do deaf studies in the global South. Instead, I explore a series of related questions and themes including: What is deaf studies?[1] What does it mean to *do* deaf studies? What does it mean to do deaf studies in different and diverse locations? What happens when deaf studies travels to the global South? In asking and responding to these questions, my goal is to problematize both "deaf studies" and "the global South" as stable categories. Going forward, I first discuss deaf studies and I then discuss the global South, using recent work in disability studies and the social sciences as a way to spark discussion. I then consider current deaf studies and social science work in, and in relation to, the global South. After this literature review, I move to a broader discussion of the stakes of doing deaf studies in the global South.

From the outset, we cannot ask what it means to do deaf studies in the global South, or countries without or with less access to political economic resources, without also asking what it means to do deaf studies in the global North, or countries with access to and control of such political economic resources. The global South includes countries in Africa, South and Southeast Asia, and Latin America, for example. The global North includes countries such as the United States and European

---

[1] In this essay, I write the names of all disciplines, including deaf studies, with lower cases. In addition, for the sake of simplicity, I attempt to consistently write deaf in the lower case except for when I mention concepts or terms that are typically written with capitalized Ds. Apologies for any inconsistencies that may exist; hopefully readers will see these inconsistencies as productive.

countries, for example.[2] The global South and global North exist in relation to each other and scholars have argued that the global North has created the global South through establishing political economic structures that privilege the global North. Similarly, deaf studies must be emplaced geographically and temporally. The discipline emerged in a specific time and place; it is not a "view from nowhere," or what feminist scholar Donna Haraway (1988:581) very provocatively calls "the god trick." By "the god trick," Haraway is foregrounding the ways that certain kinds of "scientific" knowledge are rendered authoritative, objective, and universal, removed from the context in which they are produced. As Haraway (ibid) stresses, all knowledge is situated knowledge that is produced by people in specific times and places. Similarly, the discipline of deaf studies is a form of situated knowledge (ibid) that exists in relation to other forms of situated knowledge. Deaf studies has its own epistemologies and ontologies bound up within it.

To be clear, what I am calling deaf studies in this essay is the academic and activist discipline that emerged in the United States in the early 1970s, accompanying the recognition of signed languages as languages like any other and ideas of deaf people having their own social and cultural practices.[3] This is a very specific epistemology about what deaf people are and how they should see themselves and their place in the world. It is an epistemology that was born in a particular political economic moment in the United States and the United Kingdom in which disability became a category in relation to other kinds of categories such as race and ethnicity, and deaf people felt the need to stake out a position in relation to this category (H.D. Bauman 2008). A call for deaf people to see themselves as a cultural and linguistic group was not just a scholarly move; it was also a political move in response to conditions in the United States in the aftermath of the Civil Rights movement, during which time groups were using various axes of difference to demand rights and recognition. We cannot consider deaf studies' present and future then without considering its past. And we must be mindful of where this past was situated as we move forward in thinking about what it means to do deaf studies in the global South—a very different context.

In addition, in relation to the question of what does it mean to *do* deaf studies, we also have to ask what does deaf studies *do*? That is, what does it do—as an analytical and methodological framework and as a mode of engagement with deaf people around the world? Indeed,

---

[2] Note that these are quick working definitions of complicated and increasingly contested categories.

[3] Other authors in this book, and deaf studies scholars more broadly, have different definitions of what deaf studies is and should be.

disciplines, with their theoretical and methodological orientations, do things to the world and make certain kinds of knowledge possible or impossible. Disciplines offer up ways of seeing the world, a road map of sorts. Just as deaf studies purports to be interested in *other* deaf peoples' epistemologies and ontologies, such as people who live outside the global North, it also needs to consider its own.

As a collection of essays by deaf scholars on deaf scholarship, this book raises the question of what is unique about deaf peoples' own ontologies and how this uniqueness effects and affects the production of scholarship. The book, therefore, heralds an "ontological turn" in deaf studies, and this moment is happening at a time when increased attention in deaf studies is being devoted to deaf experiences in the global South. I argue that these two moves, or turns, must be examined in relation to each other and that they can yield productive insights. Just as this book, extremely broadly, asks and analyzes what deaf people *do* when they do research on and with other deaf people, here I want to ask what deaf studies does when it travels elsewhere in the world.

By "ontological turn," I draw from recent work in the discipline of anthropology that has attended to questions of how anthropologists construct the very objects that they are studying. The "ontological turn" is concerned with how people construct and populate worlds with other subjects and objects; more broadly, it is concerned with how world-making happens and how anthropologists themselves create worlds in writing people and objects into being (for more on the ontological turn in anthropology, see Holbraad and Peterson's [2014] introduction as well as the other articles in the *Cultural Anthropology* series devoted to the topic).[4] Similarly, deaf studies scholars also create worlds through their work.

I give some examples of what I mean by the world-making that happens in deaf studies by drawing upon some foundational concepts in the discipline, such as "Deaf culture, " Deaf identity," "Deaf community," and "Deafhood," which are used to analyze and situate deaf peoples' experiences. Using these concepts means that we come to see the world with them as a lens, and we look for these things—culture, identity, community, Deafhood—as we encounter diverse deaf people. These concepts are, however, teleological in that the goal is to end up with a "capital D" Deaf culture and Deaf identity, to become a member of the Deaf community, and to actualize a sense of Deafhood. These concepts are written in the singular, there is very little or no discussion of Deaf cultures, identities, and Deafhoods, for example. They thus presume that there is one kind of Deaf culture, identity, and Deafhood. In analyzing deaf peoples' experience through these concepts, there is

---

4 See http://culanth.org/fieldsights/461-the-politics-of-ontology.

the assumption that they are relevant for all deaf people in the world; and that if they are not currently relevant, they will be. As such, these concepts are prescriptive ones that create normative d/Deaf worlds.

TRAVELING CONCEPTS AND A SEGUE INTO DISABILITY STUDIES

It is one thing to use these concepts and create these kinds of deaf worlds in the global North, where deaf studies has been situated. It is, however, an entirely different thing to produce these worlds in the global South. Because deaf studies scholars are increasingly interested in conducting research in and learning more about deaf experiences elsewhere (as I discuss further on in this chapter), it is important for such scholars to interrogate critically what tools, frameworks, and methods they are bringing to the table. Here, I draw from work done in the discipline of disability studies: Although deaf studies and disability studies have been (e)strange(d) bedfellows largely as a result of deaf studies scholars' and deaf lay people's uneasy relationship with the category of disability (e.g., Burch & Kafer 2010), recent trends in disability studies are productive to consider, especially in light of its engagement with the global South. In 2014, a new journal titled *Disability in the Global South* was launched in order to attend to and shed different light on issues of disability and development. The editors, Shaun Grech and Karen Soldatic (2014:2), note in their introduction to the first issue of the journal:

> ...the field of disability and development seems to us to remain epistemologically frozen within its own Northern framing as well as uncritical, and many issues are too often left out or intentionally ignored as they give rise to processes of theorization beyond the Northern discursive structures of categorization.

I want to flag Grech and Soldatic's comment about the field of disability and development being "epistemologically frozen" as a result of its attachment to a specific (Northern) place and time. In what ways is deaf studies similarly epistemologically frozen? What moves can deaf studies scholars engage in to "thaw" this epistemological freezing?

Elsewhere, Soldatic and Grech (2014) raise an important point about the lack of universal salience around the category of disability and the ways that it has been adopted as an unmarked and taken-for-granted category. In considering the history of disability studies, it becomes clear that disability is a category that emerged in the global North in order to address the political and social positioning of people with impairments (Barnes & Mercer 2010): Northern-based disability studies scholars have very productively created medical and social model frameworks to analyze the experiences of disabled people. While the medical model locates disability in the individual, the social model examines how disability is created through interactions between an individual's impairment and social, political, and economic structures. An embrace of the social model also has led to disabled people (mostly) in the global North attempting to resignify the category of disability and turn it into a positive identity marker and a means for social and political organizing (ibid).[5]

Soldatic and Grech (2014) argue that the language of "disability" perhaps obscures more than it reveals about specific experiences in places. Because their concern is with creating a space for justice and rights for and on behalf of disabled people, specifically those in the global South, they call for a return to the language of "impairment" because it ". . . symbolizes the ongoing suffering that is embodied, memorialized and incarnate of the corporeal pain that remains a marker of the violated body and mind." What they mean by this is that impairment often is caused by structural violence and global inequalities, something that Northern disability studies scholars often ignore in their focus on positive disability identities and social organization.

Although Soldatic and Grech (ibid) are not necessarily calling for a return to the medical model, they are problematizing the adequacy of both the medical and social model in encapsulating the complexity of impairment and disability experiences. I find this point to be useful in thinking about the salience of deaf studies concepts in the global South and what such concepts might obscure. Deaf and disability studies share a commitment to certain concepts, such as identity and community. As in deaf studies, (celebratory and positive) concepts such as disability identity and disability community are quite prominent in disability studies. In their move to foreground impairment and background disability, Soldatic and Grech (ibid) push us to interrogate critically the universal salience of such concepts as identity and community. Fundamentally, they are arguing that "disability" is not a universal category.

Indeed, elsewhere in disability studies and in studies of disability in other academic disciplines, scholars have moved away from the concept of disability. Julie Livingston (2005:7) uses the concept of *debility* in her research with physically impaired people in Botswana, because she sees this as a less politicized and more experientially near way of analyzing her interlocutors' experiences. She writes: "Disability is a biosocial identity that is at once biologically grounded and socially parsed, an umbrella term that denotes different things in different places at different times." Livingston purposely refuses to use

---

5 But see Shakespeare (2013) for a critique of the social model of disability and its failure to consider the body's material reality.

"disability" because she thinks it "has special meanings in terms of identity and capacity..." (ibid) (see also Puar 2011, Fritsch 2015). And in the global North, there has been a surge in "crip studies" in which the concept "crip" has become both politically empowering and an analytically productive way of thinking about bodily difference and the role of language in establishing discursive realities (e.g., Kafer 2013, McRuer 2006).

In addition, seeking additional disciplinary delineations and distinguishing markers, disability scholars also have proposed "critical disability studies," which presumably goes beyond (unmarked) disability studies in its attention to the role of power, privilege, and political economic realities in everyday disabled lives. Crip studies and critical disability studies share concerns about how the foundational models in disability studies—the medical and social models—do not go far enough in capturing the complexity of lived experience and present scholars with analytical dead ends. As such, these new strands of disability studies aim to interrogate and unpack foundational principles. What would it look like if we did this in deaf studies? Fernandes and Myers (2010), for example, have called for an "inclusive deaf studies" that approaches deaf peoples' experiences with increasing fluidity and an awareness that the current concepts in use are U.S.-centric. I, too, support such a move, although I would not use "inclusive" here in light of all the controversy around the concept of inclusion in deaf worlds (i.e., Kusters et al. 2015), and it would be more appropriate to call the concepts Northern-centric instead of U.S.-centric.

In the discipline of deaf studies, there seems to have been little attention paid to resignifying deaf beyond a move toward Deaf (and a move away from terms such as hearing impaired). These discussions around whether one should use a lower-case or capital D in their orthography are important in that what is at stake is the inadequacy of written language to capture what is meant in signed language, which has no written form.[6] Unfortunately, however, what often happens in these discussions is that "Deaf" comes to take on a specific meaning attached to identity, community, and Deafhood and is, therefore, limiting. The concept of "Sign Language Peoples" (Batterbury et al. 2007) was recently proposed as a way to think of deaf people as a de-territorialized collectivity unified in its use of signed languages. In addition, many deaf people—academics and lay people alike—have drawn inspiration from George Veditz and categorized deaf people as "people of the eye" or

---

[6] Because sign languages have no written form, deaf studies faces unique challenges in rendering important signed concepts into written language. Although glosses have productively been used, as in Ladd's (2003) discussion of DEAF and in Lane et al.'s (1996) concept of DEAF-WORLD, the complexity of such concepts is difficult to translate into written English.

"visual people." Deaf studies, however, still has much work to do in interrogating its foundational concepts (and here I think about Grech and Soldatic's frozen epistemologies).

Not only do deaf studies scholars need to interrogate the foundational concepts within the discipline, scholars would do well to explore the concepts that our interlocutors use in specific contexts. In addition to analyzing the discursive work of categories and carving out a space for more nuance in how we use them, we also must attend to concepts and categories used in various contexts for disability and deafness. Work by anthropologists provides an excellent guide for this: Instead of using the universal category of disability, such scholars attend to local naming practices and explore what these practices signify and mean. For example, in Ghana, Kathryn Geurts (2015) writes about how disabled people are fondly called "disables," while in China, Matthew Kohrman (2005:61–62) discusses the etymology and meaning of the concepts of *canji* (disabled) and *canfei* (crippled) as he argues that both concepts have strong sociopolitical and moral meanings. Livingston (2005) writes about *bogole* instead of disabled people, again, stressing that bogole does not map onto disability. These discussions of naming and labeling practices offer a rich arena for exploring on-the-ground systems of signification and meaning making and the role of disability and disabled people within them. Through engaging with these categories, scholars come to understand how impairment and bodily differences are known and experienced in specific worlds instead of rendering them into a universal experience through utilizing the (universalized) category of disability.

In studies of deaf experiences and worlds, such engagement with language use in context is emerging: In a 2014 linguistic anthropology dissertation, Mara Green discusses two different ways of calling someone deaf in Nepal—*laato* and *bahaara*—and she discusses the stakes of these terms in that laato is associated with being senseless and not having the capability to engage in sense- and meaning-making, while bahaara does not have these connotations. In my 2015 book, I write about deafs and normals, using the concepts that my interlocutors in urban India use, and I argue that these are both normative concepts that create valid ways of being in the world in relation to each other (Friedner 2015:13). I argue that these concepts create worlds of their own and I attempted to understand and analyze these worlds. I encourage other researchers to attend to the language used to categorize, signify, and represent deaf people elsewhere in the world. This emic, or locally produced and used, language can reveal significant details about what deafness means in specific places and how it relates to other categories of being in the world.

BIOLOGY AS A WAY FORWARD?

Elsewhere in my work (2010a), I have argued for the existence of what I have called "Global Deafness" or a normative way of being deaf in the world that is espoused by international institutions and organizations such as the United Nations, the World Federation of the Deaf, and international nongovernmental organizations (NGOs). I received less than positive feedback, however, about this concept, its phrasing in particular, as colleagues told me that they found the use of "deafness" to be inappropriate because it is a medical/ized concept. In response, however, I argue that it is actually this phrasing that I find productive because (the biological state of) deafness is still seemingly at the root of everything in which Deaf Studies is interested. I wonder, too, thinking of Soldatic and Grech's (2014) work as discussed earlier, if deafness (as opposed to deaf/Deaf) can become a shared platform for organizing, affiliation, and social justice.[7] To be sure, I do not want to fetishize biology; on the other hand, here it is biology that provides the conditions of possibility for shared epistemologies and ontologies among deaf people to emerge.

Biosociality, or social formations based upon shared biological experiences, is thus an important concept for deaf studies scholars to consider. Although embracing other aspects of Michel Foucault's work on power, deaf studies has largely stayed away from the concept of biosociality, which Rabinow (1996) defines as "nature becoming culture," or the production of social relationships because of shared biological traits. Although biosociality can potentially be problematic in its implication of medical knowledge and forms of expertise, it also can be seen as inclusive, in that it moves us away from teleological deaf studies concepts. Exploring deaf people's relationships with one another through the analytic of biosociality allows us to consider the role of biology in deaf people's affinities and sense of belonging (see also Friedner 2010).

A biological turn in deaf studies would, therefore, be a productive counterpart to the ontological turn proposed in this book. Deaf studies scholars are increasingly attending to the biological: Ben Bahan (2014) writes about deaf peoples' unique sensory orientations, and movements in deaf geographies and deaf architecture privilege the ways that deaf people move through space as deaf and deafblind people (H. Bauman 2014, Sirvage 2012). Similarly, the National Science Foundation-funded Visual Language and Visual Learning labs at universities around the United States and the Rochester, New York-based National Technical

---

[7] I do not think that deaf studies must be concerned only with questions of rights and justice. Just like in disability studies and other disciplines that have close relations to activism, there can be many streams of scholarship and intervention.

Institute for the Deaf's Deaf Studies Lab are invested in understanding the biological underpinnings of deaf peoples' cognition and learning processes, among other things (see also Hauser & Kartheiser 2014).

Attending to biology thus allows deaf studies scholars another way to analyze deaf peoples' experiences in the world, one that is not based upon seemingly universal ideas of culture, identity, community, or Deafhood. Although, remembering Haraway's (1988) admonition about situating knowledge, we also need to remember that (scientific) studies of deaf peoples' cognition, visual capacities, or sensory orientations also are emplaced and situated.

PRODUCING AND ENGAGING WITH THE GLOBAL SOUTH

Returning to deaf studies and what it does in the global South, I now provide some (inexhaustive) background on deaf studies work in the global South. It is also important, however, to consider the role of deaf studies in producing the global South as a rhetorical space of analysis. Eunjung Kim (2011) writes about the discursive creation of disability heavens and hells in attempts to justify judgment and intervention (see also Friedner & Kusters 2014). For example, when international NGOs seek to intervene in a country, they might represent that country as a space of lack. In returning to the teleological concepts associated with deaf studies, it is possible to see how countries in which deaf people do not have strong "Deaf identities" might be considered by international institutions or development organizations operating according to Deaf-centric principles to be backward or undeveloped (see also Friedner & Kusters 2014, Moriarty-Harrelson 2015). Looking at these spaces only through Northern-developed concepts, however, is misleading. Deaf people in these countries might have other affiliations, identities, and sites of belonging that are less than visible to the eyes of foreign researchers.

The global North typically refers to countries in Europe and North America with access to resources and with political power on an international level while the global South refers to countries without (or with less) access to resources and power. Many of the countries considered to be in the global South have been colonized by those in the global North. Indeed, Meekosha and Soldatic (2011:1383) write: "we use North–South terminology as shorthand for a complex of inequalities, which ... are embedded in historically set socio-relations of global power." As such, the concepts of the global North and global South are laden with issues of power and privilege. What is important to stress is that these are also political concepts: They were created as a way around thorny and value-laden concepts of development and un/der-development. As critical development scholars (e.g., Escobar 1995, Gupta 1998) have argued, these concepts—development and un/der development—function as discourses that create ways for people to identify as being advanced and developed or backward and behind. In contrast, the framework introduced by the concepts of the global North and global South can be seen as attempts to resist thinking of the world in terms of development and its lack. This framework is also antiteleological (that is, it does not argue that all countries should become like those in the global North). As such, doing deaf studies in the global South entails commitments that are different from, say, doing deaf studies in the Third World, or, doing deaf studies in developing countries. These commitments include attending to questions of economics, power, and privilege as well as being aware of how countries exist in relation to one another.

We must also nuance what we mean by the global South: Although the global South and global North as concepts are attached to countries as a result of their political economic conditions, within these countries there are significant variations and there are, of course, elite upper-class deaf people in countries in the global South. There are also cases where deaf people living in countries in the global South are more mobile than their hearing counterparts. For example, in November 2014, a cadre of deaf people from North Korea visited deaf associations in Finland and Germany, a trip difficult to imagine for anyone in North Korea because of political economic sanctions and restrictions on travel, yet these deaf people were able to travel because of the international NGOs to which they were connected. In another instance, deaf people from North Korea attended the 2015 World Federation of the Deaf (WFD) congress in Istanbul, Turkey. During my fieldwork in urban India, I met deaf youth who frequently traveled to neighboring states to attend deaf sports and cultural functions; a few also were able to travel internationally because of support received from deaf organizations, corporations, and charitable entities. Indeed, there are delegations of deaf people from developing countries at WFD conferences and congresses and many of these deaf people are the first in their families to travel abroad. Deaf peoples' experiences in urban areas of the global South may be very different from those in rural areas (see Green 2014a for research in both urban and rural Nepal and Kisch 2012 on research in Bedouin communities in Israel that are simultaneously urban and rural) and both settings offer their own possibilities and constraints. In addition, some townships and other settlements can be considered neither rural nor urban. As such, while the categories of global South and global North provide useful framing and a productive way to discuss political economic inequalities, the categories need to be rendered nuanced and specific. Locations, histories, and contexts *within* the categories of global North and global South must be considered.

The importance of specific political economic contexts cannot be overstated. The same is true for academic concepts used to analyze and theorize different peoples' conditions that have emerged from and in specific times and places. Several key scholars and texts in deaf studies, however, have utilized concepts and frameworks "borrowed" from other disciplines, such as postcolonial studies, critical race studies, queer studies, and feminist studies, just to name a few. Paddy Ladd (2003), for instance, argues that deaf people are "subalterns" (a concept taken from South Asian Studies-based subaltern studies scholarship) and that they have been "colonized" by hearing people and medical/audiology institutions. In his work, Ladd also makes comparisons and analogies between deaf people and people of color and Native peoples. However, as Soldatic and Grech (2014) note:

> Disability theorists . . . have noted that, too often, disability is drawn upon as a metaphor by (post)colonial theorists, while for disability theorists, colonization has become a key metaphor to describe experiences of oppression, marginalisation and exclusion to which disabled people are often subjected.

Drawing on the work of other disability studies scholars, they call for attention to the specific locations and places in which disabled people live. Indeed, concepts such as colonialism, while rhetorically powerful, should not be used as metaphors (see also Myers & Fernandez 2010, Ruiz et al. 2015, Sherry 2007).

To be sure, oppression, discrimination, and unequal power relations have marked deaf people and deaf experiences. Colonialism, however, refers to a very particular set of processes that cannot be applied to deaf experiences. As other scholars have argued, it can only function as a (very problematic) metaphor when applied to deaf contexts. For example, in a critique of Harlan Lane's work in which Lane equates paternalistic hearing professionals with colonialists, Mark Sherry (2007:12) argues: "Lane does not examine what makes colonialism a unique form of power, nor does he clearly differentiate 'colonialism' from various forms of power over bodies . . ." Similarly, Meyers and Fernandez (2010:42) note: "Evoking the metaphor of colonization in present historical conditions to describe the institutional relationship of deaf and hearing people actually may impede progress toward the more comprehensive theoretical understanding that we need to guide both Deaf Studies' understanding of deaf/Deaf lives and political activism on behalf of deaf people's rights in all walks of life."

Important questions thus become: What are deaf peoples' lives like under and within specific political economic regimes? What were the experiences of deaf people under colonial states?[8] How does deafness

---

[8] Ironically, in India for example, it could be argued that deaf people fared well during the colonial period because this was when many of India's deaf schools were established and there was an influx of religious and secular social service workers and educators who worked with deaf children and deaf people.

intersect with other axes of difference under different rationalities of rule? In appropriating the concept of colonialism and employing it to write about deaf experiences in countries that have not been colonialized, we erase the experiences of deaf people under colonial regimes. Frank Bechter (2008) called for the importance of developing new concepts within deaf studies as opposed to borrowing them from other disciplines; as he argues, deaf studies is uniquely situated to offer the world new theoretical interventions based on deaf peoples' embodied positioning as deaf people (see also Humphries 2008, Sanchez, this volume). As such, instead of removing concepts such as colonialism or subalterns from the contexts in which they were developed, it would be fruitful to develop new concepts or expand upon these to explore what is specific to deaf experiences.

DEAF STUDIES WORK IN THE GLOBAL SOUTH

Although there has been a range of work on international deaf mobilities and travels both in the present (Breivik et al. 2002) and historically (Murray 2007), it is only more recently, that there has been work on deaf experiences in the global South (although Owen Wrigley's 1997 book is an outlier in its critical discussion of deaf development organizations in Thailand). The best-known intervention is perhaps Leila Monaghan et al.'s *Many Ways to be Deaf: International Variation in Deaf Communities,* which, in 16 chapters set around the world, explored the history and diversity of deaf communities. In the preface, the editors write: "Commonalities among the authors include that we all ... value the roles that history and culture play in the formation of Deaf cultures and signed languages" (Monaghan et al. 2003, x). The editors also note that the title for the book was inspired by the Deaf Way conferences held at Gallaudet University in 1989 and 2002—although it was slightly modified to account for diversity and variation not represented at these conferences. They state: "The challenges faced by those in Sweden are quite different from those in Nicaragua and are set on a common global stage" (Ibid, ix). This book is a foundational one in its stress on the diversity of deaf experiences, although it does not critically engage with political economic inequality (as we can see from the phrase "common global stage" in the aforementioned quote). Most likely, this is a result of being written during a time period when scholars did not foreground such issues.

The growing concern with deaf experiences outside the global North at this current moment exists in relation to increased globalization and development interventions in the arena of disability and development. These have both preceded and come as a result of the United Nations Convention on the Rights of Persons with Disabilities (CRPD) and corporate and charitable initiatives in the arena of disability. Deaf studies scholars have traveled to the global South to both work on and in relation to these initiatives (as in the case of Goedele De Clerck's [2011] work on empowerment projects in Cameroon, discussed later). Indeed, concepts from deaf studies appear to have been adopted by the international disability and development apparatus, as can be seen in the CRPD's articles about deaf education and deaf peoples' linguistic rights. And there have been new academic programs in deaf studies, such as Gallaudet University's Masters Program in Deaf Studies, which includes a track in Language and Human Rights, that have come into being in order to further promote the human rights of deaf people—using deaf studies language (see Friedner & Kusters 2014). It is interesting to note that there is a close relationship between concepts and analytics created by and used in deaf studies and those used by international development practitioners and advocates with the latter directly adopting concepts from the former. This phenomenon is in need of further study. As such, in the process of this internationalization of discourses, it is crucial to consider how deaf studies concepts travel and are adopted and adapted by people elsewhere; as they are utilized, they may come to take on new meanings and resonances and researchers must attend to this as well. That is, Deafhood might come to mean something entirely different in deaf clubs in urban India than in the United Kingdom, for example.

Thankfully, however, a growing body of scholarship addresses this gap. Goedele De Clerck (2011) has written about her empowerment projects with Deaf Cameroonians and their conceptions of development and emancipation. In the process, she outlines the political economic constraints that they experience and she calls for attention to what she terms "indigenous epistemologies" (see also De Clerck 2010). Perhaps this call for attention to such "indigenous epistemologies" represents a move away from the "frozen epistemologies" about which Soldatic and Grech (2014) caution us. Annelies Kusters (2010) has written about deaf peoples' experiences in Mumbai's train compartments for passengers with disabilities and how these compartments are spaces for deaf encounters and deaf space formation that may serve to increase hearing peoples' understandings of sign language and deaf people, given that deaf people are quite visible in these compartments and on the station platforms. More recently, Kusters (2015a) has published an ethnography on deaf space in Adamarobe, Ghana, wherein she provides a rich description of deaf peoples' lives in the village as they interact with hearing people and with one another. My 2015 book, *Valuing Deaf Worlds*, looks at deaf peoples' social, moral, and economic practices as they aspire toward deaf development in urban India. Audrey Cooper (2015) has published a book about deaf Vietnamese peoples' attempts to establish sovereignty, and she closely connects deaf peoples' aspirations and trajectories to those of the nation-state (see also Nakamura

2006, in which the author very carefully situates developments in deaf worlds within Japan's political economic development). There also have been increasing numbers of doctoral dissertations, mostly in the field of anthropology, on deaf experiences in the global South (see Green 2014, Kisch 2012, Kusters 2011, and Lee 2012, for examples).

DEAF STUDIES, ANTHROPOLOGY, AND MANAGING UNCERTAINTY

The majority of these dissertations were written for anthropology departments/programs and the publications and monographs were written using anthropological and ethnographic methods. Anthropology traditionally has involved long-term fieldwork and draws from a host of methodological approaches, including phenomenology, discourse analysis, and participant observation. The discipline is perhaps best known for what Clifford Geertz (1973) has called "thick description." Lisa Stevenson (2014:2) more recently wrote that "Anthropology as an act of listening for what is, what has been, or what will be, regardless of whether it makes sense, blurs any easy distinction between the epistemological and the ontological, the methodological, and the ethical." Indeed, Stevenson's point about the blurring of boundaries is especially germane in this discussion of how to do deaf studies in the global South. I am not arguing that everyone should become an anthropologist, nor am I glossing over the discipline's problematic history and implication in colonialist projects, but I do think that there are important tools, methods, and orientations from which deaf studies researchers working in the global South can draw. Current research in anthropology (and many other disciplines) has attended to questions of change, flux, and movement, not to mention questions of power. These are issues with which deaf studies, too, should be concerned. In addition, deaf studies also should be concerned with the meaning of emic categories and knowledges about deaf people and how they relate to other kinds of social, political, and economic meanings. And, perhaps most importantly, returning to the "ontological turn" in anthropology discussed at the beginning of this essay, it seems to me that it is important to analyze how deaf studies scholars might construct certain kinds of deaf people and deafnesses in their work.

It is important to stress that some scholars (i.e., De Clerck 2010) have focused on "indigenous" deaf epistemologies and ontologies in other locations without exploring their own situated knowledges, or their own epistemologies and ontologies, which have developed as a result of being enmeshed in a specific place and time. This is not just a matter of reflecting upon the researcher's positionality; it also involves being aware of how knowledge (and worlds) can be coproduced by researchers and research subjects. In addition, researchers also need to explore what these local epistemologies and ontologies exist in relation to. Take this as an example: In Friedner and Kusters (2014), we discussed how numerous researchers and activists present their research or advocacy work by utilizing a template that foregrounds specific kinds of knowledges and obscures others. These presentations usually begin with a map of a country that features the location of specific sites in the country, and subsequently the location of deaf associations or deaf schools. By showing this map, the researcher/presenter presumes that she or he has emplaced the research or project and made it intelligible. However, physical and geographic boundaries and the location of deaf schools and organizations do not necessarily reveal anything substantive about the actual political economic structure and day-to-day life that deaf people experience—although these maps do reveal the presenter's orientations toward valuing clear geographic boundaries and certain kinds of deaf institutions. There is no critical engagement, however, with what it might mean to foreground this particular set of optics and what knowledge it reveals. In addition, we not only need to learn more about deaf peoples' ontologies and epistemologies but also what political economic and social contexts these exist in relation to. This means that we require more data about lived experience, history, and political economy: We must go beyond geographical information and facts about deaf institutions.

It is also essential to tend to questions of intelligibility and the lack of it when conducting research with deaf people—whether in the global North or global South. (Interestingly, this issue seems to come up more in the global South, perhaps because we provide analytical space for it to do so.) Green (2014b) conducted research with rural deaf Nepalis who use natural sign, a category that she differentiates from home or village sign in that she locates it within specific ecologies. In her research, she interacted with a deaf woman named Parvati who attempted to tell her a story, possibly about someone slapping her. Green could not understand her and when she asked Parvati's children and others nearby if they could interpret or help her possibly understand, they also did not understand. And so the story that Parvati was trying to tell was presumably unintelligible to Green and to others, something that Green found to be very productive because it allowed her to think more broadly about what it means to make sense within specific social worlds and how people actively work to create meaning together. Although this interaction could be an extreme example of not understanding (and the possibility of violence here renders it especially poignant), it is entirely possible that there will be utterances, statements, and discourses that we in the global North (or anyone) find to be unintelligible or incommensurable (even if we are "DEAF SAME" as our research subjects).

Questions of intelligibility and comprehension come up in all research settings, deaf and hearing alike. However, although hearing researchers often discuss and elaborate upon what they do and do not understand during their research (e.g., Stevenson 2014), it is possible that deaf researchers do not foreground lack of comprehension in their focus on being "DEAF SAME" with their research participants. It is also important to consider how working with deaf people and communities in different contexts might bring unique challenges as a result of lack of access to formal education and delayed language development. How do we carve out a space to discuss lack of intelligibility and comprehension without resorting to narratives of lack, pity, or the need for development intervention?

Our work can never be as neat and as easy as simply finding and categorizing local ontologies or epistemologies. Our interlocutors often make contradictory and inconsistent statements; there are gaps in what they choose to share with us, and, as Kusters (2015b) argues, they can engage in "language games" in which language is strategically employed to have a desired effect and to produce specific worlds. How do we, therefore, allow space for these ambiguities and uncertainties in our work? Stevenson (2014:2) calls for research "which persistently disrupts the security of what is known for sure. This entails taking the uncertain, the confused—that which is not clearly understood—as a legitimate ethnographic object." The value of uncertainty and confusion seem to me to be strong reasons to move away from some of the concepts, such as Deaf culture, Deaf identity, Deaf community, and Deafhood, that we have held so dear in the discipline of deaf studies up to now: These concepts do not allow for such uncertainty, or for complexity, in that they are monolithic and prescriptive.

CONCLUSION: DEAF STUDIES, DEAF SAME, AND THE GLOBAL SOUTH

It is important to consider the phenomenon of "DEAF SAME," or feelings and discourses of deaf similitude, and what this means when doing deaf studies in the global South. Indeed, "DEAF SAME" often enriches and complicates research conducted with deaf people elsewhere and also complicates ideas of shared biology. For example, at the 2015 Deaf Academics conference held in Leuven, Belgium, deaf researchers continually stressed their "insider" status when conducting research with deaf people elsewhere; in the process they backgrounded social, cultural, educational, class, and geographic differences among others. In our (2015) edited volume titled, *It's a Small World: International Deaf Encounters and Spaces,* Annelies Kusters and I, along with the chapter contributors, problematize ideas and ideals of "DEAF SAME." As we demonstrate, deaf-same is shot through with and exists alongside "deaf-different," or what Erin Moriarty Harrelson (2015) calls "deaf SAME-SAME but different." Similarly, Elena Ruiz et al. (2015) argue "My deaf is not your deaf." Do deaf peoples' shared biological, embodied, and other characteristics render the distinction between global South and global North obsolete? I argue that they do not, although as others have demonstrated they result in additional complexities.

Friedner and Kusters (2014) illustrate that deaf foreign travelers in Adamorobe were received with (marginally) more enthusiasm than hearing travelers. Similarly, Kusters was aided in her research by Adamorobees because she was "DEAF SAME" (Kusters 2015). And Arlinda Boland et al. (2015) demonstrate that it can be easier to build rapport with deaf people living in the global South while doing development projects when the researcher or development worker is also deaf. To be clear, these feelings of sameness are experienced and explored by scholars in other domains including gender (Mohanty 2003) and sexuality (Boellstorff 2012). However, there can be something to be said for what this means in imagining, making, and participating in deaf worlds because of deaf peoples' unique horizons of communication and language use (although, see Lee 2012 for an account of deaf Tanzanians who were not interested in meeting foreign deaf people). In addition, deaf researchers come to feel attached to and responsible for those whom they are conducting research with and on, because of these unique horizons. This is not to imply that hearing researchers do not also feel these bonds and this sense of responsibility. It is only to imply that these might be especially heightened for people who have shared biological and sensory experiences, especially those who are marked as being outside the norm or as "other."

And what of the global South? I have argued that doing deaf studies in the global South requires that researchers analyze their own epistemological and ontological frameworks and that at this particular moment in time, "doing Deaf Studies" comes with a host of political and scholarly commitments to be unpacked (i.e., Lee 2010). In addition to an ontological turn in deaf studies, which requires us to analyze our own epistemologies and ontologies about ourselves as researchers, we also need to consider what we mean by categories such as "deaf," "Deaf," and "the global South" and how these categories have become salient. As such, I argue that doing deaf studies in the global South requires that scholars radically re-envision what deaf studies is and should be.

REFERENCES

Bahan, B. (2014). Senses and culture: Exploring sensory orientations. In H-D. L. Bauman & J. Murray, Eds., *Deaf Gain: Raising the stakes for human diversity* (pp. 233–254). Minneapolis: University of Minnesota Press.

Batterbury, S., Ladd, P., & Gulliver, M. (2007). Sign Language Peoples as indigenous minorities: Implications for research and policy. *Environment and Planning, 39*(12), 2899–2915.

Barnes, C., & Mercer, G. (2010). *Exploring disability.* Cambridge and Malden: Polity Press.

Bauman, H-D. L. (2008). Introduction: Listening to Deaf Studies. In H-D. L. Bauman, Ed., *Open your eyes: Deaf Studies talking* (pp. 1–34). Minneapolis: University of Minnesota Press.

Bauman, H. (2014). DeafSpace: An architecture towards a more liveable and sustainable world. In H-D. L. Bauman & J. Murray, Eds., *Deaf Gain: Raising the stakes for human diversity* (pp. 375–401). Minneapolis: University of Minnesota Press.

Bechter, F. (2008). The deaf convert culture and its lessons for deaf theory. In H-D. L. Bauman, Ed., *Open your eyes: Deaf Studies talking* (pp. 60–79). Minneapolis: University of Minnesota Press.

Boellstorff, T. (2012). The politics of similitude: Global sexuality activism, ethnography, and the Western subject. *Trans-Scripts, 2,* 22–39.

Boland, A. S., Wilson, A. T., & Winarczyk, R. E. (2015). Deaf international development practitioners and researchers working effectively in deaf communities. In M. Friedner & A. Kusters, Eds., *It's a small world: International deaf spaces and encounters* (pp. 239–248). Washington, DC: Gallaudet University Press.

Breivik, J., Haualand, H., & Solvang, P. (2002). *Rome—a Temporary Deaf City! Deaflympics 2001. A Publication within the Anthropological Project: 'Transnational Connections in Deaf Worlds'* [online]. Bergen University, Norway. Available from: http://www.ub.uib.no/elpub/rokkan/N/N02-02.pdf Accessed September 17, 2011.

Burch, S., & Kafer, A., Eds. (2010). *Deaf and Disability Studies: Interdisciplinary perspectives.* Washington, DC: Gallaudet University Press.

Cooper, A. (2015). *The state of signed language and deaf cultural belonging in Vietnam.* Washington, DC: Gallaudet University Press.

De Clerck, G. (2010). Deaf epistemologies as a critique and alternative to the practice of science: An anthropological perspective. *American Annals of the Deaf, 154*(5), 435–446.

De Clerck, G. (2011). Fostering deaf people's empowerment: The Cameroonian deaf community and epistemological equity. *Third World Quarterly, 32*(8), 1419–1435. doi:10.1080/01436597.2011.604516.

Escobar, A. (1995). *Encountering development: The making and the unmaking of the Third World.* Princeton, NJ: Princeton University Press.

Fernandes, J.K., & Shultz Myers, S. (2010). Inclusive Deaf Studies: Barriers and pathways. *Journal of Deaf Education and Deaf Studies, 15*(1), 17–29.

Friedner, M. (2015). *Valuing deaf worlds in urban India.* New Brunswick, NJ: Rutgers University Press.

Friedner, M. (2010). Biopower, biosociality, and community formation: How biopower is constitutive of the Deaf Community. *Sign Language Studies, 10*(3), 336–347.

Friedner, M., & Kusters, A. (2014). On the possibilities and limits of "DEAF DEAF SAME": Tourism and empowerment camps in Adamorobe (Ghana), Bangalore and Mumbai (India). *Disability Studies Quarterly, 34*(3).

Fritsch, K. (2015). Gradations of debility and capacity: Biocapitalism and the neoliberalization of disability relations. *Canadian Journal of Disability Studies, 4*(2).

Geertz, C. (1973). *The interpretation of cultures*. New York: Basic Books.

Geurts, K. (2015). On the worlding of Accra's Rehabilitation Training Centre. *Somatosphere*. Retrieved May 19, 2015 from <http://somatosphere.net/2015/04/on-the-worlding-of-accras-rehabilitation-training-centre.html>

Grech, S., & Soldatic, K.M. (2014). Introducing disability and the global South (DGS): We are critical, we are open access! *Disability and the Global South, 1*(1), 1–4. Accessed at https://disabilityglobalsouth.files.wordpress.com/2012/06/dgs-01-01-015.pdf.

Green, E. M. (2014a). Building the Tower of Babel: International sign, linguistic commensuration, and moral orientation. *Language in Society, 43*, 445–465.

Green, E. M. (2014b). *The nature of signs: Nepal's deaf society, local sign, and the production of communicative sociality* (Unpublished doctoral dissertation). University of California at Berkeley.

Gupta, A. (1998). *Postcolonial developments: Agriculture in the making of modern India*. Durham, NC: Duke University Press.

Haraway, D. (1988). Situated knowledges: The science question in feminism and the privilege of partial perspective. *Feminist Studies, 14*(3), 575–599.

Hauser, P. C., & Kartheiser, G. (2014). Advantages of learning a signed language. In H-D. L. Bauman & J. Murray, Eds., *Deaf Gain: Raising the stakes for human diversity* (pp. 133–145). Minneapolis: University of Minnesota Press.

Holbraad, M., & Pedersen, M. A. (2014). The politics of ontology. *Fieldsights—Theorizing the Contemporary, Cultural Anthropology Online.* Accessed from http://culanth.org/fieldsights/461-the-politics-of-ontology on December 22, 2014.

Humphries, T. (2008). Talking culture and culture talking. In H-D. L. Bauman, Ed., *Open your eyes: Deaf Studies talking* (pp. 35–41). Minneapolis: University of Minnesota Press.

Kafer, A. (2013). *Feminist, crip, queer*. Indianapolis: Indiana University Press.

Kim, E. (2011). "Heaven for disabled people": Nationalism and international human rights imagery. *Disability and Society, 26*(1), 93–106.

Kisch, S. (2012). *Deafness among the Negev Bedouin: An interdisciplinary dialogue on deafness, marginality and context* (Unpublished doctoral dissertation). Amsterdam Institute for Social Science Research. University of Amsterdam. Accessed at http://dare.uva.nl/record/433414.

Kohrman, M. (2005). *Bodies of difference:Experiences of Disability and Institutional Advocacy in the Making of Modern China*. Berkeley: University of California Press.

Kusters, A. (2015a). *Deaf space in Adamorobe: An ethnographic study in a village in Ghana*. Washington, DC: Gallaudet University Press.

Kusters, A. (2015b). Peasants, warriors, and the streams. Language games and etiologies of deafness in Adamorobe, Ghana. *Medical Anthropology Quarterly, 29*(3), 418–436.

Kusters, A. (2010). Deaf on the lifeline of Mumbai. *Sign Language Studies, 10*(1), 36–68.

Kusters, A., & Friedner, M. (2015). DEAF-SAME and difference in international deaf spaces and encounters. In M. Friedner & A. Kusters, Eds., *It's a small world: International deaf spaces and encounters* (pp. ix–xxix). Washington, DC: Gallaudet University Press.

Kusters, A., De Meulder, M., Friedner, M., & Emery, S. (2015). On "diversity" and "inclusion:" Exploring paradigms for achieving Sign Language Peoples' rights. Max Planck Institute for the Study of Religious and Ethnic Diversity. Working Paper. Accessed from http://www.mmg.mpg.de/publications/working-papers/2015/wp-15-02/.

Ladd, P. (2003). *Understanding Deaf Culture: In search of Deafhood.* Clevedon: Multilingual Matters Ltd.

Lane, H., Hoffmeister, R., & Bahan, B. (1996). *A journey into the DEAF-WORLD.* San Diego, CA: DawnSignPress.

Lee, J. C. (2012). *They have to see us: An ethnography of deaf people in Tanzania* (Unpublished doctoral dissertation). University of Colorado at Boulder.

Lee, J. C. (2010). "What not to pack:" Conducting research among deaf people in Tanzania. In S. Burch & A. Kafer, Eds., *Deaf and Disability Studies: Interdisciplinary perspectives* (pp. 48–66). Washington, DC: Gallaudet University Press.

Livingston, J. (2005). *Debility and the moral imagination in Botswana.* Bloomington and Indianapolis: Indiana University Press.

McRuer, R. (2006). *Crip theory: Cultural signs of queerness and disability.* New York: NYU Press.

Meekosha, H., & Soldatic, K. (2011). Human rights and the global South: The case of disability. *Third World Quarterly, 32*(8), 1383–1398.

Mohanty, C.T. (2003). *Feminism without borders: Decolonizing theory, practicing solidarity.* Durham, NC: Duke University Press.

Monaghan, L., Schmaling, C., Nakamura, K., & Turner, G.H. (2003). *Many ways to be deaf: International variation in deaf communities.* Washington, DC: Gallaudet University Press.

Moriarty-Harrelson, E. (2015). SAME-SAME but different: Tourism and the deaf global circuit in Cambodia. In M. Friedner & A. Kusters, Eds., *It's a small world: International deaf spaces and encounters* (pp. 199–211). Washington, DC: Gallaudet University Press.

Murray, J. (2007). *"One touch of nature makes the whole world kin": The transnational lives of deaf Americans, 1870–1924* (Unpublished doctoral dissertation). University of Iowa.

Myers, S. S., & Fernandes, J. K. (2010). Deaf Studies: A critique of the predominant U.S. theoretical direction. *Journal of Deaf Studies and Deaf Education, 15*(1), 30–49.

Nakamura, K. (2006). *Deaf in Japan: Signing and the politics of identity.* Ithaca, NY: Cornell University Press.

Puar, J. (2011). The cost of getting better: Suicide, sensation, switchpoints. *GLQ: Journal of Lesbian and Gay Studies, 18*(1), 149–158.

Rabinow, P. (1996). *Essays on the Anthropology of Reason.* Princeton: Princeton University Press.

Ruiz, E., Burke, M., Chong V.Y., & Chainarong, N. (2015). "My deaf is not your deaf": Realizing intersectional realities at Gallaudet University. In M. Friedner & A. Kusters, Eds., *It's a small world: International deaf spaces and encounters* (pp. 262–273). Washington, DC: Gallaudet University Press.

Sirvage, R. (2012). Navigational proxemics of walking signers: A paradigm shift in methodology. *Deaf Studies Digital Journal.* Issue 3. Accessed at http://dsdj. gallaudet.edu/index.php?view=contributor&issue=4&contributor_id=85.

Shakespeare, T. (2013). The social model of disability. In L. J. Davis, Ed., *The disability studies reader* (pp. 214–221). New York: Routledge.

Sherry, M. (2007). Chapter 1: (Post)colonising Disability. Wagadu. 4.

Soldatic K.M., & Grech, S. (2014). Transnationalising disability studies: Rights, justice and impairment. *Disability Studies Quarterly, 34*(2).

Stevenson, L. (2014). *Life besides itself: Imagining care in the Canadian Arctic.* Berkeley: University of California Press.

Wrigley, O. (1997). *The politics of deafness.* Washington, DC: Gallaudet University Press.

6

Rejecting the Talkies: Charlie Chaplin's Language Politics and the Future of Deaf Studies in the Humanities

Rebecca Sanchez

EXPANDING THE FIELD

One of the foundational assertions of literary and cultural Deaf Studies is that the embodied and social experiences of deaf people are sources of unique insight into language, culture, and relationality, and that such insights have the potential to influence how we conceptualize all human interaction in and through language, as well as the ways these interactions and languages inform artistic practice. Since its inception, the field has been framed in terms that highlight this universal relevance. The introduction to *Open Your Eyes: Deaf Studies Talking* (2008), for example, insisted that "Deaf Studies is relevant not only to members and allies of this community," and positioned the collection as a kind of sales pitch for the discipline: "this book ... intends to compel a variety of audiences to listen" and to "consider new ways of listening" to the perspectives that emerge from deaf ontologies (Bauman:3).

Similarly, in a chapter titled "Deafness and Insight," in which he explores the idea of deafness as a theoretical paradigm, Lennard Davis (1995) argued that a consideration of deafness and disability

> in relation to social processes and cultural production can ... lay bare the cultural assumptions at the very base of artifacts such as plays, novels, [and] poems ... [and reveal] the epistemological bases and dialectical relations inherent in any notion of aesthetics. (124)

"Rather than being a marginal and eccentric focus of study," that is, Deaf Studies "goes to the very heart of issues about representations, communication, language, [and] ideology" (Davis 1995:124). By inviting a reconsideration of concepts such as silence and voice and challenging received ideas about how we interact with language, Davis explained, Deaf Studies productively deconstructs the assumed relations among reader, author, and text, relationships that are central to the analysis of any literary or cultural work. Christopher Krentz made a similarly compelling case in his 2007 book, *Writing Deafness*, for the significance of what he, building on W.E.B. Du Bois, described as a "hearing line" between deaf and hearing people and cultures. Linking this contact zone to "every speech act, every moment of silence, every gesture, and every form of human communication," he argued that the "discourse over the hearing line pertains to all people and is ulti- mately as pervasive as discourses about race, gender, sexuality, class, and disability" (5).

These diverse accounts of literary and critical Deaf Studies demon- strate the extent to which claims of its broad implications have been a central and consistent component of the field's development.[1] Such gestures outwardly function not as attempts to move away from spe- cific deaf ways of knowing or being, but rather, to borrow Paul Lauter's description of experimental modernism, invitations to "reconsider what we normally understand by the center and the margins," to rec- ognize the absolute centrality of "minority" experiences and represen- tations, in ways that have disciplinary as well as political and ethical implications (2014:1312).

Despite the compelling nature of these assertions, however, the vast majority of the scholarship in literary Deaf Studies has focused on the recovery of work by deaf authors, the analysis of deaf characters, and/or the interrogation of language and tropes surrounding deafness (whether, for example, deafness is being used in a text to signal a char- acter's vulnerability or alienation); in other words, on cataloguing and evaluating texts that have an obvious and literal link to deafness. This work has been absolutely vital.[2] Drawing attention to the significant contributions of deaf writers introduces understudied works to broader

---

[1] Critical Deaf Studies, following the use of "critical" in fields such as critical race theory, emphasizes a self-reflexivity about methodology; in this case, the consideration of the devel- opment of deaf epistemologies and ontologies, and the ways that deafness can function not only as identity or culture, but also as what Davis referred to as a "critical modality" (Davis 1995:100).

[2] In addition to Christopher Krentz's *Writing Deafness*, which provided readings of 19th-century texts by or about deaf figures, but which also gestured toward what a broader literary Deaf Studies might look like, other crucial contributions to the field in English have been Jennifer Esmail's 2013 *Reading Victorian Deafness: Signs and Sounds in Victorian Literature and Culture*, which explored what we can learn about Victorian culture by examining the treatment of deaf characters in 19th-century British literature; Cynthia Peters's 2000 *Deaf American Literature: From Carnival to the Canon*, which used the concept of the carnival as a way of tracing developments in ASL literature; Trent Batson and Eugene Bergman's 1986 *Angels and Outcasts: An Anthology of Deaf Characters in Literature* (and Edna Edith Sayers's 2012 *Outcasts and Angels*, which updated the collection); and the seminal 2006 collection, *Signing the Body Poetic: Essays on American Sign Language Literature*.

consciousness, while highlighting deaf characters in more canonical texts invites a productive re-examination of works with which readers have long been familiar. And tracing references to deaf subjects and deaf-related language and themes provides a fuller picture of the ways that ideas about deafness circulate in the cultural imaginary.

The success of such methodologies in Deaf Studies to this point has, however, produced a downside. Focusing exclusively (or near-exclusively) on texts with explicit biographical or thematic connections to deafness can function to reinforce the idea that Deaf Studies is a niche field, of significance only to those interested in deafness (or, even more restrictively, to deaf people themselves). For researchers whose critical methodologies emerge from deaf ways of being in the world, engagement with issues of embodiment, language, and normativity in any context are always informed by that deaf insight. Scholarly and creative work that makes these connections for readers who are not approaching a particular object of study from that perspective can both illuminate the work itself in new ways and expand how audiences think about deafness.

Our understanding of literatures and cultures is incomplete whenever it is not sensitive to the experiences, representations, and perspectives of the diverse groups that make up those cultures. And our understanding of the position of deaf people within cultures is similarly lacking without accounts of texts that do not explicitly address deafness (or that do so in problematic ways), but which might provide insight into other kinds of physical difference, minority politics, or embodied language. Having compellingly established the logic of Deaf Studies' broad relevance, it is important that scholarship in the field more frequently enact this relevance by performing critical readings in unexpected contexts. In addition to continuing to build on the important work of bringing to light under-represented deaf authors and identifying texts that explicitly engage with the idea of deafness, this chapter will argue that one of the ways in which the next wave of literary Deaf Studies might distinguish itself from its predecessors is by drawing on deaf insight to engage in these kinds of readings.

Such insight has been referred to elsewhere as Deaf Gain, a phrase that reverses the popular idea of "hearing loss" by directing attention to the linguistic, social, cultural, economic, and biological benefits of deafness (Bauman & Murray 2014). Work exploring this concept has been incredibly important to the field of Deaf Studies in recent years, but while "Deaf Gain" helpfully challenges commonly held perceptions of deafness as lack, it also establishes a binary division between gain and loss, suggesting that to access deaf insight one cannot understand one's own biological deafness or the social realities surrounding it as anything other than advantageous. To avoid this bifurcation, this chapter will refer to perspectives that might elsewhere be described in terms of Deaf Gain as deaf insight or deaf epistemology.

The following pages will serve as an experiment into what these insights contribute to our readings of texts that do not explicitly engage with deafness and how, in turn, these texts enhance our understanding of deafness through a reading of Charlie Chaplin's 1940 film, *The Great Dictator*.[3] The film is best remembered today for both its prescient engagement with European fascism and for being Chaplin's first full-length spoken dialogue picture, a combination that makes it particularly useful for analyzing that era's broader push to regulate bodies and languages, and which deaf insight helps us to recognize not merely as two separate facts about the film but as utterly interconnected components of its meaning.

LANGUAGE DEBATES

The assumption of the superiority of speech and the notion that it should be imposed on everyone were developments that led to significant changes in fin de siècle attitudes toward and policies regarding deaf people. Versions of what would become American Sign Language had flourished as methods of instruction during the early 19th century, especially after the founding of the American Asylum for the Deaf in 1817 by Thomas H. Gallaudet and Laurent Clerc, which encouraged manual communication. By the late 19th century, however, attitudes toward individuals perceived to be disabled, as well as ideas about language more broadly, had undergone a significant shift. As the country struggled to codify a unique and unified identity for itself in the wake of its civil war, the fact that so many citizens spoke languages other than English, or spoke English in non-normative ways, became a source of grave concern. In 1907, President Theodore Roosevelt railed against linguistic diversity, declaring "We have room for but one language in this country, and that is the English language, for we intend to see that the crucible turns our people out as Americans, of American

---

[3] Chaplin himself had a historical link to the deaf community. He was acquainted with the deaf actor Granville Redmond, who had small roles in several Chaplin films, and who taught Chaplin some signs. As John Schuchman noted, however, we have no evidence that Redmond directly influenced Chaplin's style of performance (his physical way of communicating had been established on stage and screen long before he encountered Redmond) or his ideas about language generally (1988:25). More to the point, as I argue throughout this chapter, while these kinds of facts are certainly interesting, they are not necessary as justification for putting texts in conversation with deaf insight and, indeed, there can be a danger in relying on them in this way. In the case of *The Great Dictator*, the filmmaker's sustained interest in and experimentation with non-normative modes of physical and visual communication provide ample reason for engaging the film from the perspective of deaf insight.

nationality, and not as dwellers in a polyglot boarding house" (as cited in Crawford 2000:8).

This linguistic nativism, coupled with the investment in homogenization that emerged from eugenicist philosophy, were registered in the context of deaf education by a dramatic shift away from educating children through either signs or a combination of signs and speech and toward a philosophy known as "oralism," which involved speech training and lip-reading and prohibited the use of signed languages. Because the ascendency of this pedagogical philosophy had been achieved through broad public and philanthropic support—indeed, as Jennifer Esmail (2013) has documented, it is difficult to account for the widespread interest in 19th-century deaf education outside of the context of these broader cultural anxieties—it is easy to overlook the ways in which individuals at the time attempted to reject the logic of assimilation. Works such as *The Great Dictator* serve as reminders that not everyone was comfortable with calls for linguistic conformity.

Although most writers and thinkers at the time were unaware of the significance of this standardization for the deaf community in particular, many did recognize the dangers of enforced communicative norms, restrictions on the ways people's bodies move through space and interact with others as they engage in linguistic activities. A great deal of modernist work explores strategies of resistance that both enhance our understanding of the complex ways language was understood during this critical moment in American deaf history and offer additional models of non-normative language use that might be productively adapted within Deaf Studies.[4] In turn, an awareness of how communicative norms were enforced within deaf education reveals the otherwise largely invisible stakes involved in linguistic resistance that open the door to new readings of texts engaged with similar questions.

THE ARRIVAL OF THE TALKIES

The Great Dictator is a particularly rich site for analysis in this regard because of the ways that it associated the fetishization of verbal speech within the context of fascist propaganda with the film industry's movement from silent to spoken dialogue pictures, highlighting the diverse

---

[4] Sherwood Anderson's *Winesburg, Ohio* (1919), for example, mapped the issue of communicative difference onto rapidly changing print culture and the desire to resist its influence on small communities. John Dos Passos's *U.S.A. Trilogy* (1930–1936) deployed a range of non-normative formal and typographical techniques both to register and insist on recognition of the nation's diversity. And Zora Neale Hurston's *Their Eyes Were Watching God* (1937), among many other vernacular works, captured nonstandardized speech forms on the page as a means of politically challenging assumptions about the relationships among language, text, and reader.

contexts in which debates over communicative modality were play-ing out at the time. At the center of the film is a consideration of the implications of the assumption of verbal language's superiority as a means of expression. These questions were deeply personal to Chaplin, who had made his name as a physical comedian, first on the stage and then in silent films in the early years of the 20th century. By the late 1920s, however, technology was dramatically changing cinematic form. Throughout the decade, short films were produced using synchronized dialogue, and in 1927, *The Jazz Singer* became the first full-length talkie.

Chaplin was, from the start, suspicious of the implications of intro-ducing spoken dialogue into film, and his status and financial indepen-dence enabled him to hold out longer than anyone else in adopting the new technology. Explaining his decision in a 1931 *New York Times* essay promoting *City Lights*, Chaplin described silent pictures as "a universal means of expression. Talking pictures necessarily have a limited field, they are held down to a particular tongue of particular races" (120).[5] In his association of spoken language with nationalism, Chaplin neatly identified one of the major ideological components that had led to the adoption of oralism. As the nonspeaking tramp character, Chaplin had become the most famous performer in the world, developing a language of pantomime and gesture that transcended verbal speech and enabled him to represent the downtrodden of all nations. Speech, Chaplin recognized, automatically positioned one in a world of specific nationalist politics from which he wanted to distance his character.

Both of Chaplin's films during this transitional period, *City Lights* (1931) and *Modern Times* (1936), incorporate questions about commu-nication into their storylines, demonstrating the filmmaker's ability to use synchronized sound while remaining ideologically resistant to it. "My screen character remains speechless from choice," Chaplin (1931) explained. "*City Lights* is synchronized and certain sound effects are part of the comedy, but it is a nondialogue picture because I preferred that it be that" (121). More than simply avoiding spoken language, both films deliberately highlight its absence. In *City Lights,* for instance, Chaplin uses musical instruments to represent the speech of characters, associating the voice with comical sounds that possessed no semantic meaning.

---

[5] To be clear, the physical communication Chaplin employed is not the same as specific signed languages, which are decidedly not universally comprehensible. His comments on the role of the body in communicative exchanges, however, particularly the bodies of marginalized subjects, are relevant to broader considerations of how attitudes toward embodiment shape perceptions and restrictions of actual signed languages. As Lennard Davis has argued, "when sign language is repressed as a signifying practice, what is repressed is a connection with the body" (Davis 1995:20). And the political and communicative role of the body always had been at the center of Chaplin's work.

Modern Times makes even more extensive use of the joke. When characters in the film do speak, it is mediated by technology (transmitted through radio or CCTV-style screens), and the content of their messages is consistently banal and uninteresting. The Tramp character communicates with his body until the very end, when he sings, but even then the song is a mesh of gibberish that is only given meaning through the gestures with which Chaplin accompanies it. Throughout the film, Chaplin aligns the pressure to produce spoken dialogue films with the standardization of workers' behaviors occurring at the time as a result of both industrialization and growing nationalist pressure. As he had to a lesser extent in *City Lights,* that is, in *Modern Times*, Chaplin makes visible the ideological underpinnings of communicative norms.

In addition to the nationalist political motives behind the philosophy of communicative homogenization was a largely unquestioned celebration of technology, which Chaplin found disturbing. The workers in *Modern Times* are driven by the rhythms of factory machinery in ways that are utterly unaccommodating to individual physical needs or preferences, and the film cleverly links this assembly line mentality to linguistic standardization and explores the pernicious effects of such regulation. Subjected to this pressure, the tramp character loses his mind, sexually harassing women and diving head first into the machinery before being confined to an asylum in scenes whose violence explodes the ostensibly comedic context.

This extended consideration of the role of spoken language within society and its parallels to other forms of enforced conformity carries over into Chaplin's first spoken dialogue film. *The Great Dictator* follows the story of a Jewish barber who is injured in the First World War while fighting for the fictional Tomania (Germany) and awakens from a coma 20 years later to find the world greatly changed. The opening section of the film introduces audiences both to the character of the barber and to the film's ambivalent attitude toward the speech its creator had been forced into adopting.

The first few minutes involve the Tomanian soldiers ineptly attempting to launch bombs at the enemy. After two shots that call attention to his body and its ability to produce comedy without speaking—the character wiggles his butt before pulling the line that will fire a missile and gestures his displeasure when he realizes that the shot did not hit its intended target—the barber delivers his first line, "Yes, sir," associating speech with subservience. The vast majority of the dialogue in these early sequences consists of empty, redundant commands. Having been instructed by his superior to examine a bomb that had failed to launch more than a few feet, for example, an officer turns to the man behind him, noting, "We better check the fuse." That soldier turns to the man behind him, repeating, "Yes sir. Check the fuse." The order is passed down the line before finally arriving at the barber (*The Great Dictator*,

1940). The repetition is played for laughs, but it highlights the hollow-ness of the kinds of information expressed verbally. This is speech for speech's sake; the need to inspect the fuse was obvious without any of the commands.

Rather than functioning as an effective mode of communication, speech here is frequently the butt of the joke. The set pieces of these opening scenes are, as they had always been in Chaplin films, the phys-ical comedy. Having been sent to examine the unexploded bomb, for instance, Chaplin creeps cautiously around it only to find that the bomb rotates itself to follow him. After engaging in this dance for several seconds, the bomb begins to smoke and Chaplin runs away. A similar sequence occurs when he attempts to throw a grenade, inadvertently dropping it down his pants, leading to another comic dance as he des-perately tries to dislodge it. Although there are moments in the film where the humor is delivered through the spoken dialogue itself—perhaps most memorably the barber's response to being questioned about his Aryan-ness: "I'm a vegetarian"—in this opening section, speech is used only for barking orders or meekly assenting to them (*The Great Dictator*, 1940).

There is a clear connection between Chaplin's critique of technolo-gies of the voice in *The Great Dictator* and his own ambivalence about making a spoken dialogue film. As Kyp Harness (2008) put it, "the opening scenes of *The Great Dictator* display the pitfalls of sound for Chaplin's art, and give plenty of justification to Chaplin's avoidance of it until this time" (165). Beyond this parallel, however, what the con-text of Deaf Studies enables us to register is that the fascism the film critiques, with its insistence on normative behaviors and bodies, was not merely a "felicitous" distraction that enabled Chaplin "to make his entry into the field [of "sound-and-dialogue film"] with little scrutiny or fanfare," but was conceptually linked to the enforcement of com-municative norms within the domestic and educational sphere occur-ring at the time (Harness 2008:163). In contemplating the ideological underpinnings of society's obsession with standardized verbal speech, Chaplin was engaging with questions whose implications were much broader than the shift in communicative modality in motion pictures. And understanding the film as being as much engaged in questions of the politics of communication as it is in the politics of Europe has a significant impact on the way one interprets the film's notoriously complicated ending.

THE STAKES OF CONFORMITY

In addition to making visible the nationalist and ableist assump-tions behind early 20th-century communicative norms, the history of deaf schools—particularly boarding schools in which children were separated from their parents and communities and were, therefore, much more directly subject to the power of the state—highlights the significance of linguistic rebellion by demonstrating the extent to which those in power were willing to go in order to achieve conformity. The psychological and educational risks of forcing children to communicate verbally regardless of personal preference or capacity and the prioritization of speech training over educational development in other areas underline the obsession with the voice. It is not incidental that such training was enabled by many of the technologies that Chaplin critiqued in these films. Indeed, these same technologies of voice, which had enabled radio broadcasts and film, had also made possible the ascendency of oralism. As Jonathan Sterne notes in *The Audible Past* (2003), "deafness was at the very beginning of sound reproduction"; many of the early developments in acoustic technology were undertaken so as to produce machines that could function as prosthetic hearing devices, making sound visible, from Alexander Graham Bell and his work on the telephone, to Charles Cros, who had developed a design for a phonograph and who worked at a school for the deaf, to the experiments of Thomas Edison, who was himself hard of hearing (41).

These technologies contributed to the fantasy that deaf people could or should be trained to entirely assimilate into the hearing mainstream, to conform to communicative norms by rendering their deafness invisible until, as Bell advocated in an 1883 lecture, social engineering would permit the eradication of the "deaf variety of the human race" (rpt. 1969). Signing was doubly problematic for such ideologies because, in addition to representing a non-normative modality of communication (reminding people that vocal speech was not the only means of linguistic expression), it also dramatically called attention to bodies that were themselves deemed non-normative, a category into which both Chaplin's tramp and barber characters, with their eccentric means of expression, also fell.

As was the case for these characters, the consequences for deaf individuals who either could not or who chose not to communicate normatively were often severe. Within oral boarding schools, as within boarding schools established for Native Americans that similarly strove to eliminate pupils' access to languages other than English, children were forcibly restricted from using alternate modes of communication.[6] As one man described in a 2008 documentary highlighting deaf boarding school practices, "Whenever teachers and dorm counselors

---

[6] See David Wallace Adams, *Education for Extinction* (Lawrence: Kansas University Press, 1995). For connections between deaf and indigenous American boarding schools in the early 20th century, see Rebecca Sanchez, *Deafening Modernism* (New York: New York University Press, 2015).

saw that I was signing, they would whack me on the hand with a ruler. I was 4½! Can you imagine smacking such a tiny hand?" Another interview subject recalled how "[The principal] came up to me and mouthed the words 'you signed.' I had no idea what she was talking about. 'Give me your hand!' I put out my hand, and she smacked me several times. She repeated, 'You signed' and kept on whacking my hand" (*Audism Unveiled*, 2008). For vulnerable populations, these anecdotes reveal, the pressure to conform was not merely social. Communicating or moving one's body through space in ways that deviated from the national norm carried the risk of corporal punishment.

THE DICTATOR AND THE TRAMP

In situating his critique of normative verbal communication alongside his critique of fascism, Chaplin drew attention to the implications of the generally unproblematized fetishization of vocality and of new technologies of the voice. Throughout the film, he weaves such commentary into his presentation of political authoritarianism, most notably in the public speeches that bookend it. The first serves as an introduction to the character of Hynkel (Chaplin's satirical representation of Hitler) and is delivered before a crowd of thousands of eager supporters. In addition to Chaplin's physical performance, the scene's comedy derives from the slippage between the dictator's apparent meaning and the ways that meaning is rendered in speech.

The scene is framed by a radio narration that catches audiences up with the years that have passed since the barber was injured and specifically links the voice of the dictator to a loss of political rights.

> Hynkel party takes power. Meanwhile the Jewish soldier, ex-barber, veteran of the World War suffered a loss of memory and remained an inmate of the soldier's hospital for many years. He was ignorant of the profound change that had come over Tomania. Hynkel the dictator ruled the nation with an iron fist. Under the new emblem of the double cross liberty was banished, free speech was suppressed, and only the voice of Hynkel was heard. (*The Great Dictator*, 1940)

The notion that speech is something that should be met with suspicion, that it is through the voice that pernicious ideology is spread, is reinforced throughout the scene. Addressing the crowds, Hynkel communicates in what Adrian Daub (2009) has termed "Hynkel-speak," a gibberish that borrows German and English words, but which significantly does not function as a stand-in for either language (453). The words very rarely make sense; the semantic content of Hynkel's message is expressed instead through his body language.

When the dictator refers to "Da Juden," for example, the violence of his position is communicated neither through his meaningless words nor through the translator's comically understated observation that "His excellency has just referred to the Jewish people," but rather through his gestures (fist clenched, pounding into the opposite hand), movement, and facial expressions (*The Great Dictator*, 1940). After Hynkel goes on a gibberish rant, interspersed with references to "Europe," "France," "England," and "Russia," violently gesticulating to convey his intentions to the film's audience, the translator sanitizes his remarks, rendering them as follows: "In conclusion, the phooey remarks that for the rest of the world he has nothing but peace in his heart" (*The Great Dictator*, 1940). Both through the sounds Hynkel utters, the comprehension of which is unnecessary to understand his intentions, and the voice of the translator, which highlights the ways that vocality can be used to mask rather than reveal meaning, the speech highlights the irrationality that attended the obsession with vocal utterance in fascist Germany. As Mladen Dolar (2006) has argued, "it is the relationship of the voice which makes him [Hitler] Führer, and the tie that links the subjects to him is enacted as a vocal tie … the Führer's words, supported by the immediate charismatic presence of the voice, were immediately legislative" (116, 118). It is this idea of the voice as an inherently superior form of expression that Hynkel's speech satirizes.

Truth and Power

Indeed, one of the key ways that Chaplin differentiated between Hynkel and the barber, both of whom he played, was through their use of verbal language. In his 1964 autobiography, Chaplin explained the role of speech in conceptualizing the characters: "As Hitler I could harangue the crowds in jargon and talk all I wanted to. And as the tramp I could remain more or less silent" (392). This contrast is made most explicit in a scene in which the barber and Hannah, a Jewish washerwoman, go on a date. The violence perpetrated in the ghetto by Hynkel's storm troopers had temporarily quieted as a result of the dictator's attempt to appease a Jewish banker from whom he was attempting to borrow money. But as the couple venture out, Hynkel receives news that the loan has fallen through, and he reacts by broadcasting a speech to the nation railing against Jewish people and ordering new attacks on the ghetto.

Hynkel's hysterical speech, delivered largely in gibberish, is intercut with the barber's silent, physical responses as he attempts to run with Hannah back to the safety of their courtyard, jumping head-first into a barrel when Hynkel's voice rises, performing a delicate dance with his hat and cane as he attempts to avoid being captured by a soldier. As Daub (2009) noted, in the scene "the barber's body language … approaches the visual vocabulary of Chaplin's silent comedies" (467). The juxtaposition here between the more human and humane barber who expresses himself primarily through body language and the dictator barking orders has a direct parallel in *Modern Times*. In the earlier film, the tramp takes a break from his factory job to smoke a cigarette in the bathroom only to be interrupted by his boss who appears on a giant screen, exhorting him to return to the factory floor. Although the film makes much of the distinction between normative verbal language and the various means through which the tramp makes himself understood, this is the only scene in which these modes of communication are directly played off one another.

The tramp responds to the boss's command to "Quit stalling! Get back to work!" with a series of gestures, shrugging his shoulders and pointing at the sink to indicate that he was just washing up (*Modern Times*, 1936). As in *The Great Dictator*, the authority figure's speech carries the force of compulsion; the tramp and the barber are equally powerless to resist the commands. In each scene, however, both the content of those commands and the modality in which they are delivered comes under attack; the speech itself and the technology used to convey it (radio, television) are revealed as not only inessential to communication but at times actively pernicious.

The Meaning of Silence

Chaplin repeatedly returns to these ideas in *The Great Dictator* through the character of Hannah, whose speech similarly functions as a foil for alternate embodied modes of expression. Hannah attempts to serve as the emotional core of the film by speaking to the audience directly. During the temporary halt to violence in the ghetto, for example, the soldiers help Hannah up after she falls. Shocked, she delivers the following lines to camera:

> Something's happened, I know it. The storm troopers they helped me up. Wouldn't it be wonderful if they stopped hating us? If they'd leave us alone and let us go about our business like we used to? Wouldn't it be wonderful if we didn't have to leave and go to another country? I don't want to go away. With all the hardship and the persecution I love it here. Perhaps we don't have to go. Wouldn't it be wonderful if they'd let us live and be happy again? (*The Great Dictator*, 1940)

The soft lighting and close-up shot emphasize the extent to which the scene is staged to maximize emotional impact, but far more effective than the heavy-handed rhetoric are the ways that both Hannah and the barber physically respond to the storm troopers. Hannah visibly shrinks in on herself as they draw near, and the barber involuntarily recoils as they greet him. Embedded in these postures is a narrative about the realities of trauma that rings much more truthful than Hannah's platitudes.

This pattern of contrasting silent body language with speech as responses to violence is repeated as the soldiers intensify their violence. After they attack the barber's shop, he and Hannah escape to a roof where they watch the flames consume the building. Hannah's reaction is to ramble on, desperately trying to fill the space with words as the barber sits silently, his back to the audience, coming to terms with the loss of his home. And it is this silence, all the more poignant because of the contrast with Hannah's speech, that most effectively conveys the sense of helplessness the characters are experiencing. Later on, the film's most touching scene—the murder of a son as he attempts to protect his father from storm troopers, his subsequent death in his father and brother's arms—is played entirely without dialogue.

The Barber Speaks

The Great Dictator's most subtle treatment of verbal language comes in its final speech. After escaping from a concentration camp, the barber is mistaken for the dictator and finds himself leading the invasion force into Osterlich (Austria). Upon arrival, he is required to address the victorious troops:

> Soldiers! Don't give yourselves to brutes—who despise you—enslave you—who regiment your lives—tell you what to do—what to think and what to feel! Who drill you—diet you—treat you like cattle and use you as cannon fodder. Don't give yourselves to these unnatural men—machine men with machine minds and machine hearts! You are not machines! You are men! With the love of humanity in your hearts! Don't hate! (Chaplin:400)

The scene has been controversial since the film's release in part because of the speech's content—its cries for universal brotherhood were interpreted as evidence that Chaplin was sympathetic to Communism, an accusation that would be used several years later to refuse him reentry into the United States—and in part on the aesthetic grounds that it appears entirely out of character for the barber, who has not previously demonstrated the capacity for such eloquence.

The fact that Chaplin was proud of the speech, delivering it publically and reprinting it in his autobiography, has led most critics to read it as a message from Chaplin himself to his film audience. As Harness (2008) argued, "In the course of his six-minute speech, we become aware that the face intensely, solemnly speaking these words directly to us through the camera is not the face of the Barber, of Hynkel, or of the Tramp. It is not even the face of Charlie Chaplin—it is rather the face of Charles Chaplin, internationally famous celebrity and the confidant of Albert Einstein, Mahatma Ghandi, George Bernard Shaw, Aldous Huxley, and Winston Churchill" (171). The sympathetic sensibilities expressed in the speech also have contributed to audiences' desire to understand these words as the film's overarching message. Its exhortation against standardization (humans treated as cattle, as machines) matched neatly with sentiments expressed in other Chaplin films, and enabled the appealing illusion that the barber's humanity had won out over the dictator's hate, that the masses had been convinced by his eloquence and a more peaceful future had been made possible.

Whatever Chaplin's intentions, however, the speech *is* embedded within the film. The barber speaks directly to the soldiers, repeatedly referencing them and looking at them for the vast majority of the speech, only raising his eyes to camera at the end. Moreover, as engagement with Deaf Studies helps to emphasize, verbal communication has been a subject of politicization and problematization throughout the film in ways that undermine the impulse to read the barber's words at face value. Given how the speech mirrors Hynkel's opening oratory, the audience's enthusiastic response to the barber is deeply fraught. The fact that the faceless masses react in exactly the same way to both speeches suggests not that the barber's sentiments have changed their minds (such an abrupt ideological shift, even if it were possible, would not be trustworthy), but that they do not recognize (or care) about the different messages being delivered.

Rather than being naïve, then, the way the final speech operates in the context of the film as a whole is actually quite cynical. Although Daub (2009) and others have argued that "the barber liberates that voice by actually speaking," that this final speech "functions broadly as the antidote to the film's first," the cheering crowds indicate that the content of the message, whether it be Hynkel's irrational anti-Semitism or the barber's rational and impassioned pleas for peace, is irrelevant (456, 473). The obsequious response to any verbal language delivered in this way suggests the propagandistic potential of all speech. It is not only the message that needs to be altered to combat political hatred, the scene posits, but the ideological baggage associated with that particular mode of communication, all the more insidious because of the ways it is rendered invisible through normatization.

Ultimately, then, *The Great Dictator* ends with a reminder of the potential dangers of verbal speech, a point emphasized in its very last shot. After hearing the barber's speech over the radio, Mr. Jaeckel, the barber's friend who has helped Hannah escape to Osterlich, comes outside. "Hannah, did you hear that?" he asks. Hannah puts her hand up to silence him. "Listen," she commands, her eyes lifting upward to the sky (*The Great Dictator*, 1940). At this point, the barber's speech has already finished. What she is encouraging them (and the film's audience) to focus on is silence, a space filled not with political messages, even the sympathetic ones of the barber, but with the ambiguous silence that is a vital, if often unrecognized, component of the film.

CONCLUSION

By making visible the fraught nature of verbal speech and revealing the investment of authority in homogenizing communicative practice, Deaf Studies helps us to recognize the ways this final scene, rather than being an aesthetically problematic outlier, is actually integrally linked to the theme of the language politics developed throughout the film. *The Great Dictator* is a movie about fascism; it is a movie specifically about Hitler, but as deaf insight helps to reveal, it is also a movie about communication in the modern world, and the implications of fetishizing and normativizing particular communicative modalities and the technologies used to spread and enforce them. In addition to adding to the ways we can engage the film, recognizing the links between Chaplin's critique of totalitarianism and his attitudes toward talkies enables a fuller understanding of each of these historical developments.

Beyond the specific context of the film, what I have hoped to demonstrate is the relevance of Deaf Studies and insight beyond situations in which a deaf artist or character is present. Chaplin's accounts of the production of *The Great Dictator* gave no indication that he was thinking specifically about the relationship between its critique of enforced conformity and deaf communities while making the movie. But that does not mean that the two cannot be mutually illuminative. Just as Deaf Studies provides new ways of reading the film, so, too, does the film offer productive insight into the cultural contexts shaping deaf lives in the early 20th century. Arguments about the broad implications of Deaf Studies have always been a part of the way the field has positioned itself. As it continues to develop, it will be increasingly important not only to continue making these claims in general terms, but also to provide specific readings that make good on them by bringing Deaf Studies into unexpected contexts. In demonstrating what it might look like to do so, this chapter has attempted to make a case for the expansion of the field and the continued development of deaf insight as a critical paradigm.

REFERENCES

Bahan, B., Bauman, H. L., & Montenegro, F. (Producers). (2008) *Audism unveiled.* United States. Dawn Sign.

Bauman, H. L. (2008). Introduction: Listening to Deaf Studies. In H.-D. L. Bauman (Ed.), *Open your eyes: Deaf Studies talking.* Minneapolis: University of Minnesota Press.

Bauman, H. L., & Murray, J. (Eds.) (2014). *Deaf gain: Raising the stakes for human diversity.* Minneapolis: University of Minnesota Press.

Bell, A. G. (1969). *Memoir upon the formation of a deaf variety of the human race.* Washington, DC: Alexander Graham Bell Association for the Deaf.

Chaplin, C. (1931/1995). A rejection of the talkies [rpt]. In D. Robinson (Ed.), *Charlie Chaplin comic genius* (pp. 120–121). New York: Harry N. Abrams.

Chaplin, C. (1936). *Modern Times.* United States. United Artists.

Chaplin, C. (1940). *The Great Dictator.* United States. Charlie Chaplin Studios.

Chaplin, C. (1964). *My Autobiography.* New York: Simon and Schuster.

Crawford, J. (2000). *At war with diversity: US language policy in an age of anxiety.* Clevedon, UK: Cromwell.

Daub, A. (2009). "Hannah, can you hear me?"—Chaplin's *Great Dictator,* "schtonk," and the vicissitudes of voice. *Criticism, 51*(3), 451–482.

Davis, L. (1995). *Enforcing normalcy: Disability, deafness, and the body.* London: Verso.

Dolar, M. (2006). *A voice and nothing more.* Cambridge, MA: MIT Press.

Esmail, J. (2013). *Reading Victorian deafness.* Athens, OH: Ohio University Press.

Harness, K. (2008). *The art of Charlie Chaplin.* Jefferson, NC: McFarland & Company

Krentz, C. (2007). *Writing deafness: The hearing line in nineteenth-century American literature.* Chapel Hill: The University of North Carolina Press.

Lauter, P. (2014). Modern period: 1910–1945.In P. Lauter (Ed.), *The Heath anthology of American literature* (Vol. D) (7th ed.) (pp. 1311–1340). Boston: Wadsworth.

Peters, C. (2000). *Deaf American literature: From carnival to canon.* Washington DC: Gallaudet University Press.

Sanchez, R. (2015). *Deafening modernism: Embodied language and visual poetics in American literature.* New York: New York University Press.

Sayers, E. (Ed.) (2012). *Outcasts and angels: The new anthology of deaf characters in literature.* Washington DC: Gallaudet University Press.

Schuman, J. (1988). *Hollywood speaks: Deafness and the film entertainment industry.* Urbana: University of Illinois Press.

Sterne, J. (2003). *The audible past: Cultural origins of sound reproduction.* Durham, NC: Duke University Press.

SECTION II

Deaf Ontologies

7

A Dialogue on Deaf Theology:
Deaf Ontologies Seeking Theology

Hannah Lewis and Kirk VanGilder

This chapter employs a strategy of grounding theological construction in deaf ontologies by exploring deaf theology through a dialogical conversation between two deaf scholars with PhD degrees in theology. This approach highlights the tendency for deaf people to engage with ideas through conversation and social connection rather than isolated individual thought (Ladd 2003:360). By writing dialogically, we hope to show how our thought is shaped not only by ourselves as authors, but also in conversation with other deaf people in academic, church, and everyday settings.

Our move to ground theology in deaf ontologies highlights a key methodological issue for all theology; that the content of theology—summarized as the study of the relationship between humanity and God—is inextricably tied up with the form and the way in which it is done. Traditional systematic theological methods may examine what biblical texts might have meant in their original languages and contexts and how they may be interpreted today, or engage in philosophical discussions of how Jesus Christ might be both God and man. Such traditional theological activity has developed largely in a context of power and privilege. This context is the domain of people in authority in the Christian Church who have been concerned with establishing the boundaries of authentic Christian faith in the midst of a plethora of competing ideas. Over the centuries, this method of theological enquiry evolved to meet new challenges, including the growth of rationalism in the European Enlightenment and the development of sciences; but it always evolved within the context of power and privilege in the academy and among the authorities of various Christian denominations and always with the aim of keeping Christian discourse within orthodox bounds. In the 20th century, however, new approaches to theology began to emerge. These approaches arose from the context of people living with oppression and discrimination every day who began to question the concerns of mainstream theology as something that did not relate to their experience. For example,

Latin American Liberation theology arose in response to the systematic exclusion of the poor in matters of faith and life. Latin American
liberation theologian Leonardo Boff argued that Christian scripture
held a "preferential option for the poor" because people experiencing socioeconomic disenfranchisement were much closer to the social
status of people in the New Testament than were present-day middle-
class and upper-class people (Boff & Boff 1987). This similarity means
that the poor of today interpret scripture in ways that are much more
likely to align with the original meanings and import of these pas-
sages than are the interpretations of those with privilege and power.
Similarly, African Americans such as James Cone approached Black
theology as intrinsically tied to the African American struggle for
human dignity and equal treatment under law (Cone 1970). Feminist
theologians, including those in Africa, such as Musimbi Kanyoro, and
Latin America, such as Maria Isasi-Diaz, have worked to develop theology from a postcolonial feminist perspective by engaging women
in discussing the meaning of scriptures in communal and collaborative settings that arise from their interaction as women in the village
life of their respective cultures (Kanyoro 2002, Isasi-Diaz 1996). These
theologians redefined theology as something anyone could do, ideally in dialogue with others in the academy, professional clergy, people "in the pews," and people "on the street." This dialogue also can
be between the theory and the practice of theology, as the effect of
theological ideas on people's lives modifies those theological ideas in
an ongoing dialogue (Bevans 1992).

   Although our dialogue on deaf theology has affinities with the methodologies of these liberation theologians, we contend that deaf theology
needs to prioritize concerns that arise from deaf experiences. Whatever
parallels exist in the dynamics of oppression and liberation between
Black people, women, and the people of the developing world (for
example) and deaf communities, we cannot help but wonder whether
there might be ways in which deaf people find ourselves marginalized,
oppressed, and disenfranchised that are unique to our being deaf. For
example, the disenfranchisement of poor people in Latin America may
be based on economics tied specifically to how various ethnicities or
social classes are viewed in those Latin American societies. The disenfranchisement of deaf people in many societies is, in part, rooted in a
medical view of hearing loss and deaf people as people who are unable
to do certain essential tasks. Although both situations lead to economic
disenfranchisement, the means of oppression are quite different and,
therefore, may give rise to differing strategies for liberation and different expectations of what is liberating. In that vein, there then might
be unique ways that we envision liberation from a variety of material,
social, and spiritual forms of oppression. We need to clarify what we
mean by oppression—which may cover a whole range of experiences,

including ignorance, discrimination, marginalization, audism, and paternalism. All of which—however benevolent they are in intention—have had (and still have) a disempowering effect on the deaf community and deaf individuals and which, therefore, need to be resisted. We need to identify how deaf people define liberation—recognizing that there may be more than one understanding. But again, liberation will have a wide range of meanings that extend beyond simply resisting oppression and branching into the right to flourish without the burden of having to continually defend our existence as deaf people with our particular perspectives and experiences. Although it is worthwhile to talk of our journeys from oppression to liberation in relation to those of other minority oppressed groups, we fear it may be too easy to fall onto a well-trod path made by others and overlook how our own experiences might shed light on defining what liberation means in social and theological terms.

Deaf theology has emerged into the light of academic theology as a response to marginalization. *Deaf Liberation Theology* argues that ordinary deaf people have been "doing theology" for years in the sense of reflecting on the <check>bible, and their relationship with God in the light of being deaf (Lewis 2007). One of the founding principles of liberation theologies in general—and deaf theology in particular—is how we do theology in a way that privileges deaf perspectives, questions, and experiences and also is undertaken in a way that relates to the fact that much of it is carried out in sign language. This is one of the reasons we have opted for a dialogical format for our chapter. This format seeks to preserve our differences, retain our distinctive viewpoints, and relate to the deaf cultural patterns of collective storytelling, in which people absorb ideas through discussing them with one another (Ladd 2003:360). Cornel West and bell hooks employ a dialogical format to discuss Black intellectual thought in order to capture the spirit of testimony that hooks calls "an integral part of the Black religious tradition." hooks explains a need for dialogue in writing by stating, ". . . the spirit of testimony is a very hard spirit to convey in written text, . . . it struck me that dialogue was one of the ways where that sense of mutual witness and testimony could be made manifest" (hooks & West 1991:1). Myles Horton and Paulo Freire, two prominent liberationist hearing scholars also employ dialogical methods, which Freire describes as follows: "Instead of writing a book, we speak the book, and afterwards others can transcribe it" (Horton & Freire 1990:4). Freire goes on to explain that this process better captures the movement and feel of natural conversation, which, therefore, makes it more readable and approachable for the poor he worked with in Brazil.

Our process for creating this chapter of scholarly dialogue between the two of us and a variety of other sources was primarily facilitated through written English using Internet-based collaborative writing tools. We found the mutual gap between ASL and BSL vocabulary limited our ability to discuss theological topics in depth over video chat technology. We did, however, benefit from using such technology to converse in written English while retaining the facial expressions and varied attempts at each other's signed language. We began by identifying some areas of interest and each of us started an opening paragraph or two to begin conversation. We then responded to each other's writing and produced some very lengthy conversations! From that point, our task was to identify what would be the best material for making our points regarding deaf ontologies and editing the conversation to suit an audience that might not be familiar with the terms and concepts of theology.

One final comment on the use of dialogue: It is important for both of us that our dialogue partners for this chapter are deaf. Sutherland and Rogers argue that there is a difference between hearing people and deaf people in research within the deaf community. Good research is more than being able to sign well, rather, "Deaf researchers ... have a lifetime of knowing what it is like to be misunderstood; issues of trust and common cultural values are very important here" (Sutherland & Rogers 2014:276). This shared ontological experience means that a deaf person can "get" what another deaf person is trying to say in a way no hearing person can. Sutherland and Rogers adduce the parallel of research within ethnic minority groups, or when gender is the issue. We do acknowledge that engaging in dialogue with the scholarly work of hearing people may allow for better understanding between deaf people and those who hold power and privilege in our larger societies. Engaging with hearing sources in scholarly dialogue has an important role and place within the formulation of a deaf theology, but it is not what we wish to explore here by rooting our theological dialogue in deaf ontologies. Our dialogues here consist of the following topics: the positive valuation of being deaf, deriving theology from deaf experiences, theology as expressed in signed languages, and deaf theology in a transnational context. These topics are only a selection of the many topics we could have pursued. We saw them as highlighting particular examples of theology rooted in deaf ontology. Even though deaf theology is a young subject in the academy, with only a handful of published books, chapters, and peer-reviewed articles emerging in the past 30 years, there is much more that we could have covered, and much that is still in development.

FRAMING AND NAMING DIALOGUE PARTNERS

Hannah M. Lewis [HML]: Before beginning our exploration of our topics, we should introduce ourselves and discuss the various other authors and sources we engage with and some we do not engage with in our dialogue and why we've made the decisions we've made. We have different perspectives as male and female, USA and UK, ASL and BSL, United Methodist and Anglican as well as other differences I am sure. We can celebrate what we have in common, too. We both became deaf after acquiring a great deal of spoken and written English; we were educated in English, and came to sign language and deafhood as adults—we remain two of still very few deaf PhDs and ordained deaf people in the world. We are a good example of the complicated web of similarities and differences within the deaf world that makes it a fully rounded community that can't be reduced to a single issue.

In our theological work, we are both very much deaf theologians who also embody a variety of other interests and influences. You, Kirk, are influenced by your interest in missiology, which is the study of how Christianity is transmitted across cultures, and your experience in Zimbabwe, Kenya, and other places. I am influenced by the theory and practice of being a priest in active ministry and consequently in pastoral theology, which relates the theory and practice of theology, as well as my involvement in campaigns for women's ministry within the Church of England, again among many other strands.

Kirk VanGilder [KVG]: I agree, while we don't embody the fullness of the complexity of the deaf community as we are both white, academically trained, and Christian, we do begin to capture some of the varieties of deaf experiences in both our personal lives and our professional and social contact with others. Another important difference that we embody in this dialogue is that you are currently serving in local deaf ministry in Liverpool, England, and I am teaching in an academic setting at Gallaudet University in Washington, DC, in the United States.

HML: My doctoral thesis turned book, *Deaf Liberation Theology,* was the first deaf-authored publication of deaf theology. In the intervening eight years, the line most discussed in conversational responses and reviews by both deaf and hearing people has been as follows: "I am really not interested in what hearing people, however involved with deaf people they might be, have said about what deaf people think and what a theology of deaf people might look like" (Lewis 2007:6). To be honest, I find the focus on this sentence fascinating. At the time, it was included as part of the explicit statement of who I am and where I am coming from that is essential to a theology of liberation with no intention of being either particularly provocative or particularly empowering, which is how it seems to have been understood.

KVG: That this line has become the most discussed line from your book is quite revealing of our shared commitment to privileging deaf ontologies when doing theology. When using *Deaf Liberation Theology* to teach a graduate-level class of hearing students, this was a line that generated a great deal of discussion. Some students found it unnecessarily exclusionary of the viewpoints and experiences of hearing people. They weren't able to see the strategy here in privileging deaf viewpoints and experiences as an attempt to ground deaf theology in the ontology of deaf people. We are both less interested in "theology about deaf people" as found in works by Wayne Morris (2008) and Gill Meller (2011). However helpful these insights "about us" might be, we are more focused on what deaf people are saying ourselves given the paucity of attention given to deaf contributions to theology in academic literature. Interestingly enough, some of the hearing students in this class were able to understand reasons for favoring African American contributions to Black theology in the United States but seemed unwilling to extend the same strategy to deaf theology.

HML: That's interesting; in the UK the strongest response has come from deaf people excited by this line because it established space for thinking theologically on their own terms instead of being told what was correct by hearing people. Ladd identifies a fundamental difference between deaf studies and other minority studies, and that is that because of literacy issues deaf studies has been historically instigated and run by hearing people who are of the majority (2003:449). And although such hearing-led research has been well-meaning and valuable, the result has been a critical imbalance in such research, which has focused on topics such as linguistics, psychology, and education and omitted subjects found in other minority studies. Other such subjects include the study of communities and cultures, which would include the study of religion, spirituality, and theology within that culture. Ladd suggests this imbalance means that we deaf people feel we are still objects of analysis rather than empowered subjects engaged in a common task. This is why, in this chapter, we do not engage in depth with the works of hearing people writing about the deaf community. Privileging deaf perspectives and the work of deaf people, as we seek to do in our work in general, is seeking to redress this imbalance and make visible the theological stories deaf people have been telling each other over the years. This is grounds for constructing a specifically deaf theology as part of the wider deaf project of "creating a space and a climate for reflection upon and a shaping of the re-emergence of their own communities" (Ladd 2003:450).

This decision presents specific challenges for our work; for example, very little written work by deaf people has been published, therefore, we have had to draw on nonacademic sources if we wish to access what has been said in the past. Church magazines from the late 19th century up until the present day contain articles, sermons, and poems by deaf people in varying standards of English expressing their theology. *Deaf Liberation Theology* (Lewis 2007) contains a number of examples. The deaf community has been constructing theologies for a long, long time—not necessarily in a systematic way, but through reflecting on the word of God as it relates to their experience in their time and their place.

KVG: Yes, I, too, think there's a wealth of information out there in what could be called the "folk theologies" of deaf communities. All communities of faith have this dynamic among them where there is a groundswell of ways of thinking and talking about one's faith and being that is very intimately tied to their lived experience. They are often rich and compelling and yet somewhat elusive to document. Much of what contemporary academic theology attempts to do in constructing theologies has its origins in these sorts of conversations and experiences. From an academic point of view, this elusive nature of deaf theology might arise from methods for recording conversations in signed languages, which either forces a translation to written forms of other languages or requires a formalized video recording that often takes away from the spontaneity of folk discourse. Although similar issues can arise between spoken languages and their written forms, it may be a more pronounced issue when working with signed languages. This could change, however, with the rise in popularity of video blogging in some deaf communities. As more and more "casual reflection" and "random thoughts" are captured and exchanged in this sort of manner, we might be able to better document and reflect upon the folk theologizing that happens in deaf communities. This perhaps necessitates a different role for academics in deaf theology where our work becomes more about recording and revealing what's happening in deaf communities in relation to theological thoughts, rather than constructing and systematizing thoughts of our own.

HML: Deaf people—whether identified as Christian or not—express beliefs about themselves and their relation to the world, to others and to God in different ways in addition to magazine articles and vlogs, which can be used as sources for theological reflection. For example, I have begun to utilize the work of De'VIA artist Nancy Rourke whose work explicitly explores themes of celebration, resistance, and liberation in deaf culture and deaf lives (Rourke 2015). Her most obviously religious painting is titled David vs. Goliath (Rourke 2012). In this picture, she uses the story of the little boy defeating the big giant with God's help[1] to depict George Veditz, former president of the National Association of the Deaf in the United States, who spearheaded efforts to preserve and promote ASL, beheading Alexander Graham Bell, a famous and wealthy inventor who advocated for oral methods that forbade ASL. Reflecting on her work in dialogue with a class of deaf

---

[1] The full story of David and Goliath is told in 1 Samuel 17.

ministry students, we found it inspired a discussion along the lines of, "What does it mean for God to be on the side of an oppressed minority such as deaf people?" Such discussions can be compared with discussions around what it means for God to have a preference for the poor as referred to earlier in relation to Liberation Theology in Latin America. It would be fascinating to expand such discussions to include the artist herself and other deaf people with the possibility of some distinctively deaf theological insights emerging. This method is still very much under development—we don't have any examples yet. But one of my problems in using Rourke's work and also signed poetry and other similar things as a source is that the methodology for using them to construct theology in the academy is still not well developed and is perhaps rather unsystematic.

KVG: Far from being unsystematic, there's a growing body of theological work coming from people who experience marginalization and silencing. A large number of feminist theologians from developing nations use a variety of workshops, conferences, training centers, discussion circles, and other homegrown ways of conversing and transmitting wisdom to both ground and develop their theologies (Russell, Cannon, Isasi-Diaz & Pui-Lan 1988). These sorts of "reading with" approaches attempt to make communal readings of life, experiences, scriptures, and other forms of communication a dialogical process that enables deeper and more diverse theological exploration. I engage with some of these ideas in *Making Sadza with Deaf Zimbabwean Women* (VanGilder 2012). I, too, think it's a very fertile approach to developing deaf theologies. Wayne Morris explores some of these ideas as well in *Theology Without Words* (2008). Although Morris is hearing, he observes many instances where deaf people read themselves into scriptures, such as a retelling of the story of Moses leading the Israelites to freedom through the Red Sea[2] from the point of view of "...two imagined deaf Israelites walking through parted waters..." (Morris 2008:110). In analyzing this observation of deaf use of scripture in the United Kingdom, Morris also references many of the Third World feminist scholars who come to my mind as well. I'm far more interested, however, in what deaf people think they're doing with scripture and why. To me, this would lead us closer to understanding how deaf ontologies ground deaf theology.

DIVERSITY, DIFFERENCE, AND GOD

KVG: The pluralism of deaf communities is a vital aspect to keep in mind. A key question for Christian theology is to explore how the

---

[2] Full story in Exodus 15.

diversity of human experience can be reconciled with the concept of a unified global Christian faith. Exploring our similarities and differences is a good illustration of how our individual dialogue partners, both actual people and general interests, influence and shape our theological thinking. We arrive at subtle yet important differences as to what makes us deaf people and how we live and express those differences in our conversation here. Writ on a larger scale, attention to how deaf people maintain, honor, and celebrate diversity while retaining a sense of similarity as deaf people is a very intriguing potential contribution to exploring how human diversity can coexist within a unified, but not uniform, global Christianity. It also could offer insight as to how interfaith and nonreligious communities can be built that allow for common ground and common understanding to be a cohesive foundation for global interaction.

HML: One common thread within the wide diversity of deaf experiences is that being deaf is essentially a good thing. Being grounded in the way deaf people experience ourselves, this can be a fruitful starting point for deaf theology. The essential goodness of being deaf is most visible in a scriptural quote from the book of Exodus used by many deaf people in deaf liberation movements, whether they claim to be religious or not. For example, the "Charter of the Rights of the Deaf" published by the (non-religiously affiliated) National Union of the Deaf in London in 1982 quoted from the book of Exodus: "Who taught the people to speak in the first place? Who makes them deaf or mute? Who makes them to see, or be blind? Who, if not I YHWH?" (Exodus 4:11, Priests for Equality.[3] Discussed in Lewis 2007:111). This theological claim that we are deaf because God made us that way has been used as the foundation upon which deaf people have declared they are equal to hearing people. This declaration is in direct opposition to the assertion of the 1880 Milan conference that only if we spoke properly could we be equal in God's eyes, because "speech is the light of the soul and the soul on earth is the light of the divine idea" (Lewis 2007:82).[4] I was excited to read that deaf people in the signing community of Adamorobe in Ghana also see themselves as being created deaf by God. "I like being deaf, God gave it to me." (Kusters 2015:126). Clearly this theological concept is central to deaf ontology and not just present for western Christian believers.

Another interesting angle on difference and diversity arising from the deaf gain perspective is less about the deaf gain of sign language,

---

[3] Our use of *The Inclusive Bible* translation reflects our shared commitment to employing gender inclusive language when talking of God. The quote in the National Union of the Deaf paper uses the noninclusive King James Version.

[4] This quotation is Farrar quoting Dr. Zucchi of the Royal School for the Deaf in Milan.

culture, and community and more about the deaf gain of being a "people of the eye"—which includes deaf people who do not use signed language. I was fascinated by the collection of essays in *Deaf Gain: Raising the Stakes for Human Diversity* (Bauman & Murray 2014), which included topics related to the biological experience of being without hearing—but approaching it in a completely different way from traditional texts—with a focus on deaf gain rather than hearing loss. For example, some people have argued that deaf people gain in visual processing skills (Dye 2014) or an increased tactile ability (Napoli 2014). Dye points out, however, that although from a deaf perspective these enhanced skills are seen as a deaf gain, from a medical/rehabilitory perspective these skills would be seen as compensatory changes that are a hallmark of deficit (Dye 2014:206). This medical/rehabilitory perspective has its theological parallel in what has been called the perspective of the "travesty of the divine image" (Eiesland 1994), which argues that disabled people can't be created in the image of a perfect God because they are a deviation from the norm.[5]

The deaf gain perspective in theology argues this view of being deaf really seems to add to the understanding of a well-known verse from the <check>bible: "God looked at all of this creation, and proclaimed that this was good—very good" (Genesis 1:31a, Priests for Equality). Just as enhanced sensory skills can be celebrated as an example of the wonderful diversity of human beings, so we can also celebrate deaf (and disabled people) as truly made in the image of God who created humankind in all its wonderful diversity and sees all people as good—very good. The human need in God for true acceptance of self is an ongoing struggle for many people, and I feel that the deaf struggle toward deafhood and a positive deaf identity has a lot to reflect on and contribute in this area.

KVG: My theological thought also has been influenced by this declaration of creation as inherently good. For me, it was reading the work of Matthew Fox, including *Original Blessing* (2000), which traces the history of Christian theology in a way that emphasizes the inherent dignity of all creation. I've always read deaf people as a part of that creation. In the book of Exodus, when Moses protests against God's choosing him to lead because of his slow speech and "wooden tongue," God's response, as quoted earlier from Exodus 4:11, names God as the creator and originator of human diversity in relation to speaking, hearing, and seeing. Although a hearing-centered reading of this verse might want to couple this with the notion of God as a giver of judgment and punishment, my deaf-centered eyes see something else at work. I would connect it with this "original blessing" that all creation

---

[5] This concept is discussed from a Deaf perspective in Lewis (2007:68).

is declared "very good" and thus deaf people—including our experiences, cultures, and languages—carry this imprimatur of divine goodness and value, not just for us, but for the wholeness of creation. That this verse from Genesis 1:31 is even cited as a justification for deaf liberation by deaf people who are not seeking to make explicitly religious claims, such as the National Union of the Deaf as you've noted, shows that there is a powerful resonance between this verse and deaf ways of experiencing ourselves as good.

DERIVING THEOLOGY FROM DEAF EXPERIENCES

HML: I want to describe a couple of examples of constructing theology with a deaf-centered worldview and using deaf experience I have encountered to illustrate how deaf experience and theology can dialogue to create new perspectives. These examples are intended to be working examples to demonstrate the methodology we are discussing in this chapter rather than a fully worked out systematic deaf theology. The first example took place on a residential weekend conference. A bible study led by two hearing priests who could sign asked deaf delegates to get into groups to talk about their experiences of homesickness as a prelude to exploring a biblical text. Each group fed back to the whole room afterward—and group after group said that they never really got homesick—what they had experienced was being "schoolsick" for the communication and community of their deaf boarding schools during the school holidays at home with their families. Even those who had attended a day school or mainstream school, but had experienced times with the deaf community as a child, understood that longing. This is an example of the concept of "deaf diaspora"—the longing of deaf people to be together because most of them are born into hearing families (Emery 2015). I later undertook some theological reflection on this discussion with a tutor group (of deaf and hearing participants training for ministry with the deaf community) where we discussed how this shared experience might be likened to the longing of the human heart for heaven—for the Kingdom—the Community—of God. Although this longing for heaven is not unique to the deaf community, it was eloquently described by the ancient theologian Augustine in his *Confessions* as, "Our hearts are restless, until they can find rest in you" (Chadwick 1998). I would argue that the experience of the deaf community gives a concrete insight into what this means.

KVG: This sense of "schoolsick" resonates with my reflections on serving at a deaf church in Baltimore, Maryland. The ways that deaf parishioners spoke of the value of the church in their lives and how they practiced being the church for one another was done with an air of "homecoming" each week. Not only was there a worship service, but it was followed by an affordable lunch. Donated baked goods often were available to those in the community who struggled to make ends meet financially. Informational exchange happened in formal presentations such as those on healthy living or financial planning as well as in informal conversations where people expressed their problems and gained advice from the experience of their friends. This exemplifies Ladd's identification of information exchange as a significant aspect of deaf cultural discourse (Ladd 2003:360). Also, if local professional sports teams were playing, the social aspect of "after-church" would linger around the fellowship and conviviality of cheering on the teams. All of these practices share a sense of togetherness and community care that embody the principles you mention and served as a respite from a week in the world of work, school, and neighborhoods that were predominantly hearing-centered and composed of hearing people. This experience of "deaf sociality" creates powerful bonds for deaf people, as noted by Friedner in deaf churches in Bangalore, India (Friedner 2014). Such bonds can be reflected upon theologically to explore more deeply what we mean when we claim as Christians that our only true home is in heaven.

HML: A second example of theology based on deaf experience I would like to refer to is an encounter with an individual—a deaf man who was training for the ministry and who preached a sermon on Jesus healing the deaf man in Mark's gospel. As he preached, he referred to the healing of the deaf man as being a "coming out of his shell" and recalled how he himself had had a similar experience of being called "out of his shell" to serve God in his ministry. Again, as I reflected on this sermon, I realized that it was immaterial to this reading whether the deaf man had been made to hear or speak or not—the focus was on the confidence and the vocation the encounter with Jesus gave to the deaf man. This same reading has been dramatized by a deaf priest working with his deaf congregation in the United Kingdom to create a drama that treats this healing miracle from two different perspectives. First of all, in a scene that is spoken—regardless of whether the actors are deaf or hearing—the meaning is made obvious through gesture rather than through words; the healing is that the deaf man is made to hear and speak. In a second scene—exactly the same story but this time acted through sign language—the healing is that the deaf man is given by Jesus the ability to sign and discovers the deaf community. Unlike the first example cited, in which deaf experience adds an additional strand to an ongoing theological discussion, this is a radically different perspective from that of hearing theology. No one within mainstream biblical studies has ever questioned that the healing of the deaf man meant the man was made to hear and speak. From the perspective of the dominant model that to be deaf means to be unable to hear, it is simple common sense that Jesus simply gave the man what he didn't have. The deaf reading is based on a deeply rooted (although unexpressed and unexamined) concept of deaf gain, as well as the belief that everything Jesus does is good. It would be valuable to compare this with Kusters (2015), who describes the struggle of deaf people in Adamorobe with this biblical story—they didn't want to become hearing but at the same time they said that anything Jesus does is good in itself. Other views are explored in Lewis (2007:145–149) where I discuss the various ways deaf people have interpreted this passage over the years.

THEOLOGY IN SIGNED LANGUAGES

HML: Scholarly discussions of deaf gain often explore the benefits of using signed languages as a means of communication. We could look at some of the ways that this concept creates the basic assumption that sign language theology by deaf people adds something that other contextual theologies may not have. The use of sign language and deaf experience makes clear that speech is not the sum total of language (Petitto 2014:72) and that the tongue and hands are two equal modalities for expressing language. For me this challenges the way in which we translate the Greek term *logos* as Word (as in the Word of God) as I've discussed a bit in *Deaf Liberation Theology* (2007). *Logos* is God's deep desire to communicate with humanity—and not just through speech and writing. Louise Lawrence, a hearing researcher in the field of biblical studies who has observed (via an interpreter) deaf people discussing bible readings makes some interesting observations relevant to this point. She argues that "sign language as a medium needs to be valued" for two reasons; firstly, because of the great contribution it makes to the visualization of biblical texts and, therefore, to our understanding of what they mean. Secondly, Lawrence discusses how sign language is a representative language of a collective culture and as such may be closer to the original context of the bible in its first century Palestinian tradition of stories that are transmitted by being retold "orally" many times before they are written down (Lawrence 2009:102).

   KVG: A practical theological example of this concept is how the relative economy of signed languages in using directionality and location in grammatical ways often can convey theological ideas with a grace and fluency when spoken and written languages seem to struggle. I was recently part of a team working to translate theological terms into American Sign Language (ASL) for the website of The United Methodist Church. We were wrestling with how to concisely communicate the term "justifying grace." After a lengthy theological discussion between a hearing interpreter and myself, it was a native deaf signer from a deaf family who had been observing our discussion who came up with a rather elegant and accurate sign combination for us to use. It begins with the ASL sign for "forgive" starting from above, where God is located in ASL, and ending near the signer's chest; It then smoothly transitions to make the ASL sign for "connect" or "join" moving from the signer's chest back up to the space where God is located. In addition, the signer's facial expression should convey a sense of pleading as the sign for "forgive" is produced, then shift to acceptance as it draws near the chest, then transitions to a joyous expression as one gazes upward during the production of the sign for "connect."[6] In this way, a very rich theological understanding of justifying grace as the moment at which one's sins are forgiven and one becomes reconciled with God can be communicated with an economy of signs.

In sharing this sign with hearing people, even those who were not fluent in ASL, some of them expressed an appreciation for how this sign offered them insight into what "justifying grace" meant within our church's theological tradition. Again, we see a collaborative effort of dialogue, and a privileging of deaf ontologies in this translation process that embodies Ladd's remarks about how deaf communities engage in the exchange of information and development of ideas (2003:360). Creative use of signed languages, as Sutton-Spence (2014) argues, "pushes signed languages so far beyond their normal boundaries that we need new ways to understand communication" (458). This creative use of signed languages, found in art forms such as sign language poetry, is a familiar aspect of how sign language users come to understand and express complex ideas. Using this process as a means of developing deaf theology can be a rich and meaningful addition to understanding theological terms. This sort of language play need not be conceived of as an exchange between written/spoken languages and signed languages. Both of us have encountered theological creativity in moments where multiple signed languages were being used.

THEOLOGY IN TRANSNATIONAL CONTEXTS

HML: Moments of transnational worship offer an opportunity to look at the unique way in which the global sign language community can establish communication with one another. In September of 2014 over one hundred deaf and hearing pastors (both ordained and lay, mostly from various Lutheran and Anglican churches) working with deaf people met in Nuremberg, Germany.[7] It was a diverse group with participants from 10 different nations. The majority were northern European but the group included three (hearing) delegates from Madagascar and

---

6 The video for Justifying Grace can be viewed at https://www.youtube.com/watch?v= RoX5crQNp9w

7 IEWG—International Ecumenical Working Group of pastors among Deaf People conference. http://www.deaf-iewg.org/

one (deaf) delegate from Nigeria, along with the signed languages of their own countries. For the conference sessions, the common language was spoken English and sign language interpreters were present to facilitate communication between the spoken English and one of six sign languages. When presenters were deaf, they signed in their own national sign language, which was then translated into spoken English by their own interpreters and, thereafter, into the other national sign languages. It was a very complex setup but necessary for the intellectual level of communication required because few of the delegates were familiar with international sign. Much of this complexity disappeared, however, during times of worshipping together. Interpreters were asked to not interpret as different national groups took turns leading worship in such a way that everyone could access it. This was done for two reasons: First, using interpreters would have made it necessary to render the signed worship into spoken English and then into the various signed languages present. This would have been difficult because much of the worship—created and led by deaf people in their own countries' signed languages—would have required a great many words to express and a great deal of meaning from the placement and facial expressions would have been lost. The second reason is that worshipping via interpreters is experienced by deaf people as an obstacle in the way of their ability to worship God directly in their own language (Shrine 2011). These acts of worship relied on a mix of communication through actions (such as lighting or extinguishing candles in a very measured and ritualized manner as a way to begin and end the act of worship), signed poetry and sign language (in the national sign language of the group leading worship), mime, and drama.

Conversations afterward indicated a varying level of success in the attempts to be transnational in the communication during acts of worship. Occasionally, some people felt they understood everything; other times and other people felt the atmosphere of prayer and worship was all they could access—a sense that something profound was being communicated without fully understanding what was being said. In my experience, a lot of the acts of worship were somewhere in the middle—some parts instantly clear in their meaning, others harder to follow without knowing the national sign language of the participants. It is interesting to reflect on and analyze some of the most successful moments in attempts to communicate and worship together across transnational boundaries. Why did these moments work? Do such experiences say anything about deaf ontology in a religious setting and combining the shared knowledge of bible stories with the visual/iconic nature of signed languages?

One example of a successful moment, beyond actions such as lighting and extinguishing candles as described earlier, was dramatized bible readings—acted out largely through mime and gesture. It was usually clear within the first few seconds which bible story was being acted out. And when it reached this point of recognition the congregation could sit back and enjoy the unfolding of a well-known story and sometimes improvise upon a role as actors in the drama; for example, by playing the crowd in the miracle story of Jesus feeding 5,000 people with five loaves and two fish.[8]

It is clear that a key feature of successful transnational communication in worship lies in the context and the audience. Within the framework of an act of worship certain things are understood to be happening. For example, with the dramatized/mimed bible readings, there is a shared expectation that an act of worship will include a bible reading, therefore, the congregation is open to recognizing it when it happens. Identifying the particular bible story being dramatized, which was key to fully understanding what was being represented, was made possible by the selection of extremely well-known stories and the biblical literacy of the congregation.

Was this experience of being able to share in the act of worship across different cultures and languages an example of deaf gain (Bauman & Murray 2014)? In other words, would an international hearing conference be able to worship together in the same way even if they couldn't understand each other's languages? My experience of worshipping in non-English language spoken contexts (e.g., attending Mass in Poland and worshipping with Urdu and Punjabi speakers in the Handsworth area of Birmingham, UK) suggests that although there is some generic sharing—I could deduce many of the elements of the Polish Mass through the actions being performed and I could guess the Urdu or Punjabi choir were leading us in a song of praise from their facial expressions and actions—the sharing of worship across spoken language barriers operates at a far more basic level than the sharing of worship across signed language barriers. Also, such sharing remains dependent on visual signals such as rituals, gestures, and facial expressions. The sharing of worship across international boundaries of people who are fluent in their own signed language operates at a much deeper level of being able to understand and participate in particular items with full understanding of the meaning of those items.

The experience of being able to establish communication with deaf people across linguistic barriers isn't of course unique to theological conferences in sign language. International deaf arts events, in particular, establish mutual communication across many barriers—and I believe deaf worship has much to gain and offer in dialogue with signed poetry and deaf arts—but there is something ontologically unique in my experience of sharing in signed worship in that we are

---

[8] Matthew 14:13–21.

not only referencing common humanity and shared deaf experience but also a shared belief system.[9]

KVG: These reflections seem to point toward commitments we make about what it means to be a deaf person, reflections that are grounded in our experiences of sameness as deaf people. Such commitments can be understood to be ontological in nature inasmuch as they provide a foundation from which we might build liturgical elements that are truly rooted in the experience of being deaf rather than in a translation of elements inherited from hearing cultures. For example, rather than a liturgy driven by music, chanting, or the cadence of spoken words, liturgy can be driven by visual elements of both linguistic communication and meaningful gesture. I've led a service of Holy Communion with a mixed hearing and deaf congregation this way with minimal use of actual sign vocabulary but plenty of visual gestures. It remained clear and meaningful to everyone while being firmly rooted in how deaf people experience our world through visual cues.

HML: Yes, deaf ontological themes to be detected as we analyze this experience of transnational deaf worship include the concept of togetherness/unity as a signing community before a God who clearly understands signed language and the use of storytelling in dramatic form. The bible is used as a rich source of shared stories that can be communicated across signed language barriers to illuminate our unity, and to learn from different perspectives on those familiar stories. Jesus Christ is clearly important—his name sign is one of the few signs that everybody could understand. The use of the "God-space" and heaven and earth in sign placement had sufficient shared usage to enable them to be used. Through our common understanding of and use of facial expressions it was possible to identify and share joy and solemnity, lament and peace. All of these areas would bear further investigation and research.

KVG: I, too, have experienced moments where deaf ways of doing things served as a conduit for better collaboration and collegiality between participants in international deaf gatherings. In 2013, the World Federation of Deaf Methodists met in Nairobi, Kenya in a diverse gathering of people. A majority of the participants in this conference were Kenyans, but we also had participants from other African nations as well as a large delegation from the United States, a smaller delegation from Korea, and representatives from Sri Lanka, and the United Kingdom. We, too, struggled with the array of interpreting and found a variety of creative and fun ways to work with multiple signed

---

[9] The Blue Ribbon Ceremony at the 1999 World Federation of the Deaf conference in Brisbane, Australia is another example of how a ritualized expression of shared oppression and hope can express deaf ontologies. The Blue Ribbon Ceremony can be viewed at http://www.joeybaer.com/?p=142. The English text is found as Appendix 2 in Ladd (2003:469).

languages in sharing songs, dances, and bible dramas, in both simultaneous translation and alternating translation. Although we didn't intentionally attempt to eschew translation during worship and devotionals, in practice, our exchanges often seemed to become something like what you've described at your conference in Nuremberg. Nor did we turn to something like International Sign as a means of bridging the linguistic gaps, given that there was insufficient knowledge of International Sign among the participants to communicate effectively. We also were uncomfortable with the use of ASL as a conference language despite many people at the conference knowing a fair amount of ASL. Instead, we wanted to honor the dignity and place of each participant's signed language. This perhaps reflects our languages and our being as God given gifts, as affirmed in our reading of the creation story previously mentioned.

We had set aside celebration times in which delegations or representatives from various countries took turns in sharing something their churches did in worship or devotions. In one example, the Korean delegation shared a popular song from their churches, which, although it had linguistic meaning in Korean Sign Language, also involved a good deal of playful hopping, dancing, and waving of arms and legs. It was an instant hit, and all of us began, not by watching our respective signed language interpreters for linguistic meaning, but by copying the Korean Sign Language of the song. Although one member of the delegation from Korea was a deaf man fluent in both Korean Sign Language and American Sign Language, they left the presentation of the song solely in Korean Sign Language. This was due, in part, to our shared goal of experiencing one another's cultures and languages. It was during socialization time much later that everyone was coming up to the Korean delegation to express appreciation and enrich our enjoyment of the song by learning its linguistic content. In subsequent uses of this song during devotional times, gathering times, and other moments we were able to enjoy both the energetic nature of the song and its theological message as we discovered that this exchange had facilitated the learning and appreciation of another signed language.

This was a breakthrough moment for the conference because the presence of ASL in many African countries produced a "contact variety" that created quicker mutual comprehension between African participants and those from the United States. Also, participants from the United States had just spent 10 days in service-based mission work with deaf schools and churches in Kenya and had learned a substantial amount of Kenyan Sign Language in preparation and practice just prior to this conference. So, the arrival of the Korean participants introduced a radically different signed language, and only one member of their delegation had familiarity with American Sign Language. Understanding this Korean Sign Language song first through learning the signs and motions without regard to meaning, and secondly through becoming curious about what the signs meant, facilitated the inclusion of the Korean delegation in a way that was organic and natural to how deaf communities gather. Rather than relying on a mutual signed language such as International Sign, effort was given to learning a portion of one another's signed languages. On a practical level, this is a result of most of the participants not knowing International Sign, but perhaps also the influence of Christian theological thought regarding the value of all languages arising from the story of the Pentecost in the second chapter of Acts, in which God's spirit caused the disciples to preach in myriad languages, all used by people present in Jerusalem.

CONCLUSION

This conversation between two deaf theologians set out to be an exploration of various ways that deaf theology can be grounded in deaf ontologies. By exploring the various facets of deaf viewpoints and experiences, we hope to establish some new spaces for conversation. Our first area of discussion sought to explore the positive valuation of being deaf as experienced and expressed by deaf people. A sense of purposeful creation as deaf people infuses deaf theology with self-worth that can counteract the effects of views of deafness as a deficit or flawed form of being. We pointed to possible theological insights about community and belonging that derive from deaf experiences with sociability. The use of signed languages was a third area where we see the potential for unique ways of expressing theological concepts that spoken languages may struggle to communicate. Lastly, deaf theology in transnational contexts provides exciting and invigorating ways for deaf people to explore the possible theological meanings of our unity amidst our diversity as deaf people. In privileging the viewpoints and experiences of deaf people as dialogue partners, we have sought to identify new theological insights that perhaps exist nowhere else but among deaf people. In doing so, we believe that deaf people have significant and meaningful contributions to provide to larger Christian dialogues about theology and the practice of faith. In "talking back" to the larger church in theological terms grounded in our own deaf ontologies, we contribute to our own liberation as deaf people by providing our theologically grounded perspectives on the positive value of being deaf. Yet, there are benefits beyond those for deaf people. Bishop Nicholas Holtam of Salisbury, a hearing man who is the current lead Bishop on deaf issues in the Church of England has realized through visiting deaf churches that deaf people and deaf theology have a lot to offer the church. He shares his reflections on worshipping with deaf people by saying, "Communication by signing was vivid and I would come away much more physically animated than usual. It made me think about St. Irenaeus saying that the glory of God is a person fully alive" (Holtam 2014). Deaf theologies, therefore, not only benefit those of us who are deaf but also the wider church by expanding the range of expression of Christian theology well beyond the spoken and written word, incorporating a richly visual means of communication, and bringing in the ontological experience of and engagement with the world that is very different from that of the hearing majority. The implications of exploring and understanding what deaf ontology brings to the wider discussion of theology in the Christian tradition also brings new avenues to deaf studies for exploring how we articulate and justify the uniqueness of our being in light of religious traditions that often have been sources of oppression and exclusion. In addition, our exploration of using dialogue to frame our chapter illuminates the tension that faces deaf studies when dealing with questions of deaf ontology: How do we balance working in sign language with the fact that the written word is still the most effective way to disseminate and discuss complex ideas? And how can we reflect the collaborative nature of the deaf community in individual writings? Theology is a subject that always has had the freedom to explore how its ideas are expressed through a variety of forms (e.g., poetry, art, sculpture, and architecture in addition to the convention of a written essay). Deaf theology, therefore, in bringing this freedom to the area of deaf studies may assist in the formulation and exploration of this relationship between form and content. Finally, the contribution of deaf theologies also can be an avenue for the further exploration of how ritual, whether it be religious worship or secular ceremony, can be a creative avenue for expressing our community bonds and aspirations for liberation, as well as for healing the traumas of oppression.

REFERENCES

Bauman, H.-D.L., & Murray, J. J. (Eds.) (2014). *Deaf Gain: Raising the stakes for human diversity*. Minneapolis: University of Minnesota Press.

Bevans, S. B. (1992). *Models of contextual theology*. Maryknoll, NY: Orbis Books.

Boff, L., & Boff, C. (1987). *Introducing liberation theology*. Maryknoll, NY: Orbis Books.

Chadwick, H. (Trans.) (1998). Saint Augustine's *Confessions*. Oxford: Oxford University Press.

Cone, J. H. (1970). *A black theology of liberation*. Philadelphia, PA: Lippincott.

Dye, M. (2014). Seeing the World Through Deaf Eyes. In H.-D.L. Bauman & J.J. Murray (Eds.). *Deaf Gain: Raising the stakes for human diversity* (pp. 193–210). Minneapolis: University of Minnesota Press.

Eiesland, N. L. (1994). *The Disabled God: Toward a liberatory theology of disability*. Nashville, TN: Abingdon Press.

Emery, S. D. (2015). A Deaf Diaspora? Imagining Deaf Worlds Across and Beyond Nations. In M. Friedner & A. Kusters (Eds.), *It's a small world: International deaf spaces and encounters* (pp. 187–198) Washington, DC: Gallaudet University Press.

Fox, M. (2000). *Original blessing: A primer in creation spirituality: Presented in four paths, twenty-six themes, and two questions.* New York: Jeremy P. Tarcher/Putnam.

Friedner, M. (2014). The church of deaf sociality: Deaf churchgoing practices and "sign bread and butter" in Bangalore, India. *Anthropology and Education Quarterly, 45*(1), 39–53.

Holtam, Nicholas. Bishop Nicholas. *Signs*, May 1, 2014, 8–9, https://docs.google.com/viewer?a=v&pid=sites&srcid=ZGVmYXVsdGRvbWFpbnxk ZWFmYW5nbGljYW5zfGd4OjNiYzUxMWFhZDg0Y2ZiNmQ (accessed October 28, 2016).

hooks, b, & West, C. (1991). *Breaking bread: Insurgent black intellectual life.* Boston, MA: South End Press.

Horton, M., & Bell, B. (1990). *We make the road by walking: Conversations on education and social change.* Philadelphia, PA: Temple University Press.

Isasi-Diaz, A.-M. (1996). *Mujerista theology: A theology for the twenty-first century.* Maryknoll, NY: Orbis Books.

Kanyoro, R. A. (2002). *Introducing feminist cultural hermeneutics: An African perspective.* Cleveland, OH: Pilgrim Press.

Kusters, A. (2015). *Deaf space in Adamorobe: An ethnographic study in a village in Ghana.* Washington, DC: Gallaudet University Press.

Ladd, P. (2003). *Understanding deaf culture in search of Deafhood.* Clevedon, England: Multilingual Matters.

Lawrence, L. J. (2009). *The Word in place: Reading the New Testament in contemporary contexts.* London: SPCK.

Lewis, H. (2007). *Deaf liberation theology.* Aldershot, England: Ashgate.

Meller, G. M. (2011). *Believing, belonging, and being deaf: The role of religion in Deafhood* (Unpublished doctoral dissertation). University of Bristol, England.

Morris, W. (2008). *Theology without words: Theology in the deaf community.* Aldershot, England: Ashgate.

Napoli, D. J. (2014). A magic touch: Deaf Gain and the benefits of tactile sensation. In H.-D.L. Bauman & J. J. Murray (Eds.), *Deaf Gain: Raising the stakes for human diversity* (pp. 211–232). Minneapolis: University of Minnesota Press.

Petitto, L.-A. (2014). Three revolutions: Language, culture, and biology. In H.-D.L. Bauman & J. J. Murray (Eds.), *Deaf Gain: Raising the stakes for human diversity* (pp. 65–76). Minneapolis: University of Minnesota Press.

Priests for Equality. (2007). *The Inclusive Bible: The first egalitarian translation.* Lanham, MD: Rowman & Littlefield Publishers.

Rourke, N. (2012). Nancy Rourke paintings — David vs. Goliath. February 3, 2012. Accessed from http://www.nancyrourke.com/davidvsgoliath.htm September 30, 2015.

Rourke, N. (2015). Nancy Rourke paintings—Biography. July 21, 2015. Accessed from http://www.nancyrourke.com/biography.htm September 30, 2015.

Russell, L. M., Cannon, K. G., Isasi-Diaz, A. M., & Pui-Lan, K. (Eds.) (1988). *Inheriting our mothers' gardens: Feminist theology in Third World perspective.* Philadelphia, PA: Westminster Press.

Shrine, B. (2011). *The church and the deaf community: A liberation perspective from a linguistic-cultural minority.* Cambridge, UK: Grove Books.

Sutherland, H., & Rogers, K. D. (2014). The hidden gain: A new lens of research with d/Deaf children and adults. In H.-D.L. Bauman & J. J. Murray (Eds.), *Deaf Gain: Raising the stakes for human diversity* (pp. 269–284). Minneapolis: University of Minnesota Press.

Sutton-Spence, R. (2014). Deaf Gain and creativity in signed literature. In H.-D.L. Bauman & J. J. Murray (Eds.), *Deaf Gain: Raising the stakes for human diversity* (pp. 457–477) Minneapolis: University of Minnesota Press.

VanGilder, K. (2012). *Making Sadza with deaf Zimbabwean women: A missiological reorientation of practical theological method.* Gottingen, Germany: Vandenhoeck & Ruprecht.

8

Sign Language Peoples' Right to be Born: The Bioethical Debate in Karawynn Long's "Of Silence and Slow Time"

Rachel Mazique

[. . .I don't think you truly understand what is involved here, what you are risking.] . . .
[The government takes its Child Protection Acts very seriously.]
"No. Believe me, I know exactly what is at stake here."
[Then why? Why do you want this so badly?]
She looked at him, surprised and a little angry. "I'm Deaf," she said. "You never really
understood what that means. I have not, as everyone seems to assume, lived my whole life
wishing to be a part of the hearing world. . . . Deaf is my identity, my culture. It is a whole
community, with its own customs and a language that is graceful and unique and expressive
of ideas your English can never contain. And the government," . . . "has decided that we are
'defective' and must be exterminated."

—Jeff and Marina, "Of Silence and Slow Time"

The risk that Jeff cautions Marina against in this epigraph: violating the Child Protection Acts, and the high stakes that Marina is fully aware of: wanting to conceive and give birth to a deaf baby in a state that has made these acts a crime, arise in a conversation that involves a "digital interpreter" (represented by the brackets) through which Marina, the Deaf protagonist, reads Jeff's spoken English words (brackets original, Long 2012:254–255).[1] At the time of this writing, it has been a little

---

[1] I, like Long, capitalize Deaf to not only refer to deaf people who value the many signed language(s) of Sign Language Peoples (SLPs), but also to signify the ethnic qualities of "Deafnicity." Deaf Literature is then comparable to literary canons such as African American Literature, British Literature, and so on. In defining the parameters of Deaf Literature, I take the broadest view and include literature written by deaf and hard-of-hearing authors, sign language literature, as well as literature by hearing authors (such as Karawynn Long) who have written pieces with deaf and hard-of-hearing characters. Generally, in "Of Silence and Slow Time," Long uses "deaf" when Jeff is speaking. When Marina is speaking, the text more often reads "Deaf"—referring to their different perspectives on what it means to be D/deaf. Further,

191

over two decades since Spectra, the science fiction division of Bantam Books, published Karawynn Long's "Of Silence and Slow Time" in their anthology, *Full Spectrum 5*, and four years since its reprint in the 2012 anthology of *Outcasts and Angels: The New Anthology of Deaf Characters in Literature*. This chapter's analysis of "Of Silence and Slow Time" synthesizes research from cognitive literary studies, Disability Studies, Deaf Studies, and human rights to answer a question inspired by Mark Bracher (2013): How might reading Deaf Literature promote social justice?

As an intersectional minority Deaf scholar working within departments of English, I engage with Deaf Studies and other disciplines to seek out strategies that support social justice. I offer the study and critique of Deaf Literature through schema criticism as one potential strategy. Schema criticism is a method of social criticism that interrogates social justice issues through key findings from cognitive science; these findings include the identification of eight schemas—four of which cause social harms and four of which are conducive to social justice (Bracher, 2013). Stories of deaf ontologies (such as those that Long depicts) raise significant and pertinent social concerns deserving of scholarly inspection, analysis, and discussion. Although "Of Silence and Slow Time" (henceforth "Of Silence") is not a well-known or widely discussed text, Long's story has the potential to engender social change. It not only has the power to bring recognition to a political group with legitimate claims in order to correct structural injustices via a Deaf bioethics, but, through this recognition, it also has the power to prevent the unjust denigration of signed languages (Brotherton 2008:para. 9–11).

A number of literary accounts of deaf ontologies, or deaf ways of being, portray a Deaf bioethics, as in Long's short story "Of Silence" (1995); these include Nick Sturley's *Milan* (2003), Ted Evans's *The End* (2011), and Donna Williams's "When the Dead are Cured" (2013).[2] A Deaf bioethics promotes both a consciousness of bioethical issues and consideration of approaches to bioethical debate from the perspective of Sign Language Peoples (SLPs). SLPs constitute a social group that requires self-determination in the domains of educational, linguistic, and cultural protection; this grouping is thus political (Batterbury, Ladd & Gulliver 2007:2899, Kusters, De Meulder, Friedner & Emery

---

because I define a Deaf bioethics as one that approaches bioethical debate from the perspective of SLPs, "deaf" is capitalized to denote a bioethical perspective specifically from those who experience the ethnic criteria of Deafnicity (language, community, and ontologies). Following the editors of this volume, I use the lowercase deaf to represent the many ways to be deaf. In this case, my usage of the lowercase deaf is *inclusive* of Deafnicity, those who identify as hearing-impaired, and the range of every other possible deaf identity.

[2] Of these four authors, only Long is American; she originally wrote the story from Chicago, Illinois. Sturley, Evans, and Williams are Deaf British authors.

2015:8).[3] Multiple areas of bioethical debate such as those involving genetics, reproduction, the desire for deaf babies, and the value of deaf lives affect SLPs. The formulation of a Deaf bioethics is not value neutral, but inherently political, just as the "taken-for-granted values inherent in dominant accounts of bioethics and biomedicine" are *not* value neutral but "framed and structured by the dominant community of the hearing public" (Newell 2006:276). Moves toward a Deaf bioethics have emerged as a response to biomedical advances since the rise of cochlear implantation; they are generally led by deaf activists and scholars who advocate for the rights of SLPs and work to promote a bioethical consciousness that takes deaf ontologies into serious consideration (Komesaroff 2007, Emery, Middleton & Turner 2010, Schwartz 2011, Blankmeyer Burke 2011). Bioethical inquiry (for both deaf and hearing peoples) is interdisciplinary—involving ethical examinations of how the nature of biotechnology and biomedical advances have moral implications for both our individual and common humanity (The Center for Bioethics and Human Dignity).

SLPs and non-signing readers alike are likely to benefit from reading "Of Silence." This foreboding story presents a futurist state in which scientific ethnocide, or the intentional and systematic destruction of an ethnic group through genetic cleansing, prevents any chance of a deaf baby being born. The story allows for recognition of a deaf self and one's sociopolitical group on the one hand; on the other, it enables the recognition of a Deaf Other in need of hearing allies to advocate for and correct social and political harms (alongside of SLPs). Because Long presents the bioethical concern of genetic manipulation as a eugenic campaign, readers who practice schema criticism can identify schemas that lead to this eugenic drive. The transformative potential of schema criticism, in contrast to traditional social criticism, lies in its targeting of the cognitive processes that underlie oppressive social positions and beliefs (Leake 2014:554). Identifying problematic cognitive schemas, or schemas that lead to injustice, becomes key to promoting a bioethics that values the presence of SLPs. Understanding SLPs globally, as cultural-linguistic groups that simultaneously fit the criteria for ethnic groups (Eckert 2010), lends to their self-definition as collectives whose members share the "physical and metaphysical aspects of language, culture, epistemology, and ontology" (Batterbury, Ladd & Gulliver 2007:2989). Ethnicity in relation to SLPs becomes "Deafnicity" (Eckert 2010). Eckert (2010) defines ethnicity by the social scientific criteria for

---

[3] To elucidate, I point to the authors who coined this term in their (2007) article "Sign language peoples as indigenous minorities: Implications for research and policy"; Batterbury, Ladd, and Gulliver's marking of SLPs as indigenous minorities is not value-neutral, but is a political effort to impact policymaking that affects the lives of SLPs around the world.

recognizing ethnic groups; these include (among others) an expression of self and community, which involves an emergent and situational process of external ascription and self-identification; a community of origin with shared language and ontologies; and a strategic process involving a rationale choice (317).[4]

In the following sections, I explain how Long's story makes claims to human and group rights, define the harmful cognitive schemas, and explain how literary portrayals of Deafnicity illustrate the complexities of Deaf politics' grappling with the group identities of both disability and ethnicity. My analysis of the representation of Deafnicity in "Of Silence" shows how the cognitive schemas of autonomy and atomism adversely affect SLPs and their claims to human and group rights; it also shows how the story depicts SLPs' claim to the right to be born through the schema of solidarity. In the last half of the chapter, I analyze how the story's dominant and subversive threads present both the four schemas that are harmful to social justice as well as the four advantageous schemas. In contextualizing "Of Silence," I explain how the story's portrayal of the continuing legacies of eugenic campaigns encourages a reframing of bioethical debate and connect the story to current bioethical dilemmas. Finally, I review the story's depiction of violated human and group rights to argue that the story's presentation of love and acceptance in the family becomes a model for public policy—demonstrating how Deaf Literature can encourage social justice.

THE POWER OF DEAF LITERATURE

As already mentioned, "Of Silence" presents a futurist state in which scientific ethnocide prevents any chance of a deaf baby being born. The state's control over women's reproductive lives also threatens, as Marina puts it, cultural genocide (Long 2012:255). In this dystopia, no deaf baby has been born in 25 years. Marina creates a plan to conceive a "Deaf baby" and subvert the state's control over her reproductive choices and desired family (Long 2012:252). She enlists the help of her ex-boyfriend, Jeff, a geneticist, and Grant, her gay friend and roommate, who is a gynecologist and child of Deaf adults (CODA) who offers her his sperm. Although Jeff initially objects to Marina's desire for a Deaf baby, by the end of their argument, he agrees to help (and takes the embryos that Marina has brought to their meeting) because of the love that he has for her. By the story's end, however, readers learn, along with Marina, that Jeff did not keep his end of the agreement; after

---

[4] See Lane, Pillard, and Hedberg's (2011) *The People of the Eye: Deaf Ethnicity and Ancestry* for more on the shared communities of origin.

months of appearing to go along with Marina's subversive plan, Jeff reveals that he changed his mind and did not select the embryos with the deaf gene(s).

In this story that imagines "The End" of Deafnicity and SLPs, Long raises bioethical and group rights concerns about linguistic genocide, cultural genocide, and ethnocide. Group rights are rights held by a people as a political unit, or a group (Jones 2008:1). SLPs' group rights involve two bioethical claims: (1) the "right to be born" and (2) protection from eugenics (or the genetic manipulation that results in scientific ethnocide) (Kusters, De Meulder, Friedner & Emery 2015:22). SLPs also make group rights claims for (3) the preservation of signed languages, or protection from linguistic genocide and, as we see in Long's story, (4) protection from cultural genocide. In doing so, "Of Silence" also considers the implications of what Disability Studies scholar Tobin Siebers (2008) calls the ideology of ability, or the preference for able-bodiedness; this ableist ideology necessitates the eradication of deafness in the medical industry's centuries-long search for a "cure"—a cure that some may say has been achieved by cochlear implants and that others say is achievable with genetic engineering advancements (Loeb in Bauman & Murray 2014).

To make my underlying argument explicit, the lack of attention paid to Deaf Literature, which could transform problematic cognitive schemas to befit claims to human and group rights, is one major obstacle to a Deaf bioethics and to human rights for all people defined by standards of "normalcy." Historically, group rights have been difficult to demarcate because of the possibility that they would override individuals' human rights. Group rights and human rights are complementary, however, and may coexist (Jones 2008:sec. 8). SLPs like Marina also make human rights claims in regard to their reproductive rights, or the right to conceive without intervention from the government, as well as claims to the human right to life with dignity (United Nations Population Fund 2007:para. 2, 5; United Nations General Assembly 1948). Long's story poses bioethical human rights questions such as the mother's right to choose whether or not genetic manipulation occurs; "Of Silence" also encourages readers to grapple with human rights questions about the individual baby's right to be born as well as the baby's right to be deaf. Further complicating matters, the right to be born is not only a bioethical human rights claim; in this story, it is also a group rights claim for SLPs. It is a human right because all individuals have the right to life; it is a group right because it protects a group from targeted discrimination and extermination by the state or other individuals. Readers of Deaf Literature who practice schema criticism will be better equipped to understand that "merely recognizing the rights of individuals [. . .] will not protect the group's survival"; in other words, this chapter's premise about SLPs' right to be born agrees with fellow deaf scholars Annelies Kusters, Maartje De Meulder, Michele Friedner, and Steve Emery's argument that "group rights (in addition to individual human rights) can offer the legal protection SLP communities need" (2015:23).

As I will show, the cognitive processes involved in reading imagined dystopian futures that bring about "The End" of SLPs both express and have the potential to replace the "faulty" cognitive schemas concerning human nature (Bracher 2013:x). As Bracher (2013) emphasizes in his writings on the cognitive schemas we hold about individuals, among the several sources of the four "faulty" schemas are works of literature that are both "expressions of and apparatuses for inculcating" these schemas (94, 97). In other words, literature that solely serves the faulty cognitive schemas adversely affects perspectives on SLPs' human and group rights claims. In the end, it is my hope that this chapter provokes questions, interest in learning more, and, ultimately, inspires further reading and teaching of Deaf Literature.

SCHEMA CRITICISM, DEAFNICITY, AND DEAF POLITICS

In examining the cognitive schemas that obstruct SLPs' claims for human and group rights in bioethical debates, readers of "Of Silence" encounter both the faulty general person-schemas of atomism, autonomy, essentialism, and homogeneity, as well as the converse of these four harmful schemas. General-person schemas are cognitive schemas about human nature that we hold about *all individuals*, both members of our in-group and those who are not. Group stereotypes, however, describe *groups* as a whole and limit our understanding of those who are unlike us. Faulty person-schemas that lead to injustice for certain individuals and the group stereotypes that perpetuate discrimination are not necessarily mutually exclusive (Bracher 2013:x).

Atomism is the cognitive schema that understands individuals as fundamentally separate from and competitive with others (Bracher 2013:xi). This schema undermines our ability to criticize the "practices, institutions, or systems that are destructive and unjust," which is only possible through "our ontological solidarity—our common human nature" (Bracher 2013:125). Bracher (2013) defines the schema of *homogeneity* as the human tendency to categorize individuals as either, and simply, good or bad; it blocks our "awareness of the negative qualities of some individuals and groups (usually one's own) as well as the positive qualities of others (usually members of out-groups)" (xii). The schema of *autonomy* (a concept distinct from bioethicists' understanding of autonomy) sees individuals' characters rather than their circumstances as the primary determinant of their successes/failures in life (Bracher 2013:35). Last, the schema of *essentialism* focuses on hereditary qualities rather than formative experiences in establishing an individual's character (Bracher 2013:75). As my analysis of "Of Silence" will show, Long skillfully depicts these schemas in her story in order to show her readers how prejudice and false consciousness work within her futuristic society—and our own—adversely affecting SLPs' claims both to human and to group rights.

Further, Long's portrayal of Deaf experiences in "Of Silence" delineate what Richard Eckert (2010) calls the "nexus" of Deafnicity, a powerful sociological concept for understanding SLPs. Part of Deafnicity's power lies in its ability to counteract the schemas of atomism, autonomy, essentialism, and homogeneity. The relational nexus of Deafnicity consists of: (1) multiple forms of community (both physical and virtual), (2) signed languages, as well as (3) an existential/ontological dimension: the cognitive and cultural attitudes for understanding the world. Deafnicity and its manifestations of solidarity lend themselves to a "Deaf politics," which has bioethics as one of its central human rights platforms (Emery et al. 2010, Blankmeyer Burke 2011, De Meulder 2014). Deaf scholars and activists who seek social justice as a collective ethnic group of SLPs lead Deaf politics.[5] One aspect of Deaf politics seeks to upend the politics of bioethical debates "in which despite the veneer of reason and civility [...] nondisabled accounts continue to dominate" (Newell 2006:272). Literary accounts of Deafnicity contribute to this upending and enable readers to better imagine and understand the claims of SLPs engaged in urgent bioethical debate about the challenges of Deaf futures. From the United Nation's Convention on the Rights of People with Disabilities (UNCRPD) to SLPs' arguments against ethnocide, Deaf politics grapple with the group identities of *both* disability and ethnicity (Holmes 1980/2006). Deaf politics' grappling with two discrete group identities creates a third "in-between" space for deaf and SLP identities (Bhabha 2004, Brueggemann 2009).

POTENT LITERARY REPRESENTATIONS OF DEAFNICITY

Within this third space of Deaf politics, I find Long's science fiction story to be quite realistic; in "Of Silence," SLPs have no right to self-determination (National Association of the Deaf 2010, Batterbury, Ladd & Gulliver 2007). Long also illustrates Deafnicity throughout "Of Silence"; readers encounter the relational nexus of Deafnicity in interactions between Grant and Marina, the glosses of dialogue in American Sign Language (ASL), and in the Deaf party scene (a celebratory

---

[5] Just as "It is difficult to imagine Deaf studies as an apolitical development or a completely neutral 'project'," imagining SLPs as an apolitical group is improbable; as "The very nature of a Deaf studies discipline is political," the global grouping of SLPs is also political (O'Brien & Emery 2014:28).

gathering of SLPs at a mutual friend's house). For example, just before departing for the party, Marina signs to her roommate, ". . . with one hand, the other paused just over the door panel, [. . .] 'You sure not-want come party you?' [. . .] Grant sighed, running his fingers through his short hair. 'Yes, I sure. Very-exhausted. And I promise Paul two-of-us watch movie tonight. Say hello to mother-father, please? I call them next-week'" (Long 2012:259). With the use of hyphens joining several English words, Long represents signs that appear as one word in ASL, whether through a fluid combination of two signs, facial emphasis, or directional movement. This excerpted piece of dialogue, with its other attempts to represent ASL's unique grammar, not only serves as a gloss of the visual language, but also points to the close-knit inter-generational community of SLPs when Grant, a CODA himself, asks Marina to say hello to his deaf parents at the party. These interactions and the English glosses of ASL—textual moments that rupture stand-ard English prose—illustrate Deafnicity's dynamic nexus: language, community, and ontology.

In the scene set at a Deaf party, Long presents SLPs as oppressed to the extent that revolutionary counter-hegemonic discourse loses out to resignation; SLPs become inactive agents who only lament their fate: the end of their kind. When Marina meets Larry, a newcomer from Seattle at this party in Chicago, and they discover their mutual friend-ships, Larry remarks,

> 'Deaf small world.' 'Becoming-smaller,' Julio interjected, a sour expression on his face. His hands came together until there was almost no space between them at all. [. . .] Soon none Deaf remain-ing. Genocide.' Susan shrugged. 'Know-that,' she signed, her pos-ture expressing condescension. 'Everyone know-that.' Her gesture indicated the whole room. 'Doesn't matter. Can't change.' (Long 2012:260)

Marina, who feels that "She'd had this conversation a hundred times before," withdraws from the counter-hegemonic discourse about how to fight back to resist in her own way—covertly trying to have a Deaf baby (Long 2012:252, 261). She believes that the others at the party are repeating tired ideas for resistance against the state but will not act on these ideas; Marina "abruptly" leaves the conversation about SLPs' impending fate believing: "No one ever did anything about it. Except her" (Long 2012:261). As Long presents a dystopia in which SLPs fail to take collective action to fight the government's eugenic decree that they belong to a "defective" class that should not be part of modern society, she asks readers to imagine what it would mean to act as an individual who subversively works against the government. The Deaf reproduc-tive body becomes a figurative tool for resistance. The idea that Marina could enact political change on such a small scale highlights what she is truly frustrated with: the lack of collective action. This frustration would then be activated in readers as "Any feeling that is being experienced by someone we are attending to, including a character in a story, produces a like emotion in every attentive observer" (Smith, in Bracher 2013:115).

In the end, the failure of Marina's individual act of resistance demonstrates the flaws in the cognitive schemas of both autonomy and atomism (i.e., the ideas that individuals are responsible for their life outcomes/completely self-sufficient, or autonomous, as well as atomist prototypes that promote the belief that individuals must stand or fight on their own) (Bracher 2013:37, 135).[6] Long implies instead that systematic upheavals to the state are required. This suggestion emerges both from the Deaf party scene (when Julio proposes organizing a group to lobby Congress and argue for laws to protect the culture) and from a conversation between Grant and Marina, when Grant references the success of the gay rights movement: " 'You know, [. . .] 'when scientists prove gay g-e-n-e-t-i-c finish, gay almost become class [. . .] d-e-f-e-c-t,' he spelled, 'same deaf. Only because many many of us . . .' He looked off for a moment, then spoke in English only. 'And still the political climate could reverse again at any time' " (Long 2012:261, 265). In these scenes, the dialogue and glosses of ASL not only present the ethnic characteristics of SLPs, but also the human and group rights concerns of SLPs: the preservation of language (avoiding linguistic genocide), the maintenance of the community (avoiding ethnocide), the continuation of culture (preventing cultural genocide), and the desire for deaf children and the deaf child's right to life (the right to be born).

SIGN LANGUAGE PEOPLES' RIGHT TO BE BORN

At the beginning of the short story, Marina meets her Hearing exboyfriend, Jeff, at a restaurant; Jeff works at GeneSys as a "Senior Research Director" (Long 2012:249).[7] After Marina and Jeff catch up, Marina announces her plans to get pregnant and her desire for a Deaf baby (Long 2012:251–252). With this announcement, readers encounter,

---

[6] Bracher (2013) defines prototypes as *general* types of individuals, emotions, or images—or knowledge about the external world: "the most familiar prototypes are stereotypes" (16).

[7] In capitalizing "Hearing," I follow Blankmeyer Burke's (2014) reasoning: "In addition to following the convention of using the uppercase *Deaf* and lowercase *deaf* [. . .], I also use the lowercase word *hearing* to mark the audiological condition and uppercase *Hearing* to mark the sociolinguistic cultural community of spoken-language users." Blankmeyer Burke's distinction between the audiological condition and the sociolinguistic cultural community not only draws parallels between the usage of deaf and Deaf, but also reframes what it means to be a hearing person. Capitalizing "Hearing" draws attention to its ontology—rather than leaving it as a

simultaneously, the state's control over the reproductive lives of women and an objection against the idea of deaf lives as desirable. When Marina astounds Jeff with the declaration of her desire, he "incredulously" replies that Marina's deafness puts her in

> ... a high-risk group for genetic defects.] Marina started to protest, but he shook his head and kept talking. [As soon as—I'm sorry, but most people *will* see it as a defect. As soon as your ob-gyn confirms you're pregnant—and legally, you know, you have to see a doctor within five weeks of a possible or suspected pregnancy—she'll take an embryonic sample and have a full workup done. Furthermore, again because you're in that high-risk group, they're going to want to know who the father is, or at the very least a short list of possible fathers, and they're not going to take 'I don't remember" as an answer. And if you tell them a name that doesn't match with the gene typing, you're in big trouble]. (brackets original, Long 2012:252–253)

The state's demand that women know who the fathers of their babies are—especially if in a "high-risk" group—preempts the possibility that a woman really may not know who the father is—especially if impregnated after rape. Marina's subversive plan, however, does not involve withholding the name of her baby's father. Jeff then has difficulty contemplating how a person besides Marina could approve "That his baby will be deaf"—showing how he essentializes and homogenizes deafness (Long 2012:253).

Because the law in this state will not allow a deaf baby to be born, randomly selecting an embryo that Grant (in his capacity as an ob-gyn) fertilized in vitro, and allowing nature to determine whether their baby is deaf or hearing is not an option (Long 2012:254). Without Jeff's assistance, even if Marina happened to conceive a baby who tested positive for the deaf gene markers, the law against giving birth to a deaf baby would require a medical professional to "'perform replacement therapy on the fetus'" and Marina would "'have a hearing child anyway'" (Long 2012:253). Marina thus pleads Jeff to screen, select, and give Marina the embryos that test positive for the deaf gene(s)—purposefully marking them as having tested negative for these genes (Long 2012:253, 254). The only way Jeff can fathom Marina's desire for a deaf baby is if the father is deaf as well. Marina explains that the prospective father, Grant, is a hearing CODA with a Deaf sister—someone whose genetic contribution would likely carry deaf gene(s) (Long 2012:253). As an individual member of SLPs, Grant, although hearing, values Deaf lives just as much as Marina does.

The unique relationship between roommates Grant and Marina, a loving, yet nonsexual one, one in which they agree to bring a child into the world through in vitro fertilization (IVF), presents a counterexample to the failed heterosexual relationship of Jeff and Marina. Although

Jeff and Grant are ontologically similar in that they are both hearing men who love Marina, Grant dismantles the dichotomy between deaf and hearing people. For Marina, Grant, and other SLPs, the lives of SLPs and deaf children are desirable and invaluable (Bauman 2005); for them, the rejection of such lives equates to a desire for an ethnic cleansing. The genetic cleansing, or ethnocide, of SLPs rests on the belief that deaf lives are a burden on the state and that no more such children should be conceived or born (Häyry 2004:511). It is a denial of not only SLPs' claims to the group right to be born, but also of readers' ontological solidarity—through their status as humans.

To elucidate, there is an ontological paradox in my argument about Deafnicity, or the ontologically unique status of SLPs in contrast to non-signing Hearing people, and SLPs' claims to human and group rights. Paradoxically, the ontological aspect of Deafnicity, which presents *unique*, experiential understandings of the world, also involves what Bracher calls images of *solidarity*, psychological solidarity, ontological solidarity, and practical solidarity. We see these claims to psychological, ontological, and practical solidarity when Marina appeals to Jeff for his help, and, he, out of a prevailing feeling of love for her, agrees to take her embryos and to covertly provide her with the ones that carry genes for deafness (Long 2012:257). In other words, the claim for SLPs' right to be born depends on the general-person schema of solidarity (rather than its converse: the faulty schema of atomism). The harmful nature of the schema of atomism marks SLPs as entirely distinct from hearing people—running the risk of dehumanizing them as "defective" and leading to the risk of ethnocide—as we see in "Of Silence."

Because SLPs are human too, rather than being *entirely* ontologically different from Hearing non-signers (like Jeff), SLPs (like Marina) work to enact the universal solidarity schema in their claims for human and group rights.[8] To counteract the "universalism" of the Hearing hegemony, SLPs' claim to the human right to life with dignity (e.g., Marina being allowed to give birth to a Deaf baby without the risk of the government taking him/her away to a foster home with Hearing people and putting Marina, Jeff, and Grant in jail) must also be regarded as

---

supposedly universal and natural condition that does not come with its own sociolinguistic cultural experience.

[8] Although universalist claims have "been used to dehumanize, oppress, and even exterminate people who are perceived to lack some supposedly universal human qualities or practices," the existence of a universal human nature is the crux of human rights discourse (Bracher 2013:109). To succinctly present the discourse on universal human rights, I reference Weston (2015): "Whatever their theoretical justification, human rights refer to a wide continuum of values or capabilities thought to enhance human agency or protect human interests and declared to be *universal* [emphasis added] in character, in some sense equally claimed for all human beings, present and future" (para. 1).

a group right to be born (Long 2012:252, 255).[9] As Kusters et al. (2015) explain, group rights are self-determining and would allow SLPs to put a "moratorium on genetic interventions on deafness that threaten their right to be born" (21–23). What SLPs, and other ethnic minorities object to are not claims of universalism per se, but the Hearing hegemony/ "Eurocentric hegemony *posing* as universalism" (Appiah 1992:58). The paradox, in short, resides in the tension between the atomistic and solidarity schemas. With this paradox, SLPs' status is one that is not only ontologically unique, but also overlapping and ontologically like that of hearing people. On the individual human level, SLPs do not appear very different from hearing people. As an ethnic group, however, their ontological status is distinct from Hearing people; it is their group's contribution to human biodiversity that requires the group right to the existence and maintenance of their global community (Bryan & Emery 2014:51).

With schema criticism, a close reading of "Of Silence" in relation to Disability Studies, Deaf Studies, and Ethnic Studies can contribute to a reworking of disability and ethnicity, as well as the formulation of a Deaf bioethics that marks deaf lives as valuable and essential—leading not solely to deficit, but also to gains. The reworking of disability and ethnicity in the quest to reshape bioethical discourse occurs as readers encounter the emotional debate between Jeff and Marina. Long highlights Marina's need for a covert network of supportive individuals in positions to help her work around the hegemony that prohibits the conception of deaf babies—highlighting the faultiness of both the atomism and autonomy schemas. As Bracher (2013) puts it,

> The atomism schema magnifies interindividual and intergroup distinctions and obscures our inherent sameness and solidarity with others, blinding us to the fact that each person is [. . .] ontologically overlapping and interwoven with others, such that the welfare of one person directly affects and is affected by the welfare of others. (p. 103)

Hence, the opening scene at the restaurant demonstrates the necessity of solidarity—suggesting that a strategy of resistance *requires* solidarity.

The emotional debate is one that Marina endures because she needs to convince Jeff to help her enact her plan; as she searches "for something that would make an impact, make him understand how important this was to her," she speaks to him in his language, English, and reads his words across a portable, digital "interpreter" screen (Long 2012:255, 250). Marina opines, " 'Telling me that my

---

[9] My use of "Hearing hegemony" is a continuation of previous Deaf Studies work and an engagement with Disability Studies work (e.g., hegemony of vision). It does not necessarily

child must be hearing is like—like telling a black woman that she is only allowed to bear white babies. It's wrong, Jeff. You always believed in freedom of choice, in abolishing discrimination—well, that's exactly what this is. Jeff, please . . .' " (Long 2012:255). For readers who do not share her desire, the example of Marina's deep desire for a Deaf baby works as a "secondhand exemplar," or an indirect experience acquired from others. As Bracher (2013) explains, exemplars are *specific* instances of individuals, emotions, or images—a function of our personal experiences (18–19). Although readers may not have personally experienced Marina's desire, the secondhand exemplar provided through "literature has at least the potential to make significant contributions to an individual's store of exemplars and prototypes and through them, to his perceptions, judgments, and actions regarding other people" (Bracher 2013:18). In the case of Marina, readers who originally may have thought that SLPs would never desire to perpetuate their "affliction" onto their children, are being asked to reframe their understandings of deafness and to see their original line of thinking as a matter of pathological perception and biased expectation—one that lacks understanding of diverse deaf ontologies.

Readers learn that some SLPs deeply desire to give birth to deaf babies, or, at the very least, for this potential to be allowed. In the passage quoted earlier, SLPs are contextualized in light of the human right to freedom, civil rights, morality, bioethics, and as an ethnic group. The refusal to recognize SLPs as a group who value their ontological status becomes a destructive refusal of their claims for group rights. Reading Deaf Literature such as "Of Silence" thus makes a contribution to "humanizing" SLPs' views, values, and ontologies.

DISMANTLING THE HEARING HEGEMONY? ONE WOMAN'S SUBVERSIVE ACT

As Long's story, combined with schema criticism, encourages a new understanding of "disability," Marina's desire for a Deaf baby, as well as the deaf community's desire to protect the lives and future lives of SLPs, become exemplars for the cognitive schema of heterogeneity. In other words, readers who previously saw disability/deafness as an entirely individual trait (essentialism) resulting in a life not worth living (autonomism) because disability is only and always a bad thing/undesirable (homogeneity) and completely separate from/irrelevant to H/hearing people (atomism) are challenged to reconceptualize deafness. Instead, readers learn to read deafness in terms of Deafnicity (solidarity) and Deafhood (malleability), to read the state's social construction of disability as pathological/defective as what creates life's difficulties (situationism), and to recognize disability/Deaf identity as an aspect of one's being that can be and often is cherished and desired (heterogeneity).[10]

Long's heterogeneous characterizations of SLPs in "Of Silence" show that SLPs, like Hearing people, are neither perfect nor degenerative. In contrast, the combination of good and bad traits among both Deaf and Hearing people, to the attentive reader, activates the heterogeneity schema as a way to understand *all* people as imperfect beings worthy of human rights. In Long's depiction of the importance of acceptance and love of others despite/beyond differences, readers are faced with both a Deaf woman's subversive desires and a Hearing man's ultimate denial of this desire.

In the end, the dominant narrative wins out, creating a sense of mourning in readers who have begun to identify and empathize with Marina's and SLPs' desires for deaf children. Jeff, the Hearing ex-boyfriend, the biogeneticist who has the power to choose—who agrees to subvert the dominant narrative (in the name of love)—only to renege in the end, provides the "rational" choice. After Marina gives birth to a boy, Jeff visits and "defiantly" explains that he selected against the deaf embryo and Marina's right to choose (Long 2012:264). He presents the status quo as a rationale for this denial; in essence, it is too late to resist (Long 2012:264, 265). One woman's subversive act will not dismantle the hegemony.

To avoid the homogenizing tendency that this attention to Jeff's failure seems to promote, I argue, instead, that Jeff, like Marina, is representative of larger groups of people/systems. In Jeff's case, his failure is one that indicts the hegemonic system that is already in place. He becomes representative of the Hearing hegemony. The true object of critique is not Jeff, but the overpowering Hearing hegemony, which denies SLPs their group right to be born. Although some deaf people may wish to have been born hearing, a premise that supports Jeff's counterargument that Marina's son may have grown to resent his deafness, Jeff's supporting reason points to how Marina's son would have been the last of his kind (Long 2012:264–265). Clearly, not all deaf people are SLPs and some may wish to be hearing or to have been born hearing. As Jeff indicates, though, this wish is, at times, because of the lack of community, the individual deaf person's experience of isolation when surrounded by hearing people, and/or because of the ubiquitousness

---

mark all hearing people as oppressors, but, instead, points to privilege, power, and dominance. This privilege, power, and dominance exist whether hearing people are aware of it or not.

[10] Ladd (2003) coined the term Deafhood in *Understanding Deaf Culture*. Deafhood is both a dynamic *process* of actualizing one's (culturally) Deaf identity and a counternarrative against hegemonic structures (Ladd 2003:3–4; Kusters & De Meulder 2013:431). The procedural aspect of Deafhood is a reflection of the malleability schema. Malleability is the schema that sees individuals' characteristics as malleable, or predisposed and likely to change over time or given certain situations and formative life experiences. Bracher asserts that this schema is more adequate than its converse: essentialism (2012:98).

of the Hearing hegemony. Once again, a tension arises between the individual human right to choose how a child should be born and the collective group right to protect the deaf child's right to be born (and to grow up to choose his ethnic identity).

Shortly after Jeff's revelation that Marina's son is not deaf because he gave Marina an embryo with hearing genes—after leading her to believe he was still going along with her plan to subvert the government's decree against deafness—Marina realizes that part of her motivation for a Deaf baby may have been to defy her Hearing mother who never accepted her. Long (2012) thus problematically suggests that Marina's resistance against the dominant power is not one that truly seeks to undermine the state's stranglehold on reproductive rights for *all* people, or even for her own community as a whole—but is, instead, an individual and personal narrative (266). Shortly after Marina's realization, she resolves to *"not make the mistake [her] mother did"* (emphasis original, Long 2012:266). Instead of resenting her child's difference (as her mother did), Marina resolves to, *"not try to mold you selfishly in my own image. No matter how hard it is. I will let you grow to be your own person, and take joy in that"* (emphasis original, Long 2012:266). Although Marina proclaims that Jeff had "no right" to "trick" her into "bearing a child [she] did not want" and no right to deny her choice, she is now faced with the situation that many hearing parents face when they unexpectedly bear a deaf child (Long 2012:264, 265–266). Although Marina, like most hearing parents who unexpectedly bear a deaf child, feels grief, she also knows that she does not want to withhold maternal love and take out her grief on her child (as her mother did) (Long 2012:252).

The resolution Marina makes is one that continues to work in direct defiance of her mother; it is also, however, one born of immediate love as she holds her hearing son and remembers the love that her Deaf friend and signing hearing daughter share—pointing to how many SLPs would not only love to conceive deaf children but also hearing children. While holding her "sweetly" nuzzling baby who sleeps "against her neck," Marina rests "her cheek on the top of the baby's soft head and [makes] him [the] silent promise" (Long 2012:266). Despite their differences, Marina feels a deep love for her son—one that tackles the grief over her violated human rights at the hands of a hegemonic Hearing patriarchy. The story ends with Marina turning on music, holding "her son in both arms and danc[ing] to her own internal rhythm" (Long 2012:266). This convoluted ending leaves an opening for a reading of "Of Silence" that imaginably argues for a love of different ontologies. This reading looks at how the story's serpentine ending presents love as the most important narrative—one that is more important than hearing status/sameness/difference. Although the dominant discourse of this dystopian setting is that deaf lives are undesirable—that one is better off dead/unborn/never given a chance at life than deaf—we can see that this discourse is a result of intolerance for difference. A reading of Long's *underlying* narrative that deaf lives should be welcome and desirable becomes all the more potent with schema criticism. Schema criticism allows readers to see how Long's story leans toward the humanist hope for a love of different ontologies that would then lead to an ideal image of the nation—the socially just nation—even as it simultaneously associates the failure to love difference with the origin of audism and ethnic cleansing (Ahmed 2015:139, 140). With a critique of our cognitive general-person schemas, readers can make sense of *both* the dominant and subversive narrative threads.

In short, the story's equivocal acceptance of the end of Deaf culture may create empathic mourning in readers who may, with schema criticism, be more apt to become allies to prevent such a state—refusing apathy in favor of action that promotes social justice and the human and group rights of SLPs. As such, the ambivalent nature of Marina's individual narrative, which does not really seek to serve the greater collective, and the ambivalent nature of the SLPs' resignation to the government's act of ethnocide (e.g., Susan's physical expression of indifference and her declaration that everyone knows this cannot be changed), *questions* the idea that the end of Deaf culture is acceptable (Long 2012:260). Even with failed acts to promote the reproductive and group rights of SLPs, Marina's declaration that the denial of her choice is wrong, and the SLPs' proclamation that this is genocide, challenges the lack of collective action and general feeling of powerlessness (Long 2012:255, 260).

THE CONTINUING LEGACIES OF EUGENIC CAMPAIGNS

Although Long's science fiction story is not a piece of historical fiction, it realistically illustrates the contemporary legacy of Alexander Graham Bell's 19th-century proposal for preventing the formation of a deaf race (Greenwald 2004:36–37). These eugenic legacies inform SLPs' current claims for both human and group rights. The depiction of these eugenic legacies in protest stories such as "Of Silence," which portray the eradication or curing of deafness as an act of genocide/ethnocide, seeks to move its readers to reconsider the bioethics behind such decisions. In "Disability, Democracy, and the New Genetics," Bérubé (2004) describes the shift in eugenic thinking from a "public" to a "private" eugenics, one in which the "old eugenics" categorized humans as an "aggregate of various ethnic and racial traits," while the "new eugenics," on the other hand, sees *individuals* as "aggregates of biochemical traits" (215). In both cases, certain populations or individual traits are marked as detrimental to their families or their nation(s) (Bérubé 2004:215). The shift away from marking entire ethnic or racial *groups* to marking *individual* traits points to why SLPs currently make claims to group rights and protections that recognize their Deafnicity. Successfully achieving the recognition of Deafnicity, with its unique ontologies, makes claims against scientific ethnocide stronger.

The shift from Bell's 19th-century proposal for preventing the formation of a deaf race to the 21st-century rhetoric of deaf people as "hearing-impaired," or hearing *individuals* who "happen to have" an impairment (which can be eliminated) illustrates Bell's legacy in promoting the idea that "we should try ourselves to forget that they are deaf" and treat deaf people as if they are hearing (as cited in Werner 1884:11). Bell's proposition thus sought a form of linguistic genocide—to deny SLPs their sign language and to encourage oral speech. Bell's proposals for preventing the formation of a deaf race also involved actions to prevent the formation of Deaf identities by dismantling this group and isolating individuals amongst hearing people. Doing so prevents SLPs from becoming a political *group* with the power to claim group rights. It also marks these newly designated "hearing-impaired" *individuals* as in need of intervention from the biological/medical sciences in order to take away the impairment and make them "whole" (or hearing) again. As Kusters et al. (2015) assert, "the addition of *group rights* in order to accommodate diversity would provide a much stronger basis for protection than the mere argument that SLPs are part of (and contribute to) human diversity and the emphasis on human rights (which are usually *individual* rights)" (14). In other words, relying solely on human, or individual rights, would not grant SLPs the right to be born—especially if deafness is viewed solely as an individual characteristic of impairment. The controversy inherent in the shift within eugenic rhetoric raises bioethical issues that are reflected in "Of Silence": who should/can determine what it means to be a deaf individual? Should deaf babies be recognized as members of a protected class of SLPs and raised as such? Who should/can make these decisions? Contemplating the range of questions inherent to a Deaf bioethics is essential to considering the group rights claims of SLPs.

FOREBODING DYSTOPIAN FUTURES, CURRENT REALITIES, AND THEIR CONNECTIONS TO OUR EUGENIC PAST

The value of stories like "Of Silence" lies in how they explore these bioethical and group rights concerns. In fact, "Of Silence" presaged (by seven years) a controversy that made headlines both in the United States and the United Kingdom, when a Deaf lesbian couple in the United States, Sharon Duchesneau and Candy McCullough, turned to a friend (who had a Deaf family across five generations) and attempted to have a Deaf baby with his genetic contribution. In a case that evokes Long's dystopia and Marina's desire for a Deaf baby, a sperm bank turned Duchesneau and McCullough away saying, "donors with disabilities were screened out" (Teather 2002:para. 2). This "screening out" of "disability" fails to recognize both disability as a social construct and Deaf people as an ethnic minority. This couple, like Marina in "Of Silence," had to turn to outside help because of a Hearing hegemony that would deny their choice.

The foreboding dystopia in "Of Silence" (1995) thus began to manifest itself both in this 2002 controversy in the United States and, more recently, in the United Kingdom. The sperm bank that turned away Duchesneau and McCullough—foreshadowed (and influenced) the drafting of clause 14 in the United Kingdom's 2008 Human Fertilisation and Embryology Act (HFEA), which requires the screening of embryos implanted via IVF (Emery et al. 2010, Bryan & Emery 2014, "Reproductive Medicine" n.d.). The media coverage over Duchesneau and McCullough's choice encouraged the British Government to make the act of choosing to implant an embryo that screens for a deaf gene illegal (Emery et al. 2010); the Health Minister released a letter to *The Sunday Telegraph* indicating that the Human Fertilisation and Embryology Bill's embryo-testing provisions were to "*avoid serious medical conditions* or *disabilities*, not to *create* [emphasis added] babies with desired characteristics or traits, such as deafness" (Primarolo as cited in White 2008:21–23). This provision against deafness defines it in medical, pathological terms; deafness is a "disease," a "serious" illness in the minds of these policymakers, which thus leads to their enforced demand for the *creation* of *non-deaf* babies.

Long's prophetic dystopia took these measures even further: to acts of extermination (ethnocide) and to the act of witnessing cultural genocide: "your culture dying all around you, because no children are born to carry it forward. You can't imagine it" (2012:255). Although the United Nations General Assembly's (1946) resolution on genocide could not foresee the future that we currently live in, their definition of genocide is applicable to the argument against genocide that the SLPs in "Of Silence" present:

> Genocide is a denial of the right of existence of entire human *groups*, as homicide is the denial of the right to live of individual human beings; such denial of *the right of existence* shocks the conscience of mankind, results in great losses to humanity in the form of *cultural and other contributions* represented by these *human groups* and is contrary to moral law and to the spirit and aims of the United Nations. (emphasis added, 188–189)

Marina's declaration that such a reality is impossible to imagine is exactly what Long's story seeks to refute. Long calls on her readers' imaginations as she depicts the values, ontological experiences, and human desires of SLPs. In other words, readers' cognitive processes (while imagining the story) become an act of public imagination: "an imagination that will steer judges in their judging, legislators in their legislating, policy makers in measuring the quality of life of people near and far" (Nussbaum 1995:3). In short, hearing readers of "Of Silence" are made capable of imagining the value of deaf ontologies.

Reading the prophetic "Of Silence" within the historical context of eugenics and with consideration of our current bioethical dilemmas, we can see how the crisis in the family stands in for the crisis of paternalistic state control. As Nussbaum (2006) argues, ". . . the family is a political institution, not part of a 'private sphere' immune from justice" ("Introduction"). Marina's proclamation that she "will not make the mistake [her] mother did" presents a model for state *non*-intervention, via its critique of how the government acts paternalistically by determining whose image should be made (Long 2012:266). It critiques the imposition of audist desires as it raises the bioethical human/group rights question of eugenics: Which lives are desirable? With the story's closing presentation of love as surpassing all potential grief at difference, Long shows how differences may be crossed and bonds may be made—however "tenuous" they may be (2012:266). Ultimately, in this story, love and acceptance matter most. With this maternal commonplace, "Of Silence" presents a bioethical group rights claim that deaf lives should be welcome and desirable within all families/ nations: Hearing, Deaf, or somewhere in-between.

CONCLUSION: DEAF LITERATURE AND POLITICS, SCHEMA CRITICISM, AND A DEAF BIOETHICS

With this chapter's assertion regarding the power of literature, I argue that, if, along with the influx of interest and enrollment in ASL courses in schools across the United States, Deaf Literature also was increasingly incorporated into American, British, Ethnic, and World Literature courses, there would be much more potential to replace harmful cognitive schemas with those befitting the human and group rights claims of SLPs (Brueggemann 2009:31; Florence 2015). This argument agrees with Nussbaum's (1995) assertion on literature's cognitive potency: ethical appeals to the human right to a life with dignity "will fail" unless those who are being appealed to are first "made capable of entering imaginatively into the lives of distant others" and experience the emotions of distant others through this imaginative encounter (xvi). Imaginative and emotionally compelling pieces of Deaf Literature could thus offer SLPs greater success in claiming their group right to be born.

This chapter's call to deaf scholars and their allies asks for greater attention to and exploration of a Deaf bioethics through the lens of deaf ontologies. Reading literary texts (that illustrate deaf ontologies) and engaging in schema criticism becomes a strategy for transformative social justice; cognitive research shows us that such critical reading practices lay the groundwork for successful legal changes (Bracher 2013:288). Schema criticism thus offers one way in which SLPs and their allies can enact effective social change. To echo and reinvigorate a sentiment proposed by a Deaf professor of law, Michael Schwartz (2011), "Deaf scholars and their allies in the professional academy and the world of practice" (or policymaking), must "frame the debate in terms that help advance the struggle for a better life" (872). Or, to make a stronger case for a Deaf bioethics, the debate must not only advance the struggle for a better life, but also permit SLPs' right to be born in the first place.

As threats toward communities of SLPs continue today in various shapes: developments in genetic engineering making it possible to eliminate deaf genes; some believing that deafness is cause for abortion (Middleton 2004:136); and others believing a Deaf life is undesirable—arguing that is unethical to prevent "the likelihood that one's children might be deaf," favoring, instead, laws like HFEA, or genetic screening and action to prevent deaf children from being born (Johnston 2005:426)—deaf communities often call on Deaf scholars to refute these violations to their human and group rights (Ladd 2003, Greenwald 2004, Murray 2004, Haualand & Allen 2009, Emery et al. 2010, Blankmeyer Burke 2011, Schwartz 2011, De Meulder 2014, Bryan & Emery 2014, Kusters et al. 2015). It is the voices of these Deaf scholars and their lived experiences within deaf ontologies that make their counterarguments so potent. Deaf Literature's engagement with the cognitive schemas of its readers—both Hearing and deaf—potentiates social-perspective taking in a way that can enable readers' understanding of deaf ontologies.

Literature also provides fertile ground for cross-disciplinary explorations of bioethical issues. It "emerges as the privileged site for promoting social justice by correcting the faulty cognitive structures that are ultimately responsible for injustice" (Bracher 2013:xiii). In other words, literature has the power to transform our daily interaction with others, our feelings about others, and the policies we enact that affect these "others" who are not us. I invite and hope that legal scholars, human rights scholars, bioethicists and philosophers, deaf educators, sociologists who study families or minority communities, professors of medicine and the humanities (who already explore these seemingly divergent fields through the lens of narrative), as well as Deaf Studies and Disability Studies scholars, will take up this chapter's challenge to read Deaf Literature, to analyze it in consideration of deaf ontologies, and to engage in critical debate about the rights claims of SLPs.

ACKNOWLEDGMENTS

The writing of this chapter greatly benefited from a June 2014 summer residency at the Anderson Center for Interdisciplinary Studies, funded by the National Endowment for the Arts.

REFERENCES

Ahmed, S. (2015). *The cultural politics of emotion* (2nd ed.). New York, NY: Routledge.

Appiah, K. A. (1992). *In my father's house: Africa in the philosophy of culture.* New York, NY: Oxford University Press.

Batterbury, S., Ladd, P. & Gulliver, M. (2007). Sign language peoples as indigenous minorities: Implications for research and policy. *Environment and Planning, 39,* 2899–2915.

Bauman, H-D. (2005). Designing Deaf babies and the question of disability. *Journal of Deaf Studies and Deaf Education, 10.3,* 311–315.

Bauman, H-D. & Murray, J. M. (2014). Deaf gain: An introduction. In H.D. Bauman & J.J. Murray (Eds.), *Deaf gain: Raising the stakes for human diversity.* [Kindle version]. Minneapolis: University of Minnesota Press.

Bérubé, M. (2004). Disability, democracy, and the new genetics. In J. V. Van Cleve (Ed.), *Genetics, disability, and deafness* (pp. 202–220). Washington, DC: Gallaudet University Press.

Bhabha, H. K. (2004). *The location of culture.* New York, NY: Routledge Classics.

Blankmeyer Burke, T. (2014). Armchairs and stares: On the privation of deafness. In H.D. Bauman & J.J. Murray (Eds.), *Deaf gain: Raising the stakes for human diversity.* [Kindle version]. Minneapolis: University of Minnesota Press.

Blankmeyer Burke, T. (2011). *Quest for a Deaf child: Ethics and genetics.* (Doctoral dissertation, The University of New Mexico). Retrieved from *Academia.edu.*

Bracher, M. (2013). *Literature and social justice: Protest novels, cognitive politics and schema criticism.* Austin: University of Texas Press.

Brotherton, M. (2008, April 29). Comic book writers in SFWA? [Web log post]. Retrieved from *Mike Brotherton: SF Writer.*

Brueggemann, B. J. (2009). *Deaf subjects: Between identities and places.* [Kindle version]. New York: New York University Press.

Bryan, A., & Emery, S. (2014). The case for Deaf legal theory through the lens of Deaf gain. In H.D. Bauman & J.J. Murray (Eds.), *Deaf gain: Raising the stakes for human diversity* (pp. 37–62.) Minneapolis: University of Minnesota Press.

De Meulder, M. (2014). The UNCRPD and Sign Language Peoples. In A. Pabsch (Ed.), *UNCRPD implementation in Europe—A Deaf perspective, Article 29: Participation in political and public life* (pp. 12–28). Brussels, Belgium: European Union of the Deaf.

Eckert, R. C. (2010). Toward a theory of Deaf ethnos: Deafnicity ≈ D/deaf (Hómaemon • Homóglosson • Homóthreskon). *Journal of Deaf Studies and Deaf Education, 15.4,* 317–333.

Emery, S. D., Middleton, A., & Turner, G. H. (2010). Whose Deaf genes are they anyway? The Deaf community challenge to legislation on embryo selection. *Sign Language Studies, 10.1,* 155–169.

Evans, T. (Director) (2011). *The End*. Neath Films and the BSLBT. [Film]. Available from Vimeo. https://vimeo.com/24804168

Florence, L. (2015, February 16). Study reports a decline in language enrollment. *The Daily Texan*, pp. 1, 3. Retrieved from http://www.dailytexanonline.com/2015/02/16/report-shows-decline-in-foreign-language-program-enrollment

Greenwald, B. H. (2004). The real "toll" of A.G. Bell: Lessons about eugenics. In J. V. Van Cleve (Ed.), *Genetics, disability, and deafness* (pp. 35–41). Washington DC: Gallaudet University Press.

Haualand, H., & Allen, C. (2009). *Deaf people and human rights*. World Federation of the Deaf. Helsinki, Finland: Swedish Agency for International Development Co-operation and Swedish Organisations of Disabled Persons International Aid Association. Retrieved from http://www.wfdeaf.org/wp-content/uploads/2011/06/Deaf-People-and-Human-Rights-Report.pdf

Häyry, M. (2004). There is a difference between selecting a deaf embryo and deafening a hearing child. *Journal of Medical Ethics, 30*, 510–512.

Holmes, M. A. (2006/1980). Bicultural adaptation and survival: Integration or disintegration. In R. Lee (Ed.), *Deaf liberation: A selection of NUD papers 1976–1986* (pp. 137–150). Middlesex, Great Britain: British Deaf History Society.

Johnston, T. (2005). In one's own image: Ethics and the reproduction of deafness. *Journal of Deaf Studies and Deaf Education, 10.4*, 426–441.

Jones, P. (2008). Group rights. *Stanford Encyclopedia of Philosophy*. Retrieved from http://plato.stanford.edu/entries/rights-group/#GroRigIndRigCoExiCom

Komesaroff, L. (Ed.) (2007). *Surgical consent: Bioethics and cochlear implantation*. Washington, DC: Gallaudet University Press.

Kusters, A., & De Meulder, M. (2013). Understanding Deafhood: In search of its meanings. *American Annals of the Deaf, 157.5*, 428–438.

Kusters, A., De Meulder, M., Friedner, M., & Emery, S. (2015). On "diversity" and "inclusion": Exploring paradigms for achieving Sign Language Peoples' rights. *MMG Working Papers, 15.02*, 1–29.

Ladd, P. (2003). *Understanding Deaf culture: In search of Deafhood*. Clevedon, UK: Multilingual Matters.

Lane, H., Pillard, R. C., Hedberg, U. (2011). *The people of the eye: Deaf ethnicity and ancestry*. Oxford, UK: Oxford University Press.

Leake, E. (2014). A cognitive route to social justice: Mark Bracher's radical pedagogies. *Pedagogy: Critical Approaches to Teaching Literature, Language, Composition and Culture, 14.3*, 553–559.

Long, K. (2012). Of silence and slow time. In E. E. Sayers (Ed.), *Outcasts and angels: The new anthology of Deaf characters in literature* (pp. 248–266). Washington, DC: Gallaudet University Press.

Middleton, A. (2004). Deaf and hearing adults' attitudes towards genetic testing for deafness. In J. V. Van Cleve (Ed.), *Genetics, disability, and deafness* (pp. 127–147). Washington, DC: Gallaudet University Press.

Murray, J. J. (2004). "True love and sympathy": The Deaf-Deaf marriages debate in transatlantic perspective. In J. V. Van Cleve (Ed.), *Genetics, disability, and deafness* (pp. 42–71). Washington, DC: Gallaudet University Press.

National Association of the Deaf. (2010). Vision 2020 strategic plan. *National Association of the Deaf*. Retrieved from http://www.nad.org/about-us/vision-2020-strategic-plan

Newell, C. (2006). Disability, bioethics, and rejected knowledge. *Journal of Medicine and Philosophy, 31.3*, 269–283.

Nussbaum, M. (2006). Introduction. *Frontiers of justice: Disability, nationality, species membership*. [Kindle version]. Cambridge, MA: The Belknap Press of Harvard University Press.

Nussbaum, M. (1995). *Poetic justice: The literary imagination and public life*. Boston, MA: Beacon Press.

O'Brien, D., & Emery, S. D. (2013). The role of the intellectual in minority group studies: Reflections on Deaf Studies in social and political contexts. *Qualitative Inquiry, 20.1*, 27–36.

Reproductive Medicine: Pre-Implantation Genetic Diagnosis. (n.d.). Ministry of Ethics. Retrieved from http://www.ministryofethics.co.uk/?p=8&q=7

Schwartz, M. (2011). America's transformation: The arc of justice bends toward the Deaf community. *Valparaiso University Law Review, 45*, 845–874.

Siebers, T. (2008). *Disability theory*. Ann Arbor: University of Michigan Press.

Sturley, N. (2003). *Milan*. Victoria, Canada: Trafford Publishing.

Teather, D. (2002, April 7). Lesbian couple have Deaf baby by choice. *The Guardian*. Retrieved from http://www.theguardian.com/world/2002/apr/08/davidteather

The Center for Bioethics and Human Dignity. *Bioethics*. Retrieved from: https://cbhd.org/category/issues/bioethics

United Nations General Assembly. (1946). *General Assembly resolution 96 (I) of 11 December 1946 (The crime of genocide)*. 1st sess. PDF file (pp.188–189). Retrieved from *Audiovisual Library of International Law, Historic Archives: Criminal Law*.

United Nations General Assembly. (1948). *The Universal Declaration of Human Rights*. Retrieved from http://www.un.org/en/universal-declaration-human-rights/index.html.

United Nations Population Fund (UNFPA) (2007). Supporting the constellation of reproductive rights. Retrieved from *United Nations Population Fund*, http://www.unfpa.org/resources/supporting-constellation-reproductive-rights

Werner, E. S. (1884). Proceedings in detail: Third day, June 27, President Bell in the chair, question-box. In E.S. Werner (Ed.), *Convention of articulation teachers of the Deaf, held at the institution for the improved instruction of Deaf-mutes*. Albany, NY: The Voice Press. Retrieved from *Google Books*.

Weston, B. H. (2015). Human rights. *Encyclopaedia Britannica*. Retrieved from http://www.britannica.com/topic/human-rights

White, E. (2008, May 2). *Human fertilisation and embryology bill [HL] Bill 70 of 2007–08*. United Kingdom, House of Commons Library, Science and Environment Section, Social Policy Section, Home Affairs Section. London, UK: Library Research Publications. Retrieved from http://www.mbbnet.umn.edu/scmap/HFEAbill.pdf

Williams, D. (2013). When the dead are cured. In J.L. Clark (Ed.), *Deaf lit extravaganza* (p. 146). Minneapolis, MN: Handtype Press.

9

Cripping Deaf Studies and Deaf Literature: Deaf Queer Ontologies and Intersectionality

Rezenet Moges

During my winter vacation in 2014, I was a tourist visiting a well-known progressive bookstore named "City Lights Booksellers" in San Francisco. Upon arriving at the bookstore, I marched directly to the Queer Studies section downstairs. Befuddled, I found myself standing in front of an entire bookshelf, staring at a single book. Its title, *Mean Little deaf Queer* called my name. I was convinced that someone was playing a joke on me. Up until then, I had never seen a book that represented my multiple identities displayed on a shelf at a mainstream bookstore. This brought me to the realization of the value of having Deaf Queer[1] people, a marginalized group, made visible in print. The unexpected encounter with this rare book opens this dialogue about Deaf Queer literature.

In this chapter, I will study a particular aspect of deaf ontologies by examining literature produced by the Queer-identified group within the greater linguistic minorities of Deaf people in the United States; and I will do this through the lens of intersectionality (Crenshaw 1989).

---

[1] I chose to capitalize the terms *Black, Deaf,* and *Queer,* to center the self-identified members of social groups that have been long marginalized in mainstream society and treated as having presumably distinct identities without any intersection. Although there is a growing consensus of scholars in Deaf Studies shifting from the use of capitalized "D" for "Deaf" to using a lowercase "d" for all deaf people (Kusters et al, this volume), I, nonetheless, will still capitalize these terms, following Crenshaw's (1989) capitalization of "Black." I find it necessary to maintain this convention because to me, not maintaining those conventions means dismissing the history of fighting constantly against oppression, unequal rights, marginalization, negligence, and invisibility; denying the existence of these social and political groups as collectives; and by extension, denying my identity as a Black Deaf Queer woman. Where I do not capitalize those words of deaf, queer, and black, I use the words as mere descriptors of people's deafness, sexual performance and color, respectively.

Originally feminist, the sociological theory of intersectionality allows for a study of complexities within intersectional Deaf Queer identities.[2] Adopting this volume's focus on deaf ontologies, this chapter focuses on *being* Deaf and Queer. Therefore, my own positionality as I review the literature by Deaf Queer authors is essential to maintain a Deaf-centric study. The chapter discusses the self-representation of Deaf Queer people in literature and history. This literature is significantly under-represented and under-recognized in the larger body of Deaf Studies literature. I do this literary analysis from my perspective as a self-identified Intersectional Deaf Lesbian of Color.

The term "Queer" will be used instead of LGBT (or GLBT)[3] to iden-tify political stances, sexualities, and gender variations and to provide an inclusive approach that applies a singular umbrella term for all types of sexuality and genders that differ from heterosexuality and/ or cisgender.[4] The term is comparable to using the term "Deaf" when referring to the wider community including the frequently invisible Hard-of-Hearing (HH) people (i.e., Galloway 2009). "Queer" also pro-vides a holistic perspective on both defined and fluid sexualities. For example, a lesbian could develop sexual tendencies for a man, and her fluidity of sexual attraction would still maintain her Queer identity. This inclusive term "queer" comes from Queer Theory, more specifi-cally Warner's (1999) *The Trouble with Normal*. I use the term to frame this chapter and to delineate a dichotomy between queer and hetero-sexual people, given that Queer people do not share the same privileges as heterosexual people: being Queer often leads to hate crimes, unequal treatment in employment, or lack of family support (Cohen 1997).

Regarding Deaf Queer communities, I will maintain an inclusive approach that Ruiz-Williams et al. (2015) and Friedner (this volume) use to remind us to pay heed to the diverse and plural communities and identities of people who belong to the category of "Deaf people." For example, Bienvenu (2008) came up against this when the Deaf les-bian community, of which she is a part, needed and produced their own space; heterosexual or gay male Deaf people were upset by their separation from the rest. By emphasizing the need for a Deaf lesbian space, she dismantled the idea of a monolithic and singular unified Deaf culture that overrides other specific intersectional identities. To

---

[2] I write "Deaf identities" in plural because of the variation of linguistic preferences such as users of ASL, Signing Exact English, Cued Speech, or spoken English (without any signing) and varying identifications associated with hearing levels such as Deaf, Hard-of-Hearing, Cochlear-Implanted and Late-Deafened.

[3] LGBT is an acronym for Lesbian, Gay, Bisexual, Transgender and this still leaves out other (unnamed/undefined) Queer-identified people's specific or fluid sexual orientations.

[4] "Cisgender" refers to a person who remains in the same sex since birth as opposed to a transgender body.

avoid the erasure of any nonmentioned or neglected identities, authors have proposed acronyms that enumerate a number of specific characteristics or identities, such as DDBDLVDDHHCILD[5] or DDBDDHH[6] (Ruiz-Williams et al. 2015). While acknowledging these considerations, I will use "Intersectional Deaf people" instead for all Deaf and/or any Queer/Gender/Person of Color communities for this paper. Rather than singling out particular idiosyncratic identities or standardizing one privilege equally for all individuals, the term "Intersectional Deaf people" encompasses any particular identified group in Deaf populations and it promotes inclusion and raises awareness of the *bodily, racial,* and *sensorial* diversity of Deaf Americans.[7]

The paucity of academic Deaf Queer and intersectional literature implies that Deaf Queer people are largely invisible in academia. This field has remained underdeveloped since Zakarewsky (1979) first focused on deafness and homosexuality. Three decades later, Bienvenu's (2009) grievance about the absence of any theoretical study on the intersections of Deaf and Queer identities provided the incentive for writing this chapter. Ruiz-Williams et al. (2015) encourage us to embed the study of intersectionality in Deaf cultures into a theoretical framework, rather than essentializing the experience of being a (white) Deaf Queer (i.e., Bienvenu 2009). As Friedner (this volume) warns, "frozen epistemologies" in Deaf Studies restrict (new) academic discourse from developing new understanding or analyses of the constructed identities of diverse Deaf communities.

Thus, this chapter breaks new ground. Ultimately, the goal of this chapter is to move forward, build some foundations in theoretical framework(s), and foreground some research and stories, which have focused on Intersectional Deaf Queer communities. An important part of this chapter is the analysis of Deaf Queer literature. First, I identify a theoretical framework called crip theory, relate it to this Queer-identified minority, and by cripping Deaf/ASL literature, I reframe the Deaf Queer authors' work by reclaiming their ontological experiences through the lens of both critical Disability and Queer Studies.

---

[5] DDBDLVDDHHCILD serves as an acronym, referring to the variations of deafness with some intersections of varying abilities: Deaf, Deaf-Blind, Deaf-Low-Vision, Deaf-Disabled, Hard-of-Hearing, Cochlear-Implanted and Late-Deafened people. This is based on my recollection of all varying identities within the Deaf communities that I have journeyed through over time and noticed the grievance of negligence on other unmentioned groups such as LV, CI, and LD-people. Another question to ponder about this acronym is who decides which identity to list first if not in an alphabetical order?

[6] DDBDDHH means "Deaf, DeafBlind, DeafDisabled, and Hard of Hearing peoples" (Ruiz-Williams et al. 2015:263).

[7] This chapter focuses on deaf people in the United States, thus the international aspect is beyond the scope of my research.

After covering the framework of crip theory, I examine whether the framework is adequate to explore the experiences of people living at this intersection of Deaf and Queer identities. Second, I lay out the methodology of this chapter's literary analysis. Third, the literary analysis will analyze one anthology, a memoir, and an American Sign Language (ASL) poem. The fourth part describes elicited responses from two Deaf Queer archivists who outline their struggle in preserving and/or recovering the history of this minority group. Finally, this chapter will summarize the significant contributions of Deaf Queer literature that validates and recognizes the existence and visibility of this intersectional group.

UNDERSTANDING INTERSECTIONALITY AND CRIP THEORY

Analyzing the multifaceted identity of this minority group, Deaf Queer people, demands fitting theoretical frameworks. In this respect, I use the term "Intersectionality," coined by Kimberlé Crenshaw (1989, 1991) who warned that the exclusion or misrecognition of particular minority identities was damaging and augments multiple layers of oppression. In her groundbreaking article, Crenshaw (1989) gave several crucial examples of court cases where antidiscrimination laws did not protect Black female clients from racism and sexism in the same ways as the rights of Black males or white women were protected. This arose from a legal loophole in human rights, which overlooked people with multiple identities who were not entitled to the same benefits that each individual marginalized group (women in general and Black men) received from their membership in separate and protected categories. Attending to how such identities or memberships intersect, intersectionality theory provides the foundation to analyze multiple identities of minority groups; to understand how each identity shapes the other identities and how people experiencing multiple intersections adapt to oppression in everyday life. "Intersectionality" as a concept and theory has been employed in multiple disciplines. Besides race and sex/gender, the investigation of diverse intersections has broadened its scope to include socioeconomic class, disability, sexual orientation, and nationality. Similarly, this chapter explores the intersectionality of Deaf Queer people, considering each stigmatized identity separately, as well as how they shape each other in everyday life.

Critical disability theorists have argued that disabled people are both a political group and an identity group because they are perceived as abnormal by wider (able-bodied and able-privileged) society (Sandahl 2003, McRuer 2006, Kafer 2013). If society were structured according to the principles of Universal Design, in ways that accommodated disabled people's needs, then physical disability would not be viewed as problematic. Thus, being Deaf and using sign language has subjected

Deaf people to a political and social construction of abnormality. Yet, the majority of culturally Deaf Americans reject any association with "disability," arguing that they are disabled by the medical perspective of deafness taken by wider society (Baynton 2008). The rejection of an association with "disability" within Deaf communities has resulted in the exclusion of Deaf-Disabled and Deaf-Blind people. Intersectional Deaf beings, with any ability and disability status, and their queer sexuality are considered in this chapter. Thus, this paper will remain within the purview of critical Disability Studies while applying the lens of intersectionality.

Exploring suitable frameworks to examine this intersectional group, I consider crip theory (Kafer 2013, McRuer 2006), which emerged from an interdisciplinary connection of Disability Studies and Queer Studies. Crip theory constitutes a framework for the critical analysis of collective practices in Intersectional Deaf Queer communities. McRuer (2006:71–72) proposed five principles of crip theory: (1) claiming disability and a disability identity, (2) claiming queer history and identity, (3) demanding an accessible world, (4) insisting on a disabled world, adapting to the needs of disabled bodies, and/or (5) critically questioning the cultural differences between disabled and able-bodied-people. In Principles 1 and 2, cripping practice means the reclamation of intersectional identities, the centralization of the roles of disabled people in societies, the documentation of disabled and queer lives, and the refusal to be marginalized. Principles 3 and 4 denote crip activism, a political movement that rejects separation from wider society to prevent being forgotten, neglected, excluded, or murdered. The underlying conviction is that increasing visibility, awareness, and recognition will secure employment, social group memberships, and quality of life in general. Principle 5 is the next step for crip theorists and scholars: instead of limiting Disabled or Queer Studies to the essentialized dichotomy of, for example, able-bodied or disabled people, pushing for a greater understanding of the complex and interwoven lives of people with diverse gender roles, sexualities, and sensory and bodily variations, and the role of cultural differences in those. McRuer (2006) argues that crip theory is a critique of and resistance to normativity. While Queer Theory challenges the hegemony of heterosexual ideology, crip theory further challenges the able-bodied heteronormativity narrative. Similar to queer sexualities, the arguments of crip studies are known to be fluid and flexible (Kafer 2013, Sandahl 2003). Adopting all the five principles of crip theory, cripping Deaf Studies and Deaf/ASL literature entails that both fields of study undergo a reframing process through a critical examination of the existing Intersectional Deaf Queer genre based on their intersectionality, centralizing on their existing work, and bringing attention to the (inaccessible) historical resource of this marginalized group.

A larger visibility and acceptance of Disabled and Queer identities in the general population will be paralleled by a further development of, and widespread credibility of, academic research projects. This is important because, in my observation, several Deaf Queer scholars are reluctant to do research and publish on this topic because coming out with a Queer identity can threaten their safety or jeopardize a tenure-track position due to insufficient professional support at work, or a lack of interest in their scholarly research interests. Using this theoretical frame to look at Deaf Queer literature and deaf ontologies can be enlightening, liberating, and therapeutic for Deaf Queer authors, archivists, and readers, when they attempt to justify their rightful places in Deaf (academic) communities.

The marginalization of the identities of Deaf and Queer people originates in the compulsion of homogeneity, forcing those minorities to seek a cure for either homosexuality or to attempt to acquire hearing ability and speaking skills for reasons ranging from religious salvation to social inclusion. After experiencing sexual awakening and learning about their sign-language rights (instead of being forced to speak at all times), Deaf Queer people come out twice and act politically in defiance of normativity, assimilation, and marginalization, by resisting homophobia, discrimination, oralism, and audism.[8] There is no "coming-out" for a racial identity for Deaf Queer People of Color, although for them, the oppression and micro-aggression faced on an everyday basis provides an alternative existence to that of white Deaf Queer people privileged by their race. Intersectional Deaf Queer people embody and enact their intersecting political identities (such as disability, sexuality, race, and gender) dynamically and inclusively, instead of having to pick one or another. "Compulsory heterosexuality" (Rich 1980), "compulsory able-bodiedness" (McRuer 2002), and "compulsory hearing [and speaking]" (Harmon 2010) all impose ideologies of heteronormativity in Deaf Queer lives daily. People of Color experience yet another form of coercion from the dominant race: "compulsory whiteness"[9] (Tehranian 2007), which is a conflation of White privilege and White performance, marginalizing the expression of their racial and cultural diversity. In the label "Deaf Queer," there is already an evident cripping of identity by overcoming the struggle from the compulsory hearing/speaking and heterosexuality.

---

[8] Audism is, based on individual type, "the notion that one is superior based on one's ability to hear or behave in the manner of one who hears" (Humphries 1975) or based on "corporate institution," it is a systematic oppression by "the hearing way of dominating, restructuring, and exercising authority over the deaf community" (Lane 1992:43).

[9] My gratitude goes to Dr. Lissa Stapleton for the suggestion of this frequently overlooked type of compulsion on People of Color.

With my focus on Deaf Queer in creative literature, I weigh the importance of validation and representation of literary Deaf Queer experiences in what I consider to be "survival literature." Derived from the genre of lesbian pulp fiction novels during the 1950s and 1960s, Keller defined "survival literature" as a vital resource for closeted or isolated lesbians (and Queer people) in America; those fiction novels were "coveted and treasured for their sometimes positive and sometimes awful but decidedly lesbian and decidedly available representation" (2005:386). Regardless of how sleazy or doomed the lesbian characters were in the novels, they released some kind of tension for the lesbian readers, curing their feelings of isolation due to queer sexualities. Such literature is a vehicle to give a "sense of cultural [and physical] belonging" (Dirlik 2002). Through the analysis of Deaf Queer authors' and poets' creations, I explore the ontological initiative to create stories or histories that recognized their existence, and that built "survival literature" for other lost souls to reassure them in their sense of belonging to Intersectional Deaf Queer communities.

METHODOLOGY AND POSITIONALITY

According to my consultation of a librarian at Gallaudet University Library, there is no exhaustive list of creative literature by Deaf authors. Although the Gallaudet University library does not shelve every published Deaf-authored book, it is one of the largest collections of Deaf resources in America, if not the largest. According to my calculations, the library contains over 650 Deaf-authored books. I narrowed down my search to novels, poetry, and biographies and in this collection, only 23 publications were based on queer topics, written by gay or lesbian identified Deaf authors. In total, that makes up only 4% of Deaf-authored books in general, indicating a dismal and limited number of works for this marginalized group. Even more discouraging is the infinitesimal number of texts by Deaf People of Color and by transgender and Deaf-Disabled authors who are Queer and who experience additional intersections.

A number of past studies (including hearing-authored research) have focused specifically on lesbian, gay, and bisexual people (Phaneuf 1989, Kleinfeld & Warner 1997, Neumann 1997, Bienvenu 2008, Ruiz-Williams et al. 2015). Of these publications, only the last one includes authors who are People of Color. The time-line of these published research papers aligns with the priorities of the political Queer movement for equal rights in the past decades (such as same-sex marriage, adoption, hate crime laws, and employment discrimination). Whereas there is a gradual increase in publications about Deaf Queer people in both creative and academic literature, the Deaf Queer literary collection often repeats the same topics and format of telling and retelling life stories (of whatever length, i.e., brief or book-length) without in-depth critique or analysis of these stories.

Of the 23 Deaf-authored publications on queer topics I located in the Gallaudet library, I selected Raymond Luczak's anthology, *Eyes of Desire: A Gay and Lesbian Reader* (1993) and Terry Galloway's *Mean Little deaf Queer: A Memoir* (2009) to study in more depth. The former includes works of 42 authors including poetry, biography, and literary texts, and the latter is a biography. The third published piece of Deaf Queer literature analyzed here comes in the form of an ASL poem, "Pawns" (1995), composed by Clayton Valli, representing literature coming from within the visual-centric ontology of Deaf-sighted signers, which is crucial to understanding deaf ontologies.

My analysis focuses on the authors' experience of growing up as a Deaf person and realizing their queerness, eventually gaining awareness of their sexual orientation. In addition to an analysis of Deaf Queer literature, interviews with two archivists (one independent and another affiliated with a university) are integrated into the analysis: Dragonsani Renteria, a Deaf Latino transgender man, and Bridget Klein, a white Deaf Queer woman. Renteria's multiple intersectional backgrounds propelled him to become a LGBT activist, trans educator, and a photojournalist who is currently documenting and fighting gentrification in his neighborhood in San Francisco's Mission district, which has traditionally been predominantly Latino. Klein, who presents as a butch[10] woman, comes from the older generation of a Deaf lesbian community, and has the goal of documenting the signed-stories from a fading generation of a Deaf population in New York City. My association with Renteria and Klein is based on mutual interests in Deaf Queer Archives (Renteria), which span eight years prior to the writing of this chapter, and on Deaf Lesbian Herstories[11] (Klein) over the past year. The interviews supplied me with insights into their methodology and archival journeys.

It is important to note that the majority of the selected texts are authored by predominantly white Deaf cisgender and able-bodied authors, which shows that the need for more work by Queer authors experiencing multiple intersections (such as People of Color, transgender, Deaf-Blind, Deaf-Disabled) is clear—both on the theme of intersectional identities, and in the general Deaf Studies literature where more diverse insights are needed. As an African lesbian, I was baffled after

---

[10]   A description used in a Queer culture that refers to extremely masculine women or hyper-masculinity.

[11]   "Herstory" is a female-centralized term, intended to dismantle the patriarchal discipline of history by decolonizing the term "history" from its male-association ("his-" and "story") by replacing "his" with "her" (Nestle 1990).

reading Morgan and Wieringa's *Tommy Boys, Lesbian Men and Ancestral Wives* (2005), a book that focuses on lesbians residing in six east-African countries. This book both expanded my awareness and finally confirmed my suspicions of my initial assumptions about my identities on that continent, after being taught that homosexuality did not exist in Africa but was a Western predisposition. With my intersectional background, I felt an affiliation with that book, having grown up in an African-Diaspora community, which is extremely sheltered and, like the values of my nuclear family, dramatically different from the mainstream culture of America. I grew up as a tomboy, and I would wear neckties/bow-ties on occasion but refuse to wear dresses. My masculine traits are emphasized in my marriage to a feminine wife. That is why I identify myself as a soft butch. During my early twenties, before graduate school, I recall a significant and unforgettable meeting with an older and well-known Black Deaf lesbian filmmaker, Jade Bryan,[12] an extremely intimidating veteran of Black and Deaf lesbian communities. I could not believe that I was socializing with a group of three women, including Bryan, with almost identical identities as mine in regards to gender, sexual orientation, deafness, racial background, class, education, and signing levels. At that moment, our multiple identities struck me for the first time. As a novice, I nervously asked them their views, worried that I might provoke them by saying, "You ever realize that we are placed at the far bottom of the smallest minority there can ever be?!" This statement predominantly indicates my naivety in not considering my other privileges, such as my middle-class and (recently admitted) college-educated background and my able-bodiedness. Nevertheless, that ephemeral reaction signified my perspective and limited experience of my position/status in society at that specific moment. (This was largely due to not having met other people with a similar background and different types of privilege or a greater number of minority identities.) Amazingly, they shrugged it off, simply accepting that perspective because it was our way of life, experiencing a multiplicity of involuntary struggles of loneliness and unfair treatment for being female, Black, Deaf, and Queer. This specific intersectional background has not been articulated in print until today.

During my master's study in linguistic anthropology, I became fascinated with the study of language and gender, and initialized an ongoing research project: an analysis of the masculine signing style of a specific group of Deaf masculine women. This project has been put on hold, however, due to insufficient existing work and a lack of appropriate theoretical frameworks. I want to express my concern and

---

[12] Another contributing author of the book, *"Eyes of Desire"* who was personally invited to share her poems by Raymond Luczak (personal communication with Jade Bryan, 2016).

disappointment with the neglect and marginalization of Deaf Queer people in academia, given that there are a number of Deaf Queer scholars in liberal arts fields such as anthropology, linguistics, sociology, psychology, history, and Deaf Studies who do not focus on Deaf Queer topics. It is maddeningly frustrating for me to see so little scholarly interest in Deaf Queer people. There needs to be some foundational theory on this intersectional group before I can really begin to "celebrate" Deaf Queer academia and its queer signing styles, and, I hope, continue my research project. Thus, contributing to the project of taking this Intersectional Deaf Queer group seriously in academia, I now will analyze the selected texts to examine how the authors claimed their crip identity in biographies, poems, and short anecdotes.

DEAF QUEER LITERATURE ANALYSES—LITERARY TEXTS AND SIGNED POEM

Eyes of Desire

The canonical, "*Eyes of Desire: A Deaf Gay and Lesbian Reader*" (1993), edited by Raymond Luczak, white Deaf gay male, is vital as the earliest resource to the Deaf Queer experience for multiple types of audiences, either Deaf or Deaf Queer communities. This book was published by a small press, is now out-of-print, and has not been picked up by another publishing house for a reprint or new edition. In itself, this is illustrative of the marginality of Deaf Queer literature. "*Eyes of Desire*" collected various voices in a single volume and has been used for self-help, inspiration, and as an academic guide. This anthology contains entries from 42 Deaf, Hard-of-Hearing and hearing[13] Queer authors and provides a rich diversity of unique queer lives. Most authors were U.S.-based and one author had a South African background. Although these accounts are all in textual form, the volume contains a wide range of different formats: essays, newspaper articles, poetry, interviews, and short stories. Luczak collected the entries by word-of-mouth, corresponded through fax machines, traveled to videotape some interviews, and received submissions in answer to an advertisement[14] calling for participants (personal communication with Luczak, 2015). Some entries were translated from ASL poems to written English, and some are transcripts of interviews by means of a telecommunication device (TDD), a now outdated method where two interlocutors communicate through typed conversations. Some chapters are not edited into Standard English grammar

---

[13] Only one hearing author contributed and five hearing people participated in the interviews as a spouse to a Deaf person.

[14] The advertisements were posted by a representative, Sasha Alyson, from the book's publisher company, Alyson Publications.

and are left as original in "Deaf English," or they are a word-for-word transcript directly from TDD conversations.

Instead of examining each entry, my selections illustrate the complexities of being an Intersectional Deaf Queer person. An author with a pseudonym of "Pablo" offers some astute insights into his intersectionality in "Black, Deaf, and Gay: True Identities," ordering these identities as various kinds of "disabilities": "...Since my skin color is visible, they can identify me as black. Then they find out I'm Deaf. As for being gay, it's a sticky situation [because...] my rights as a gay person, they are not quite established" (39). Tanis, as a white Deaf Disabled Dyke, reminds us that she "cannot be out in all the communities" in which she lives and each of her labels is not "mutually exclusive" (71). These two contributors' politically and socially constructed identities are a multilayered series of identities, in which these individual defend themselves from different types of oppression that they cannot single out, but instead experience all at once.

In contrast, Tom Kane insists that in a Deaf context, as a white Deaf gay man, he is "more concerned with deaf rights than with gay rights" (36). In managing his dual identity, he explains that in the Deaf community, they will "think of [themselves] as gay first, then deaf second; but in the hearing world, [they] think of [their] deafness first, [their] gayness second" (Ibid.). Missing a deeper understanding of how intersectionality functions in complex combinations, he as a Deaf person does not embrace his gay identity when participating in the Deaf political movement for language and access rights.

Many authors claim that Deaf gay people watch out for one another and consider the group to be a family (91)—implying a kind of shared bloodline/kinship of people with a Deaf Queer identity. They typically do not mention racial differences, however, so it is uncertain if the sentiments also apply to Intersectional Deaf Queer people, including People of Color.

In "*Eyes of Desire*," a large number of contributors mention two significant themes: Gallaudet University, a university oriented towards Deaf and signing people, as the main site for sexual liberation; and their constant frustration with bar or nightclub scenes as difficult sites to find both a partner (either short- or long-term) and acceptance of their deafness. Several authors discuss experiences with hearing Queer people. "Patrick" and Jack Farrell share their experiences at the bar: deafness is invisible (182), unless communication is attempted. They lament that the use of sign language prevents them from seducing potential hearing non-signing lovers. Within this context, many contributors discuss the search for a hearing lover, or as Hannah Gershon, a white late-deafened lesbian, puts it, an "interauditory" relationship (189). This perpetuates a desire for sensorial "exogamy," a committed relationship outside of a person's cultural identity or adopted family of shared identities. Due to the small population of Deaf Queer people, the number of available suitors is severely restricted because oftentimes, within this small network, many already have met, dated, fostered kinship, or damaged relationships among one another. Sometimes, it seems practical to some Deaf Queer people to venture out into a new unexplored social group with (non-signing) hearing people outside of their network of camaraderie.

Luczak grants an invaluable opportunity for readers to glimpse a wide spectrum of Deaf Queer identities and lives; yet, this is only the beginning. "Victor," a bisexual Deaf-Blind author from Boston perceptively captures the hunger for the spotlight in this minority group: "More Lights, Please!" Luczak produced a second anthology, *"Eyes of Desire 2: A Deaf GLBT Reader"* (2007) through a different press with a larger number of contributors, including more international authors. Retrospectively, when he sent out a call for poetry submissions in 2006 for that second anthology, I regrettably declined to submit my work for fear of outing myself too soon, especially as a daughter of African-immigrant parents, who grew up devaluing homosexuality. A decade later, the writing of this chapter is an act of paying my respects to Luczak and all other authors who have given back to Deaf Queer communities through their representations, despite the risk to their own personal and professional/academic lives; and an act of giving myself a second chance in this chapter to contribute my own "Eyes of Desire."

Mean Little deaf Queer

The second literary text, Terry Galloway's *"Mean Little deaf Queer: A Memoir"* (2009) offers a biographic overview of Galloway's lifelong struggle after losing her hearing at a young age, after developing English-speaking competence. The emphasis of the word, "deaf" with a lowercased "d," in the book's title emphasizes her interpretation of the lack of (American) Deaf cultural identity in her life, such as lack of fluency in ASL and lacking any Deaf social life. Galloway explains her choices not to learn sign language and to attend schools for the hearing without any access to sign language. In order to maintain her "normalcy" in her family, she declines her parents' offer to let her attend deaf institutions (76). Later in life, she was shunned from the Deaf-signing community in a cruel way, due to her lack of "Deaf" identity. Regardless of that, she does not regret her choice of picking speech over "Sign," because she is "enthralled by the effects of sounds," comparing it to "the spell of enchantment" (107). Because she relies entirely on her hearing aids and her speech skills, her life resembles that of a speaking Hard-of-Hearing person; yet her "deafness had the power to infantilize [her] then" (100) because of the hardships experienced prior to the passing of the antidiscrimination law (the Americans with Disabilities Act) that demands access for Deaf Americans today (such as provision of interpreters, captions, and phone-relay services). Galloway is known for theatrical performances that shatter the image of a meek, well-behaved hearing-impaired woman (Sandahl 2003).

The dry humor in which Galloway recounts her childhood, including discovering her emerging intersectionality and sensory changes allows some relief from the somber story of her learning to tolerate the loss of hearing ability. It was an incredible experience to read about Galloway's intersectional childhood and about her mischievous childish acts and naïve infatuation with a female adult, because I could really relate for the first time, having never felt this shared childhood experience through literature before.

> "The deep-end instructor had grabbed *me*, pulled *my* body to hers, wept over *me*. Those were *my* lips she had pressed her own against, *my* dripping body she had dried off with a towel. I've been publicly intimate with the woman, for God's sake, and art, not competitiveness, had earned me her divine embrace." (Galloway 2009:57, with her emphases)

Reading this excerpt reveals what a privilege it is to be acknowledged, and to read about these shared silly childhood moments; recognizing what it is like growing up with same-sex interests and simultaneously being deaf and taking advantage of our deafness to lure an older person of the same-sex to soothe our younger passionate queer selves.

Through another candid anecdote within the context of queering and cripping herself, Galloway details how it can get difficult to fumble with one's deafness in the dark while in a bed with a stranger. Notably, this was not mentioned in *"Eyes of Desire"* and yet, this is a common issue between Deaf and hearing sexual partners. Nonetheless, Galloway does not hold back from exposing deaf-and-queer sexual tendencies and faux pas.

> "After I discovered condoms, sex with men was always easy, and I never had to worry or work at it too hard. The women were something else. And more and more often I was finding myself in bed with them. They took work. [...] Midway into the polka, I'd become aware that the breath in my ear wasn't the random happy panting of sexual frenzy but the cadenced breath of persistent speech, which meant that my partner was probably trying to pass on some urgently needed information. [...] [B]ut we were in bed with the lights on dim, not the ideal environment for lip reading. And then, whump." (Galloway 2009:130)

The content in *"Mean Little deaf Queer"* underlines that crip theory can present valuable information about Galloway's deaf and Queer experience, a woman who struggled with compulsory normalcy by switching from unqueering or undeafening herself. In her wisdom, she elucidates her intersectional experiences, while juggling the hardships from her identities quite succinctly: "Passing as hearing took such a toll that passing as straight was a piece of cake" (101).

Pawns

The third selected piece of literature is a visual narrative with poetic structures that touches the very core of deaf ontologies, "Pawns"[15] by Clayton Valli (1995). As a nonstandard form of creative literature, sign language poetry "literally provides new space in literature to exist" (Rose 2006:13). Sanchez (2015:128) states that "Through [the] constant movement, the poem presents a challenge to ideas of the visual image (or of visual poetics) as capturing a singular moment in time." I chose "Pawns" because of its allegory depicting the unequal power relationship between governing rulers and their pawns. Valli's poem expresses an unapologetic, veracious political outcry, and a desire for us to face the sorrow, discrimination, and neglect inherent in the rise of AIDS-related deaths in the Deaf gay community. This poem exemplifies the "queer temporality" (Kafer 2013) that emerges from the AIDS crisis, symbolizing a healing period for the HIV/AIDS-stricken gay communities, who now can look forward to both a present and a future beyond the conventional life of family and child-rearing (Halberstam 2005, Kafer 2013:35). The poem is performed by Ella Mae Lentz, who shares a similar intersectional background with Valli as another white Deaf lesbian and ASL poet who engaged in ASL literature from a Deaf Queer perspective.

This dense poem is filled with metaphors and symbolic references. The spatial placement of the KING+QUEEN rulers indicates, according to Sutton-Spence (2010), a high-versus-low indexicality, which portrays the disparity of power on a metaphorical chessboard. Using this reference, the performer indicates the governing KING+QUEEN placed up high distinguishing their hierarchical status and power over the less powerful and diminutive PAWNS, representing gay activists (as shown in Figure 9.1). The fraught facial expression of the signer depicts the narrative of unexpected deaths and the shrinking group of gay activists and lack of sympathetic acknowledgment or aid from those in power. The royal reference symbolizes the authoritative power of governments and their refusal to provide timely medical resources and to formulate health safeguards against HIV/AIDS for the unprotected and sexually active gay people in the 1980s and early 1990s. The two castles imply

---

[15] This video can be seen online, https://vimeo.com/170190473 and the password for the video access is "pawns."

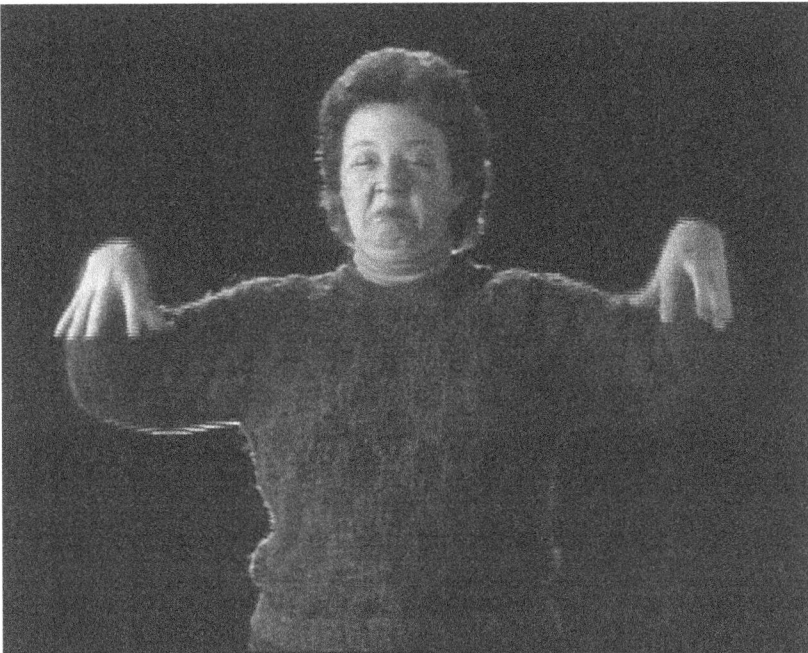

Figure 9.1 Ella Mae Lentz performs the poem, "Pawns," and indicates two castles placed high above the "pawns" in this still-image. (Reproduced with permission from DawnSignPress—Quality Sign Language Materials.)

two rival political parties, such as Democrats and Republicans, or the two houses of the U.S. Congress. In the second half of "Pawns," the poet pays homage to two deceased white Deaf gay men: John Smith and Sam Edwards.[16]

The DVD, *ASL Poetry of Clayton Valli* (1995), includes a bonus video[17] of Valli himself describing his poetic technique, including that of compounding three signs, "FLAG+DIE+LAY-DOWN" (Figure 9.2), which created a powerful metaphor of the U.S. flag and deaths from HIV/AIDS, with two hands signing simultaneously and symmetrically. This

---

[16] On a side note, to illustrate how small the Deaf Queer community is and how the dual identities of Deaf and Queer are so closely intertwined: Sam Edwards, whose name is mentioned in this poem, had been already mentioned in Luczak's book. He was remembered by "James Mackintosh" and Jack Ferrell (who also passed away from AIDS-related complications) as an immensely charming and magnificent storyteller (Luczak 1993:47 and 93–98, respectively). It was Edwards's quote that was cited, "Deafness and gayness are not my problems; they are those of people who do not accept themselves, and therefore do not accept others" (Ibid.:5).

[17] This video can be seen online, https.//vimeo.com/171608611 and the password for the video access is "pawns."

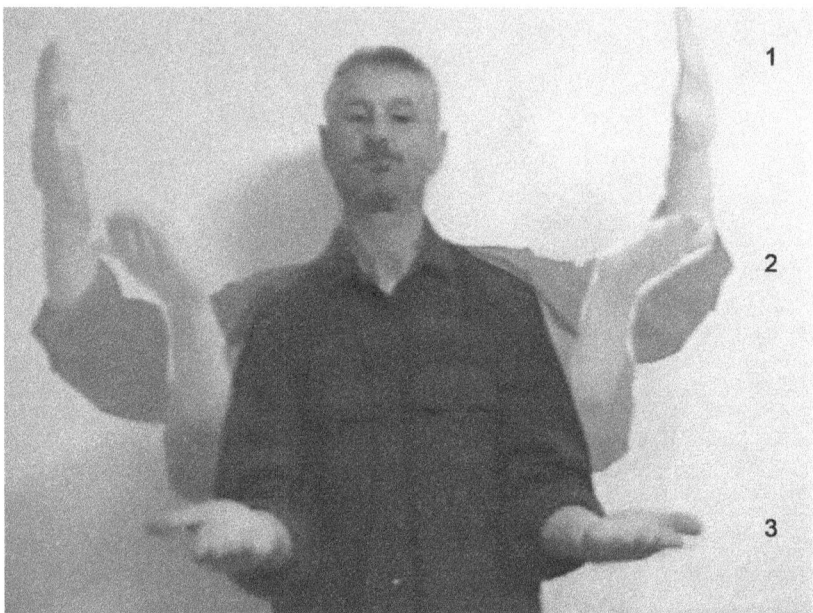

Figure 9.2 Clayton Valli demonstrates a combination of three signs. (Reproduced with permission from DawnSignPress—Quality Sign Language Materials.)

poetically conveyed the multiple and tragic AIDS-related deaths captured by the phrase "patriots gone too soon" (my interpretation). The freedom of creative expression in poetry allows Valli to exercise the "manipulation of linguistic codes" (Davidson 2008), with a great deal of flexibility to play with the words, and send out poetically dense and vivid information. The poem closes with an angrily expressed interrogative "BEAUTIFUL?!" (Figure 9.3), showing the contradiction of the multilayered complication of life and death of many, including these two deceased Deaf gay Americans, stuck in the disparity of power. Valli returned to the topic of AIDS in the Deaf gay community in a poem titled, "Wall and the Quilt" (Valli 1995).

While the poem personalized the Queer community and the national HIV/AIDS epidemic, it also served as a representation of Deaf gay men, and Deaf Queer communities within the political Deaf community, indicating that deaf ontologies can be explored through the confluence of crip theory and political Queer identity. It took a Deaf gay poet to expose and describe the dark period of the 1980s to 1990s, which was never described before in ASL literature, a significant element of a signed language culture. By doing so, Valli cripped ASL literature through his own ontological experience.

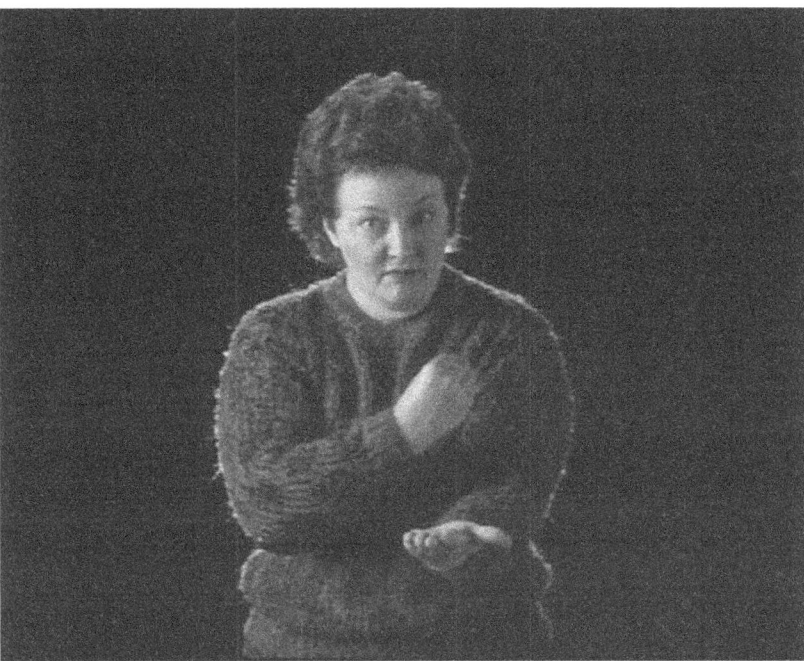

Figure 9.3 The final hold of the sign, "BEAUTIFUL,"(RH) and "BANNER+LAID-DOWN" (LH) angrily expressed by Ella Mae Lentz. (Reproduced with permission from DawnSignPress—Quality Sign Language Materials.)

Literature Analysis Summary

All of these literary accounts reflect crip theory when each Deaf and Queer author describes their experiences of compulsory hearing/speaking and heterosexuality. Considering the miniscule number of Queer-authored books available, these three accounts stood out in defiance and exhibited the intersection and negotiation of race, Deaf, and Queer realities and lives. When inquiring about sexual performance of disabled and deaf queer bodies, the imagination of able-bodied and heterosexual people is often limited when attempting to visualize how this sex works. Deaf people, including me, are frequently asked the following common question: "How do you know if s/he's experiencing orgasm, when the lights are out?" This assumes a lack of tactile ability to feel a physical response. Or, "How do you communicate if your hands are busy?" which implies a "constructed identity [of] normate" (Garland-Thomson 1997), seen as a heteronormative and ableist ideology of there being supposedly one single way of having sex. To summarize, as seen or imagined with deaf, disabled, and/or queer bodies, the extraordinary experiences by the bodies and identities of these Deaf Queer authors provide us with a "survival literature" that presents their shared struggle of being rejected and neglected, finding love in a relationship in which communication is not an issue, debating whether to have "interauditory" relationships, or mourning for (un)forgotten death of our AIDS brothers.

DERIVED ETHNOHISTORY: HISTORICAL ETHNOGRAPHY

I now shift to the two interviews with participants who provide an overview of their ongoing projects building archives of, and drawing from, Deaf Queer histories. A true protagonist in the Deaf Queer community, Dragonsani Renteria, a Deaf Latino transman (complete transition from a female-to-male body), has already dedicated 30 years (since 1986) to accruing an archival collection and recordings of interviews with Deaf Queer people for his upcoming book of Deaf Queer History. Before his transition, he also contributed to Luczak's first anthology, *"Eyes of Desire."* The second interviewee, Bridget Klein, is a doctoral student of anthropology at American University. She conducted an ethnohistory, a methodology that incorporates the ethnography of collecting histories of elderly (mostly white) Deaf lesbians, documenting their stories (manual/signed history) of the pre-Stonewall Riot era (before 1969). Through these interviews, I learned more about the ontological experience of Deaf Queer archivists, who are themselves passionate about the preservation of our history and knowledge that is often neglected in publications.

Figure 9.4. shows several journal articles from Renteria's archival collection. The "Coming Together Newsletter" (CTN) was, as Renteria described it, "the first known, independent national newsletter published by, for and about the Deaf LGBTQ community at large beginning in 1991." The photograph here, provided by Klein, shows the first yearbook photograph (Figure 9.5) of the 1987 "Lambda Society at Gallaudet University" (LSGU, the former name of the gay student club) from 1987. The image reads, "The Lambda Society of Gallaudet University was established in 1984 after a ten-year struggle for recognition from the Student Body Government." The news of the first Queer-identified president of Gallaudet University, Roberta "Bobbi" Cordano in 2016 demonstrates the gradual acceptance of those with Queer identities over four decades at Gallaudet University.

The answers on of the interview questions, "Can you describe your struggle as an archivist/historian?" indicate the difficulty of elicitation and organization of massive amounts of historical information and artifacts. Klein noticed the hesitation of her research informants to share full stories or longer version of stories. She had to ask the right questions to elicit more elaborated stories or to find more participants willing to reveal extremely personal stories. It took time to build trust; hence, her project of ethnohistory is a prolonged process of documenting stories

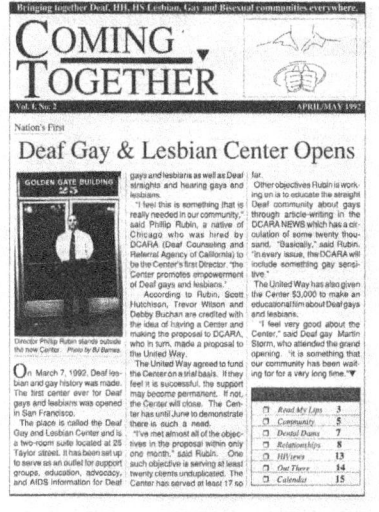

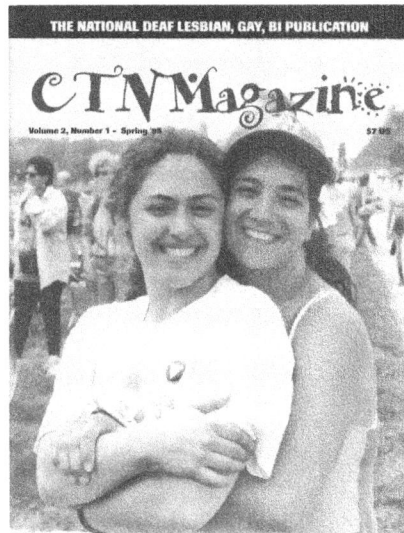

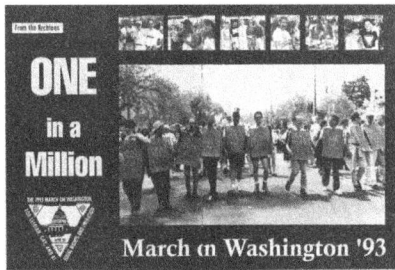

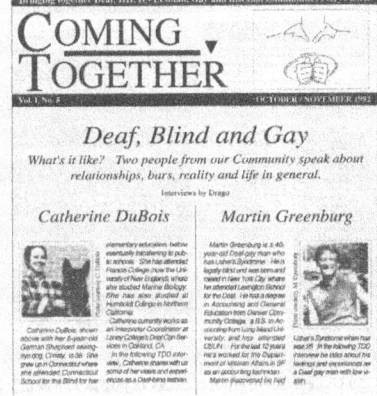

Figure 9.4 Scanned documents from National Deaf LGBT Archives; all came from the journals of Coming Together Newsletter (CTN). (Images courtesy of Dragonsani Renteria.)

over time and continued correspondence with those participants. My interpretation is that this reluctance to share their stories is possibly caused by the participants not having expected the interest in their historical narratives and life stories and the dedication to collect these. This investment contrasts with the usual neglect of the existence of their Deaf lesbian identities and histories.

Renteria stated: "I collect materials of all kinds relating to our community (T-shirts, flyers, art, books, newsletters, buttons, etc.) and often conduct [videotaped] interviews with community members [about their

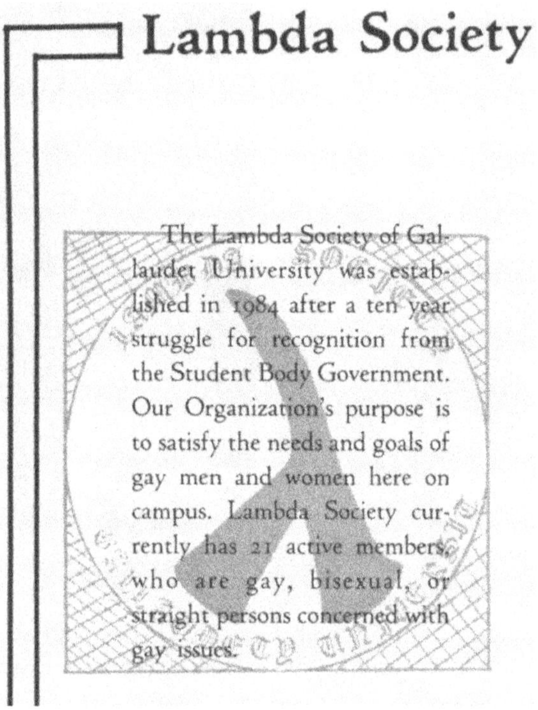

Lambda Society

The Lambda Society of Gallaudet University was established in 1984 after a ten year struggle for recognition from the Student Body Government. Our Organization's purpose is to satisfy the needs and goals of gay men and women here on campus. Lambda Society currently has 21 active members, who are gay, bisexual, or straight persons concerned with gay issues.

Figure 9.5 A cropped image of the statement about Lambda Society of Gallaudet University from the university yearbook, 1987. (Image courtesy of Bridget Klein.)

personal stories]." Accordingly, this trailblazer voluntarily founded his independent project, the "National Deaf LGBT Archives" (NDLGBTA) in 1994, which is now stored at his property. While he was Director of the Deaf Gay and Lesbian Center in San Francisco from 1992 to 1995, he created a temporary public display of the archives at that center. He also founded the Deaf Queer Resource Center (deafqueer.org), a website that provides coming-out stories in ASL, among other resources. It previously published FLASH, an e-zine (sent out through e-mail only) composed by Deaf Queer folks, which covered current events, news, and opinions. From his description of his assemblage of archival materials, they are currently "unprocessed collections," that are undocumented or unreported entries. Another technical term that refers to such inaccessible, "untapped knowledge" (Yakel 2005) is "hidden collections,"[18] which form a "scholarly barrier" (Jones 2002) that prevents researchers

---

[18] My gratitude goes to Dr. Octavian Robinson and Dr. K. J. Rawson for their historical expertise and suggestion for "hidden archives" as an appropriate technical term for archivists and librarians.

from gathering more information about the history of certain groups, which may shed light on these groups' current situations. Unfortunately, NDLGBTA is currently closed to public access due to lack of funds and inadequate staff assistance, which is frequently the case for such hidden collections. I hope that in the near future, studies on Deaf Queer will become more widely undertaken and shift away from "frozen epistemology," once Klein's hidden archives and Renteria's unprocessed collections acquire the necessary support, making these valuable archives accessible, by either digital or analog means.

The question of what impelled them both to document the life stories of Deaf Queer elicited the following response from Renteria: "With the advent of AIDS in the 80s, I especially felt this undertaking was paramount. We were losing people left and right, and with them parts of our history." This parallels Klein's urgency documenting elderly lesbians' life stories. She felt that there is a "scarcity" of representation of Deaf lesbians within literature in general. There are adequate numbers of published resources for each, Deaf and lesbian, as separate identities, but none bring them together with an intersectional focus.

There are many untold stories and undocumented difficulties that elderly lesbians went through during the pre-Stonewall Riot era. From Klein's key interviews, she shared this anecdote that illustrates the hardship of managing a secret lesbian identity at a Deaf workplace (paraphrased here):

> "ONE WOMAN FINISH EXPERIENCE SELF HESITATIVE #JOB WORK (at Deaf institute) ONE-TIME LIKE+++ ONE WOMAN (but) CANNOT TELL-HER I LIKE HER. CANNOT. BACK-OFF (Acting nonchalantly) AT BAR ENTHUSIASTIC-CHAT AHHH (5-wiggling-fingers, thumb-touching-chest) (but) AT-WORK... CANNOT INFORM-HER "YES I A-M ONE. Ah, YES." CANNOT! (If) SHE-INFORM ME (outing herself) "Okay." TELL? (No,) CONFIDENCE! Oooh (wrist flicking)." (Bridget Klein, signed in ASL on a video-interview, 2015)

In a rough translation of this signed quote, Klein narrated that one woman would not reveal her true lesbian identity at a Deaf institute, regardless of her adoration of her co-worker, and not even when others outed themselves to her. The only place that this closeted lesbian would shed her work persona and be her lesbian self was at bar scenes. Klein emphasized the value of their rich experience and stories of adversity, which she found exceptionally significant as authentic evidence about our past as Deaf lesbian communities.

Renteria remarks on why the reason for researching on past publication of the identity of Deaf Queer communities has been difficult: "Hearing queer historians and Deaf straight historians have often deemed us unworthy of inclusion in their history books." In addition, he saw "virtually no published literature produced by Deaf LGBTQ

People of Color." It is erroneous to believe that categorizing them by a single identity that excludes their other overlapping identities will suffice. Often, hearing Queer and white Deaf Queer people were guilty of doing so to Intersectional Deaf Queer people (such as Deaf Queer People of Color or Deaf-Disabled Queer people). Crenshaw's historical example of intersectionality being stuck in a legal loophole, being ignored by the two separate categories of sex and race, is an accurate appelation to describe the Deaf Queer People of Color experience, being denied recognition of their multiple identities. When we further marginalize an identity of a group, we miss out on learning opportunities based on these groups' own perspectives, which are shaped by their unique life experiences. Borrowing from Sandahl's "cripping" practice, Klein's signed histories and Renteria's archival materials essentially "crip" the history of Deaf Queer people, given that the archives can become a repository available for the "public display of sexualized bodily difference and the process of bearing witness to past and present injustice" (2003:28). Both of these archivists/historians are unsung pioneers who vigilantly preserve our histories, so we will remember what our communities have experienced in the past.

CONCLUSION—WE ARE NOT ALONE

Is crip theory adequate for framing an interdisciplinary approach to Deaf Studies and Queer Studies? Ultimately, the Deaf Queer authors and poets' ontological experiences, expressed in textual and visual literature, build a stronger sense of belonging for Deaf Queer readers in their communities. Luczak's collected contributions from a diverse range of people cover themes such as language barriers, sexual identities, and class and family crises. Galloway documented her revealing journey as a crip activist who became a theatrical star. Valli's poem exposed the raw deal, without sugarcoating, of the AIDS epidemic, which deeply affected the Deaf gay community in America in the 1980s and 1990s. To crip Deaf/ASL literature, I have elaborated the framework of both Critical Disability and Queer Studies by examining the authors' perspectives and life experiences. Indeed, the cripping of the selected textual and visual literature is evident as each author negotiates Deaf, Queer, and racial identity. Thus, I am deeming crip theory suitable for centering and mobilizing a future literary genre for and by Intersectional Deaf Queer people.

In this book chapter, I discussed several works, although in a piecemeal fashion, produced by authors from diverse racial and sexual backgrounds such as gay, lesbian, transgender, Black, and Latino. The insufficient representation of bisexual Deaf authors here is noted and needs to be investigated further. There is still inadequate published work that concentrates on varying intersectional backgrounds of Deaf-Disabled and Deaf-Blind people within Deaf Studies and in Deaf Queer literature overall, besides a brief description of intersecting white, Queer, and Deaf-Disabled identities written by Meredith Burke (Ruiz-Williams et al. 2015). Burke affirmed that she primarily focused on her Deaf-Disabled identity and not on her queerness because the significant purpose of her article was to emphasize the lack of support for Disabled students at Gallaudet University (personal communication, 2016). Ruiz-Williams et al. (2015) reveal the inadequacy and the need to explore further the complexities of negotiating Deaf-Disabled Queer identity against the backdrop of heteronormativity. Other valuable unexplored topics are, just to name a few: Deaf Queer parenting (i.e., adoption or in vitro fertilization), Deaf Queer artists, cross-cultural and cross-linguistic relationships of Deaf and hearing Queer partners, Deaf Queer visibility in media, linguistic study of Deaf Queer language use, and geographic study on urban Deaf Queer as compared with rural Deaf Queer populations and their mobility.

Each piece of literature described in this paper provided a small glimpse into the lives of Deaf Queer people. The two interviewed archivists agreed with the scarcity of our representation within the literature, which prompts the questions about our significance and visibility in dominant spoken-English hearing Queer communities and within Deaf Studies. The first published book by a Deaf Queer author, which Klein, Renteria, and myself could recall, was "*Eyes of Desire.*" This pioneering book formed a part of the mere 4% of Deaf-Queer-authored texts out of all Deaf-authored books at the Gallaudet University library. This indicates the importance and effective impact that the limited availability of Deaf Queer "survival" literature has on us, as readers and scholars, seeking any published validation of our existence. Reading Galloway's book, a first of its kind as a full-fledged autobiography of a Deaf Queer person, unlike the anthology, partially filled some of the voids I feel in my experience as an intersectionally Black, Deaf Queer woman. I know I am not alone in feeling this way, so I look forward to more works of "Pablo," Dragonsani Renteria, and other Queer-identified People of Color in both academic literature and creative textual and visual literature. With this chapter, I aim to contribute to an emergent multidisciplinary critical study on Deaf Queer identities and people. Indeed, Renteria struck a chord about our duty as scholars to record the existence of our people: "After realizing that both Deaf history books and LGBTQ history books were not documenting our history, I made a commitment to begin doing so." If we do not, who will do it and value our lives?

Heartfelt gratitude goes to my support system for making this paper a part of Deaf Queer scholarship: Paola Morales, Awet Moges, Lina Chao,

Michele Friedner, all three of my editors, both interviewees, Bridget Klein and Drago Renteria (who abhors doing interviews!), and all Deaf Queer prominent figures I have corresponded with (Jade Bryan, Meredith Burke, Ella Mae Lentz, and Raymond Luczak). Without you all, this chapter would never have happened. Nevertheless, the responsibility is mine for any error reflecting on people or identities mentioned from our Intersectional Deaf Queer communities.

REFERENCES

Baynton, D. (2008). Beyond culture: Deaf Studies and the Deaf Body. In H-D. Bauman (Ed.), *Open your eyes: Deaf Studies talking* (pp. 293–313). Minneapolis: University of Minnesota Press.

Bienvenu, M. J. (2008). Deaf as Queer: Intersections. In H-D. Bauman (Ed.), *Open your eyes: Deaf Studies talking* (pp. 264–273). Minneapolis: University of Minnesota Press.

Cho, S., Crenshaw, K. W., & McCall, L. (2013). Toward a field of intersectionality studies: Theory, applications, and praxis. *Signs: Journal of Women in Culture and Society, 38*(4), 785–810.

Cohen, C. J. (1997). Punks, bulldaggers, and welfare queens: The radical potential of Queer politics? *GLQ: A Journal of Lesbian and Gay Studies, 3*, 437–465.

Crenshaw, K. W. (1989). Demarginalizing the intersection of race and sex: A Black feminist critique of antidiscrimination doctrine, feminist theory and antiracist politics. *University of Chicago Legal Forum*. Volume 1989, Issue 1 Article 8, pp. 139–167.

Crenshaw, K. W. (1991). Mapping the margins: Intersectionality, identity politics, and violence against women of color. *Stanford Law Review, 43*(6), 1241–1299.

Davidson, M. (2008). Tree tangled in tree: Re-siting poetry through ASL. In K. A. Lindgren, D. DeLuca, & D. J. Napoli (Eds.), *Signs & voices: Deaf culture, identity, language, and arts* (pp. 177–188). Washington, DC: Gallaudet University Press.

Dirlik, A. (2002). Literature/Identity: Transnationalism, Narrative and Representation. *Review of Education, Pedagogy, and Cultural Studies, 24*(3), 209–234.

Galloway, T. (2009). *Mean Little deaf Queer: A memoir*. Boston, MA: Beacon Press.

Garland-Thomson, R. (1997). *Extraordinary bodies: Figuring physical disability in American culture and literature*. New York: Columbia University Press.

Halberstam, J. (2005). *In a Queer time and place: Transgender bodies, subcultural lives*. New York: NYU Press.

Harmon, K. (2010). Deaf matters: Compulsory hearing and ability trouble. In S. Burch & A. Kafer (Eds.), *Deaf and Disability Studies: Interdisciplinary Perspectives* (pp. 31–47). Washington, DC: Gallaudet University Press.

Humphries, T. (1975). *Audism: The making of a word*. Unpublished essay.

Jones, B. M. (2002). Hidden collections, scholarly barriers: Creating access to unprocessed special collections (White Paper). Association of Research Libraries Task Force on Special Collections, November.

Kafer, A. (2013). *Feminist, Queer, Crip*. Bloomington: Indiana University Press.

Keller, Y. (2005). 'Was It Right to Love Her Brother's Wife So Passionately?': Lesbian pulp novels and U.S. lesbian identity, 1950–1965. *American Quarterly, 57*(2), 385–410.

Kleinfeld, M., & Warner, N. (1997). Lexical Variation in the Deaf Community Relating to Gay, Lesbian, and Bisexual Signs. In A. Livia & K. Hall (Eds.), *Queerly Phrased: Language, gender, and sexuality* (pp. 274–286). New York: Oxford University Press.

Lane, H. (1992). *Mask of benevolence: Disabling the Deaf community*. New York: Alfred Knopf.

Luczak, R. (1993). *Eyes of desire: A Deaf Gay and Lesbian reader*. Boston, MA: Alyson Publications.

Luczak, R. (2007). *Eyes of desire 2: A Deaf GLBT reader*. Minneapolis, MN: Handtype Press.

McRuer, R. (2006). *Crip Theory*. New York: New York University Press.

Morgan, R., & Wieringa, S. (2005). *Tommy Boys, Lesbian Men and Ancestral Wives: Female sex practices in Africa*. Johannesburg, South Africa: JACANA Press.

Nestle, J. (1990). The will to remember: The lesbian herstory archives of New York. *Feminist Review*, Number 34, Spring, 86–94.

Neumann, T. (1997). Deaf Identity, Lesbian Identity: Intersections in a Life Narrative. In A. Livia & K. Hall (Eds.), *Queerly Phrased: Language, gender, and sexuality*, (pp. 274–286). New York: Oxford University Press.

Phaneuf, J. (1989). Considerations on Deafness and Homosexuality. *American Annals of the Deaf, 132*(1), 52–55.

Rich, A. (1980). *Compulsory heterosexuality and lesbian existence*. London: Onlywomen Press.

Rose, H. (2006). The poet in the poem in the performance: The relation of body, self, and text in ASL literature. In H-D. Bauman, J. Nelson, & H. Rose (Eds.), *Signing the body poetic* (pp. 130–146). Berkley: University of California Press.

Ruiz-Williams, E., Burke, M., Chong, V.Y., & Chainarong, N. (2015). "My Deaf Is Not Your Deaf": Realizing intersectional realities at Gallaudet University. In A. Kusters & M. Friedner (Eds.), *It's a small world: Deaf world international studies* (pp. 262–273). Washington, DC: Gallaudet University Press.

Sanchez, R. (2015). *Deafening Modernism: Embodied language and visual poetics in American literature*. New York: NYU Press.

Sandahl, C. (2003). Queering the Crip or Cripping the Queer?: Intersections of Queer and Crip identities in solo autobiographical performance. *GLQ: A Journal of Lesbian and Gay Studies, 9*(1–2), 25–56.

Sutton-Spence, R. (2010). Spatial metaphor and expressions of identity in sign language poetry. Online Journal: metaphorik.de 19/2010 http://www.metaphorik.de/sites/www.metaphorik.de/files/journal-pdf/19_2010_sutton-spence.pdf (Accessed September 2015.)

Tehranian, J. (2007). Compulsory Whiteness: Towards a Middle Eastern legal scholarship. *Indiana Law Journal, 82*(1), Article 1, 1–47.

Valli, C. (1995). *ASL Poetry: Selected works of Clayton Valli*. DVD. San Diego, CA: Dawn Pictures.

Warner, M. (1999). *Trouble with normal: Sex, politics, and the ethics of Queer life*. New York: The Free Press.

Yakel, E. (2005). Hidden collections in archives and libraries. *OCLC Systems & Services: International digital library perspectives, 21*(2), 95–99.

Zakarewsky, G. (1979). Patterns of Support Among Gay and Lesbian Deaf Persons. *Sexuality and Disability*, September, 2(3), 178–191.

10

Intergenerational Responsibility in Deaf Pedagogies

Marieke Kusters

Deaf teachers have an additional experience, a deaf experience, that they must pass on. So that the younger generations don't need to experience and pass through the same as the older generations. It has to be different for them. The good experiences can be repeated, but the barriers should not be there. [. . .] Deaf teachers are responsible for that.

Here, a deaf teacher discusses the intergenerational responsibilities of older toward younger deaf generations. During my research on the experiences of deaf teachers in Flanders, the northern Dutch-speaking part of Belgium, it appeared that intergenerational responsibility is their most important incentive to teach deaf children. For their pupils, they try to remove disabling barriers and oppressive practices in education and society and try to transmit positive experiences and attitudes with regard to being deaf. An important connection exists between intergenerational responsibility and "deaf ontologies," a concept central to this book. Indeed, my research demonstrated that deaf teachers feel connected with deaf children because they feel they are *the same* as their pupils. This ontological "sameness" informs their incentive to teach.

Ladd and Gonçalves (2012) observe that research about the experiences, practices, and knowledge of deaf teachers is extremely scarce. Several existing studies primarily focus on one single aspect of deaf pedagogies, such as classroom discourse practices (Smith & Ramsey 2004), but do not holistically connect different aspects to one another (Ladd 2013). In contrast, West (2008), Gonçalves (2010), and Ladd (forthcoming), conducted holistic research projects on the experiences and practices of deaf teachers in the United Kingdom, the United States, and Brazil. Based upon a comparison of these studies, Ladd (2012) identified cross-country, even cross-continent similarities among deaf pedagogies, which he found remarkable, because these practices emerged and existed independently of one another. This led to his hypothesis that there is a universal ontological experience related to being deaf, leading to universal Deaf(hood) pedagogies (Ladd 2013).

The research upon which this chapter is based, undertaken in 2013, focused on the experiences of three active and two former deaf teachers in Flanders, Belgium. The reason for also interviewing former teachers is that only half of the deaf people in Flanders who hold a teaching degree still work in deaf education. Investigating their experiences and (former) positions in deaf schools, I gained insight, among other things, into what workplaces they experienced as (un)supportive or (counter) productive to practicing their intergenerational tasks. As I set out later in this chapter, the findings show important parallels with those of Ladd (forthcoming), West (2008), and Gonçalves (2010). Yet this study is unique in (1) its inclusion of former teachers and (2) its emphasis on intergenerational responsibility.

Going forward, I first give a brief overview of the history of Flemish deaf education and the current situation of deaf teachers in Flanders. After that, I explain my research methods and positionality, including a reflection on anonymity and research ethics. Subsequently, I describe and analyze statements on intergenerational responsibility based on shared ontological experiences. I conclude with some thoughts about deaf pedagogies and, again, some reflections about my position as a deaf researcher.

DEAF TEACHERS: HISTORICAL SITUATION IN BELGIUM AND CURRENT SITUATION IN FLANDERS

In Belgium, from the 15th century to the 18th century, before the establishment of the first public schools for deaf pupils, education for deaf children was organized predominantly by hearing teachers who taught individual deaf pupils of wealthy families. There were exceptions though: A few of those individual teachers were deaf, such as Joseph de Caigny (1750) (Buyens 2005, Scheiris & Raemdonck 2007).

In the 18th and 19th century, many deaf schools in Europe and North America were cofounded by and/or employed deaf people. The cofounders were mostly alumni of the first public deaf school in Paris (1771), or other schools with Parisian influence. The Parisian school used methodical signs, based on the grammar and syntax of spoken French (Andrews & Franklin 1997, Scheiris & Raemdonck 2007). Yet, despite a fully fledged sign language not being the language of instruction, this approach recognized and respected the value of signs in education and the visucentric nature of deaf children. Abbé De L'Epée, the founder of the Parisian school and its method, and his followers, also acknowledged the valuable contribution of deaf adults in the education of deaf children. Successful deaf alumni of the Parisian deaf school became supervisors, teachers, and assistants in this school. At the same time though, in Germany (1778), Samuel Heinicke set up a public deaf school with another approach, which vehemently focused on the development of spoken language and lip-reading (Scheiris & Raemdonck 2007).

In Belgium, the first deaf schools were established in Liège, in Wallonia (the southern French/German-speaking part of Belgium), and in Ghent (Flanders) in 1819 and 1820, by a hearing teacher (Liège) and a canon (Ghent), with the help of Joseph Henrion (Liège) and Louis De Stoop (Ghent), both former pupils of the Parisian deaf school who brought the Parisian method to Belgium. Deaf people were employed as tutors[1] in Flemish deaf schools, allegedly because there were not enough (hearing) teachers or friars available (most Flemish deaf schools are Catholic and in the past, were run by friars) (Buyens 2005, Scheiris & Raemdonck 2007).

The "Second International Congress on the Education of the Deaf," in Milan (1880) was of enormous (symbolic) importance in the history of deaf education. At that conference, a resolution was signed stating that the use of sign languages should be forbidden in deaf education, because only speech should be used as a medium of instruction and communication. Although these resolutions affected deaf education in Flanders, the Flemish deaf schools had different approaches: In some schools sign language was not (immediately) banned, while other schools already adhered to the strictly oral approach even before the conference (Scheiris & Raemdonck 2007).

Worldwide, including in Flanders, deaf teachers were fired or were not replaced after their retirement. Baynton (1996) cited one teacher: "to make the deaf teach the deaf is but to undo our work" (Yale 1883, as cited in Baynton 1996:60). Deaf activists in Belgium were critical of hearing teachers who replaced deaf teachers: They were said to lack the skills necessary to teach deaf pupils and to lack knowledge about what it meant to be deaf. Moreover, deaf teachers represented the Belgian deaf community in the educational system, defending the community's points of view on deaf education. Most deaf adults were strong opponents of the strictly oral education system. The prevailing viewpoint was that speech lessons are not problematic in themselves, but banning sign language is. The sheer amount of time and effort invested in speech training came at the cost of a broader education, hindering successful integration in wider society rather than stimulating it. Lack of access to sign language also compromised participation in the deaf community, resulting in isolation and lack of information (Scheiris & Raemdonck 2007).

At international conferences for deaf education, deaf delegates were not treated as sources of expertise or as equal conversation partners.

---

[1] Buyens (2005) and Scheiris and Raemdonck (2007) use the Dutch word "studiementor," which refers to a person assisting pupils with studying.

Deaf professionals in Belgium began to organize conferences themselves, thus claiming their right to speak out about, and advocate for, themes that concern deaf people, including education. In these conferences, community leaders argued for deaf teachers to be re-employed in the deaf schools. Their voices did not gain enough political support, however, to lead to the changes they desired. Sign language no longer had a place in Belgian deaf education (Scheiris & Raemdonck 2007, Van Herreweghe, De Meulder & Vermeerbergen 2015). During the following century, deaf education in Belgium mainly was characterized by the use of the oral method (Van Herreweghe, De Meulder & Vermeerbergen 2015).

Later, in the 1980s, when there was a growing acknowledgment of the fact that the oral method was only partially successful, signing was reintroduced into methods of teaching, yet learning Dutch remained the priority (Van Herreweghe & Vermeerbergen 1998). In practice, a widespread method of instruction was "Nederlands met Gebaren" (Signed Dutch), using signs with the syntax and grammar of spoken Dutch (Van Herreweghe & De Maere 1998, in De Meulder et al. 2008). By way of exception to these approaches, in September 1996, the first Flemish bilingual–bicultural deaf education program was implemented in a special education setting in Kasterlinden, Sint-Agatha-Berchem (Brussels metropolitan area). The founders of this education program believed it crucial to employ deaf teachers, with Flemish Sign Language (VGT) as their first language, as bilingual–bicultural role models to the children. Because there were not enough qualified deaf teachers at the time, the program employed deaf classroom assistants (Antoons 2012), who focused on teaching VGT and Deaf Culture, and on using and learning visual communication strategies in the classroom.[2]

Things continued to change slowly: According to a report of Flemish deaf schools in 2005, each school then used a spectrum of various communication media and languages of instruction (De Meulder et al. 2008). In some schools, the spectrum only recently had widened to include VGT. The vision statements on the websites of the schools apprise viewers as to the extent to which the schools expect their teachers to learn VGT. In Flanders, no specialized deaf education training program exists, thus teachers are not specifically trained to teach deaf children. Most deaf schools require their teachers to learn VGT, but most teachers have poor signing skills. Schools typically do not (frequently) assess teachers' VGT skills, in advance of hiring them or during their employment. In each of the seven deaf schools in Flanders, the subjects Deaf Culture (including themes such as Deaf history, Deaf community events, Deaf Art) and VGT mostly are offered as isolated

---

[2] www.kasterlinden.be/gehoor

subjects and not broadly implemented across the curricula and school culture (De Meulder et al. 2008).

To this day, there are few deaf employees in Flemish deaf schools. Regular teacher training programs in higher education were (and still are) not fully accessible for deaf people due to a lack of competent sign language interpreters and a lack of governmental funding to finance these interpreters. Also, deaf students are part of a cultural–linguistic minority while the teacher-training program is designed by and for hearing majority students (Andrews & Franklin 1997). This means the curriculum, exams, and tests are not adapted to any specific linguistic and cultural needs of deaf students, leading them to experience barriers in obtaining teaching qualifications. Yet, after the turn of the millennium, a number of Flemish deaf persons obtained bachelor's-level teaching degrees.

In 2016, five of the seven Flemish deaf schools had a total of 18 deaf teaching staff among them. Kasterlinden, with its bilingual–bicultural education philosophy, proves the exception with 11 deaf employees, although only one of them has his or her own classroom. Three other schools have two deaf employees each and one has one deaf employee. Of those eighteen, six have teaching degrees, including two with a degree for teaching a vocation (such as welding). One has a degree for teaching preschoolers (aged two and a half to six years); two of them have a degree for teaching in primary school (ages six to twelve years) (but one of them actually works in secondary school), and one acquired a degree while doing an internship in the secondary school (ages 12 to 18 years) where she already worked. Three of them became teachers responsible for their own classroom and five of them teach general courses such as mathematics or history. The roles of deaf employees who do not hold a teaching degree vary and mostly consist of working as teachers' assistants, tutoring deaf pupils in mainstream education, and teaching the subjects Deaf Culture and/or VGT.

In 2013, when I conducted my research, there were four qualified active teachers (not including the teachers who taught a vocation) and four qualified former teachers. Thus, while there are only a few deaf teachers with teaching degrees, still, only half of this group is currently teaching deaf children. The reasons for this are expanded upon later in this chapter.

METHODOLOGY AND ETHICS

The research described in this chapter was conducted in 2013 and focused on how five qualified deaf teachers experienced their educational practices, their responsibilities, their role in deaf education as a whole, and their personal and professional relationship with pupils, parents, colleagues, and principals. A comparison of deaf and hearing

teachers' didactic methods was not part of the study, although participants inevitably compared themselves with hearing teachers and associated differences between deaf and hearing teachers with the existence
of deaf ontologies.

Three participants were employed as teachers (with their own classroom), while two were not employed as teachers any longer (and never
had their own classroom). Thus, I identified teachers' motives not only
for starting and continuing to teach, but also for quitting. As I will set
out later in this chapter, former teachers quit teaching because they felt
they could no longer carry out the intergenerational responsibilities to
which they felt committed.

I used purposive sampling to select the research participants, meaning I chose to include those teachers from whom I thought I would gain
the richest and most relevant data. All the participants use Flemish Sign
Language as their first language, but they had diverse backgrounds as
regards having deaf or hearing parents and the rate of exposure to sign
language when growing up. All seven Flemish deaf schools were represented in the scope of the research, in the sense of (former) teachers
having been employed or having done internships or volunteering.

My research design consisted of three parts: (1) a one-week (video/
written) diary kept by the three active teachers; (2) observation of their
teaching practices, meetings, and playground supervision (amounting
to approximately one full day per participant); and (3) in-depth semistructured interviews (one and a half to two and a half hours in duration)
with all five participants. Obviously, the former teachers looked at their
experiences retrospectively and, thus, from a certain distance, while the
active teachers were right in the middle of it. It became apparent that
emotions, views, or facts from the past can be transformed when talking about them in the present (Baarda et al. 1996).

RESEARCHER'S POSITIONALITY

As a deaf researcher, I believe it is relevant to make explicit how being
deaf impacted on my researching deaf-related issues. In both my personal and professional life, I am familiar with the topic of deaf education. I attended school in a special education setting for deaf children
from the time I was two and a half years old until I was mainstreamed
into regular education at the age of nine. I had very few encounters
with deaf adults in my leisure time and none in the schools I attended.
After finishing my Bachelor of Socio-Educational Care Work, I obtained
a Master of Science in Educational Studies, major Special Education.
I have work experience (including internships) in deaf schools and
dormitories as a Deaf Culture teacher, a dormitory supervisor, and
an educationist/pedagogue. In these positions, I exchanged experiences, concerns, ideas, opinions, insights, and knowledge about deaf

education with deaf teachers, deaf dormitory supervisors, and deaf persons in leadership functions. Their narratives often were loaded with frustration and dissatisfaction and informed my incentive for undertaking this research. With this research, I aimed to stimulate schools, hearing staff, parents, the Flemish deaf community, and deaf teachers to acknowledge, recognize, and respect the shared ontology of deaf teachers and their pupils. Thus, I have feelings of intergenerational responsibility toward deaf children in common with the teachers in this study, even though I am not a teacher myself. Instead, I want to contribute to improving the educational conditions for deaf children through my research.

The fact that the participants already knew me and my educational background possibly contributed to willingness and trust on their part. One participant commented: "It would have been different if you were hearing, because then I would have to explain everything all over. But you are deaf. You already know the basis. That's easier, and we can talk more in depth." Shared deaf ontologies were thus experienced as stimulating by the research participant. Yet, the assumption that we shared knowledge about these themes also meant that deaf teachers did not elaborate on certain important themes. For example, none of the deaf teachers explained why they thought Flemish Sign Language is important in education for deaf children. We should not readily assume that deaf researchers hold the same understanding of those matters as their research participants.

ETHICS: TO ANONYMIZE OR NOT?

Consent forms were in Dutch and explained in VGT to the deaf research participants. The principals of the schools where I observed also signed an informed consent form. A challenge arose when discussing the issue of anonymity with the participants, because there were different preferences. The two former teachers' concerns were related to the principals and the staff of the deaf schools where they were employed in the past. Indeed, both teachers quit mostly because they were not happy with prevailing norms and values in the schools where they worked. One of them wished to remain anonymous, because of not wanting to be held responsible for naming and shaming the school. The other wanted to be recognized by her former supervisor and former colleagues, and to name and shame the deaf school they worked in. This deaf former teacher expressed strong feelings of intergenerational responsibility toward the children in this school. For the most part, the three active teachers agreed with the prevailing norms and values of the deaf schools where they were employed. One of them did not mind being recognized by the principal and staff of the school, but did not want to be recognized by the Flemish deaf community, probably because in the research they had commented about other deaf teachers or deaf teacher's assistants. The two other teachers did not have specific wishes with regard to being recognizable to either the deaf community or the deaf schools.

I thus faced a dilemma between protecting the teachers who did not want to be identified and complying with the desire of the former teacher to be identified. Bachrach and Botwinick (1992:138, in Nespor 2000:561) state "An organization or institution should be considered public if its decisions and nondecisions, and indeed, its very existence, has a significant impact upon the life of the community in which it is located." Deaf schools have a noticeable impact upon the Flemish deaf community, and anonymity of the teachers and the schools could mean that my research would not lead to conceivable impact on the schools. In the end, I decided to anonymize all the participants, prioritizing the protection of the privacy of the two teachers who wished not to be identified. Because the group of qualified teachers is very small, identifying one teacher could easily result in unintentionally identifying the other teachers who wished to remain anonymous. Yet, by choosing to adopt a proactive dissemination strategy for this study, rather than choosing to identify individual teachers and schools (see discussion further on), I allow this research to have a (small) impact on deaf education in Flanders.

DEAF ONTOLOGIES AND FEELINGS OF SAMENESS

"I think they thought: 'Finally! We're both deaf: I'm deaf and the teacher is deaf'. [. . .] I think they felt like recognition, like, 'oh, a deaf person, the same!'"

Here, a deaf teacher narrated that it was quite a relief for deaf pupils when they (the teachers) arrived at the school where they taught. This shared ontological experience of being deaf, often signed as "DEAF-SAME," is "grounded in experiential ways of being in the world as deaf people with (what are assumed) to be shared sensorial, social, and moral experiences: it is both a sentiment and a discourse." (Kusters & Friedner 2015:x). As I set out in this section, this sameness is central to how deaf teachers experience their relationships with their deaf pupils.

Deaf teachers themselves feel their predominantly visual–tactile experience of the world is central to their nature, and they believe they share this with deaf pupils. Accordingly, they apply (be it consciously or unconsciously) visual–tactile-centered attention-getting techniques, teaching methods, and communication practices when engaging with pupils:

> I felt it was natural to wave at the children, and if I had their attention, I started. . . [. . .] I saw what hearing [teachers] do, they called

the children more heavily, tapped them individually [on the shoulders], were more stressed and said: "look at me, look at me!" It should happen automatically: asking for their [students'] attention, to look and wait, and when having everyone's attention, start signing. Just in a calm way ... [...] Sometimes a pupil said [impatiently]: "Come on, start signing!" Then I said: "I can't start. I have to wait till the other pupils look at me. Then I will start. If you find this troublesome, you can let him know the course is starting. This way, you can cooperate with me". [...] I'm deaf myself, I knew, I felt I need to do it this way ... It's natural ...

In addition to their visual–tactile disposition, deaf teachers and deaf children have similar experiences with regard to social life in wider society, such as with regard to barriers to communication and information.

Deaf teachers had the impression that deaf pupils seek contact with them more often than with hearing teachers. They evaluated and compared the quality of deaf–hearing and deaf–deaf pupil-teacher relationships and identified differences based on shared deaf ontologies: "I think I can understand the pupils better, because we passed through the same things." Examples include communication difficulties at home with family, feeling lonely in hearing environments, and building a healthy deaf identity by encountering deaf peers and role models. One teacher said: "I'm deaf and the child is deaf, too. A hearing person has a different life and grew up a different way. I can understand how the child develops." West (2008, 2011) also identified this ontological bond between deaf teachers and pupils.

In addition to these instances of *sameness* in experience, the *intergenerational difference* between deaf teachers and pupils was important. A first example linked to this age difference is teachers' use of authority: Facing a deaf teacher, deaf pupils cannot readily use being deaf as an excuse to escape duties such as doing homework. This was confirmed after presenting my research to a group of hearing people who attended a VGT course where I was a guest lecturer. A hearing teacher of the deaf commented: "If we move from one classroom to the other, deaf pupils walk slowly, signing all the time, as though they want to delay the start of classes. If I ask them to move faster, because class is starting again, they say: 'Oh, you don't understand, it's deaf culture, we deaf people move slower, because we sign.' It's different with a deaf teacher, pupils do listen to them." So, this hearing teacher observed that in certain contexts, deaf pupils resisted being disciplined by hearing teachers, using "deaf culture" as an argument to distance themselves from hearing teachers' authority, but they accepted being disciplined by deaf teachers.

Another instance wherein the generational difference between deaf teachers and pupils is important is when deaf teachers serve as role models to deaf pupils. In such cases, they are deaf adults in professional positions. This is important not only for students, but also for their mostly hearing parents, who realize what their child could achieve. Moreover, a teacher noted that some parents recognize the shared ontological experiences of the deaf teacher and their deaf child. One of the participants explained that at teacher–parent meetings, "Hearing teachers sometimes only give very brief accounts about children. Then [hearing] parents sometimes ask me: 'What do you think? You can assess my child better, because you're deaf yourself'."

The participants felt the need to further explore their didactical and pedagogical practices and how deaf ontologies inform their teaching practices. Being DEAF-SAME means more than just sharing similarities: DEAF-SAME constitutes a breeding ground for deaf epistemologies and certain (political) aspirations. This brings us to the next section, which describes what motivates and inspires deaf teachers to teach deaf children. Indeed, feelings of intergenerational responsibility have their roots in this specific ontological bond, characterized by feelings of DEAF-SAME.

THE INCENTIVE OF DEAF TEACHERS TO TEACH DEAF CHILDREN

"I think the most important reason why I chose the teacher training, is that deaf children need a deaf teacher."

Although DEAF-SAME and thus shared ontologies are a central motive for deaf teachers to teach deaf children, there is more to it than sharing "sameness" in educational contexts. Participants identified a number of motives to teach deaf children, which I expand upon in this section: (1) lack of sign language use in deaf schools, (2) low educational attainment levels in deaf schools, (3) historical patterns and events in deaf education, and (4) teachers' personal life histories.

(1) Participants explained that, for quality education, fluent reciprocal communication is needed in sign language. Indeed, in contrast with spoken languages, sign languages are accessible for *all* deaf children because of these languages' visual nature. According to them, the goal of deaf education should be for deaf children to become bilingual–bicultural adults "with a strong deaf identity" (as the teachers expressed it). The lack of sign language skills of staff in deaf schools worried deaf teachers: They observed that hearing teachers can express themselves in VGT to some extent, but did not have sufficient receptive skills and thus do not understand their pupils well.

(2) Impoverished communication in the classroom results in low educational attainment levels. Deaf teachers believed deaf children have the potential and capacity to learn, and because they felt the current education system did not provide opportunities to learn through sign language, they felt responsible to teach deaf children.

(3) Deaf teachers are imbued with the notion that deaf education has been governed by hearing people, which is a pattern they do not want to see repeated or continued.

(4) Participants had had negative personal experiences in deaf education and in mainstream education. None of the teachers received sign bilingual education, nor did they have VGT and Deaf Culture as a subject course, nor were they taught by deaf teachers. They explained that being taught only by hearing people did not chime with their deaf ontology. Deaf teachers who had attended mainstream education looked back with regret on their own social-emotional development during their childhood and adolescence, given that they largely had missed out on encounters with other deaf signers. Those teachers acquired sign language skills as adolescents, through encounters within the Flemish deaf community, of which they became a part.

Based on the connection they feel with deaf children, participants wished for deaf children not to confront the same barriers they had faced, and wished that they would get the opportunity to become part of the Flemish deaf community and learn VGT from an early age. Indeed, according to the participants, the best possible access to information and communication is through VGT; and, being part of the deaf community helps deaf children build a "healthy deaf identity" and provides them with social and cultural capital (see discussion later in this chapter).

ATTEMPTS TOWARD INTERGENERATIONAL CORRECTION

For the teachers included in this research, one of the most powerful motivations to become a teacher was changing deaf education. They attempted to do this by corrective microactions within the deaf schools: (1) challenging or defending school policy, (2) improving frequency and quality of sign language use, and (3) engaging in acts of advocacy aimed at hearing staff members. The extent of deaf teachers' commitment to intergenerational correction depended on the extent to which they observed and experienced injustice in the school where they were employed. Their perspectives were informed not only by their own experiences but also by studying Deaf Studies and sign language studies in adult education courses, by inspiring conversations and encounters within the Flemish deaf community, exchanges with students and colleagues in Flanders or abroad, visits to (bilingual–bicultural) deaf schools or education programs abroad, and encounters with VGT experts.

Challenging or Defending School Policy

The active teachers in my research mostly agreed with the deaf school's general approach and policy. These teachers worked in schools that were probably the most "aware" schools in Flanders. These are the only schools where deaf teachers have their own classrooms and seem to enjoy relatively equal positions as compared to hearing teachers. For some issues, there were divergences among the school's viewpoint, the wishes expressed by the teachers, and the implementation of those wishes in policy and practice. Hence, teachers agreed with some aspects of the policy and disagreed with others. As to the latter, the teachers acknowledged that such disagreements are sometimes caused by practical problems, such as difficulties finding teachers who could sign. Teachers felt a responsibility to convince new colleagues of aspects of the school policy they approved of, and to make sure it was respected and carried out in practice, such as the implementation of the bilingual–bicultural approach.

The policies of the schools where the active teachers worked were quite comparable to each other, although they differed from the policies of the schools where the former teachers had worked. The view of the former teachers fundamentally differed from the policy of the schools in which they were employed, which they experienced as oppressive, normalizing, and patronizing. These schools' approach was dominantly oral and the former teachers were obliged to use spoken language during their Deaf Culture classes. They felt that their colleagues did not understand what it meant to be deaf and experienced a taboo around using VGT. Colleagues did not acknowledge that communication in sign language gives deaf children the best possible access to knowledge. The former teachers' coping mechanism consisted of enacting a discourse different from the school policy.

> I didn't really look at that [the policy]. I somewhat ignored it. I did my own thing [. . .]. Sometimes they said I need to speak and sign [simultaneously], but I didn't do that. I just signed, that's it. Sign language is a real language. They already used spoken language a lot. It [the time that pupils have sign language as language of instruction] was just one hour a week, that's a little, that was all.

> I told them [the pupils] it is OK to, for example, write back and forth with people at a ticket window, and it is also OK to sign [. . .]. Why do you need to speak? [. . .] I actually said the opposite of what the

speech therapist said. [. . .] I taught them that accommodation should be reciprocal. The speech therapist said that [only] the deaf person needed to adapt.

In the end, these teachers failed in their attempts to change current practices in the schools they worked in. One teacher said they had been naive, that change was impossible:

It's an impossible task. Impossible. Can the policy [of the deaf school] change? It's been the same for a hundred years. Can you change that??? Do you really think that??? [tense, frustrated, laughs forcefully]

Both active and former teachers explain that it is very hard for teachers, both deaf and hearing, to carry on teaching while disagreeing with a school's policy. This is how former teachers interpret some hearing teachers' resignations, and how they explain their own.

The active teachers, on the contrary, felt they had gained respect from their hearing colleagues and their supervisors, that they had gradually acquired a valued and valuable position in their school and had obtained space to learn and develop skills and knowledge. Yet, they still felt they needed to watch over the implementation of the VGT aspects of the school policy, to defend the rights, needs, and strengths of deaf children, and to prove that deaf people can be teachers, too, and should have equal footing to hearing teachers regarding responsibilities, qualifications, function, and status. An active teacher described how they had to prove herself in the school: In the beginning, the teacher only taught the subject Deaf Culture, and started teaching without a degree. Later, she acquired a teaching degree and consequently was assigned more subjects to teach and acquired more responsibilities. Throughout the years working at this school, the teacher also had experienced a gradual increase in the trust and respect she experienced from her colleagues.

Improving Frequency and Quality of Sign Language Use

Deaf teachers think it is vital that all teachers consequently sign when there are deaf children around, including when they are in conversation with each other. Deaf pupils always fall short of information about what's happening in the immediate social environment, so deaf schools need to create opportunities for deaf children to learn social, behavioral, and conversational rules by providing linguistic access to conversations that are happening around the children. A teacher explains:

I want to pass on adult norms and values to the children. That means that they [deaf pupils] need to see and learn how agreements are made, how people quarrel—they are allowed to see that, although it depends on which words are used and which topics are talked about.

A deaf teacher told about a discussion about a school trip to a theme park, where hearing colleagues chitchatted all the time with each other, speaking, not signing, and they challenged these colleagues, who responded:

-"But it is easier to just speak."

-"For you, it is easier, but for us, it's not! I'm your colleague; I don't feel good about this, so what about the children? You work here, for the children. This trip is for the children, not for yourselves!"

- "Yes, but . . . even so, we can't sign all day. Whew!"

- "If you're not into this, you should not work here; you better leave this school. If you choose to work here, you also choose to fully engage yourself for VGT!"

Four out of the five participants chose to sign at all times to their hearing colleagues, even when children are not present and even though some of the participants are able to speak clearly. Signing with hearing colleagues was also a way to improve the latter's signing skills, to expand their lexicon, and to enrich their signing with more iconic structures. Highly iconic signing helps deaf pupils understand the subject matter better, for example, through the abundant use of metaphors and impersonations, such as when one teacher explained Hepatitis B to deaf pupils by taking the role of a mean small biting animal that eats the liver. Deaf teachers claimed that for most hearing teachers, acquiring this skill is more challenging than the acquisition of a "frozen" sign language lexicon. Yet, although deaf teachers feel that they and their deaf colleagues (if they have them), are responsible for helping hearing teachers improve their sign language skills, their willingness has its limits. One deaf teacher explained that they were prepared to adapt their style of communicating (e.g., signing slowly and clearly) to hearing teachers who cannot sign yet, but that they would not keep doing this if hearing teachers' signing skills did not improve. One participant paraphrased how they explain that, calmly, to them:

"Children don't have patience, and even I, one day, will have had enough of your clumsy signing. I know it sounds harsh, but I prefer being honest. If your signing doesn't improve, I think you should consider the question of whether you're in the right place here."

Deaf teachers admitted that at times they act more emotional, feeling angry or frustrated, and hence their remarks also can be more harsh and confrontational.

Acts of Advocacy Aimed at Hearing Staff

In some cases, deaf teachers feel responsible for defending the strengths, rights, and needs of deaf children. For example, a deaf teacher told how a school team intended to temporarily send a deaf pupil with a slight intellectual disability and behavioral disorder to a specialized therapeutic institution. The deaf teacher wondered how the pupil would communicate with other people there and was concerned that the problems would escalate because of isolation and misunderstandings. The school team had not considered this important question. The deaf teacher offered alternative solutions, such as adapting the school's expectations toward the pupil. Thus, it happens that while defending deaf children, deaf teachers project their own experiences onto deaf children.

It then depends on the situation, the individual deaf (or hearing) teacher, and the school policy whether the hearing staff accepts such suggestions from deaf teachers. Sometimes hearing teachers' ideas about the place of deaf people in society are radically different from those of deaf teachers; for example, the normalizing approach of hearing teachers (i.e., deaf children should act as hearing as possible) versus the empowering one of deaf teachers (i.e., it is OK for deaf children to communicate differently). The quote mentioned earlier about communicating with hearing people through the ticket window illustrates this. Here, conflicting values emerge: focusing on teaching how to speak (hearing speech therapist) versus how to communicate with hearing people in different ways (deaf teacher). This results in conflicts and disagreements. On the other hand, it also can happen that hearing teachers acknowledge the deaf-related knowledge and experience of deaf teachers. Sometimes the deaf teacher inspires them to modify their own pedagogical practices in order to adapt them better to deaf children. For example, one hearing teacher wanted to adopt a deaf teacher's way of creating visual didactic materials.

TRANSMISSION OF IDEAS OF "HOW TO BE DEAF"

Deaf teachers feel the need to teach deaf children "how to be deaf" in this world, knowledge that is not found in the current curriculum for deaf education, and which I call social and cultural capital. Social and cultural capital are concepts used by Bourdieu (1997) and applied by several other researchers who focus on deaf communities (O'Brien & Emery 2014, Rogers & Young 2011, Wilkens & Hehir 2008). "Cultural capital" refers to, for instance, cultural knowledge and cultural competencies, while "social capital" means, for instance, having social relationships, networks, reciprocity, trust, and shared norms and values. Here, I outline what kind of social and cultural capital deaf teachers intend to transmit to their deaf pupils: (1) navigating and negotiating society as a deaf person; (2) information about deaf clubs, events, and networks; and (3) being deaf as a way of life. These findings corroborate with the cultural holism theory of Ladd and Gonçalves (2012), which states that deaf children become complete and balanced adults when they are educated about the cultural norms and values of the deaf community and about their place in society.

Transmission of such deaf social and cultural capital happens both during regular teaching hours and outside these hours, such as when tidying up the classroom and during playtime. One way to transmit such knowledge is through narratives: stories and examples from deaf teachers' lives and the lives of other deaf people from Flanders and abroad. This concurs with Gonçalves's (in Ladd & Gonçalves 2012) identification of storytelling as a core pedagogical strategy of deaf teachers. Using real-life examples helps deaf children shape ideas of what the life of a deaf adult could look like. Another way of transmitting social and cultural capital is through performance: deaf teachers literally (consciously and unconsciously) perform ways to navigate society and present oneself as a deaf person.

Navigating and Negotiating Society as a Deaf Person

Deaf teachers teach deaf children how to be confident, to maintain a positive self-image ("I can do it!"), to be assertive, to ask for help when necessary, to be helpful toward one another, and to be independent and self-reliant; for example, by using tools and resources such as online search engines (e.g., Google) or a dictionary. Deaf teachers teach and inform deaf children about current news, both in general and in deaf communities, in order for them to have a better understanding of the world in which they live. Deaf teachers also teach deaf children about intercultural communication (Mindess 1999), by explaining general differences in communication and social regulations between deaf communities and Flemish hearing society. One teacher explained that deaf people sometimes ask direct and open questions, in ways that are not always experienced as appropriate by hearing persons. The teacher explained how questions could be formulated in a different way, in order to be able to comply with expectations within majority society.

Deaf teachers suggest strategies for communication with hearing people, such as writing back and forth, using gestures, teaching sign language, and working with sign language interpreters and speech-to-text reporters. A teacher explained, while narrating her own life story, how to communicate in important situations; for example, while getting to know the results of a medical examination at the hospital. "You can use a sign language interpreter," the teacher explained, "but I used pen and paper to write back and forth. It doesn't matter what way you choose to communicate. Most important is that you understand people when they have crucial information for you. Don't be passive if you don't understand." Being a part of the deaf community, the deaf teacher was aware that lots of deaf people lack information, remain timid and passive, and do not assertively ask for clear information and reciprocal communication. Deaf teachers also teach through their own performance: When a hearing colleague who does not know how to sign enters the classroom, they communicate by writing back and forth on the blackboard.

Another example is a situation I witnessed during a school barbecue, where deaf and hearing adults and children were present. A deaf pupil, about seven or eight years of age, asked a deaf teacher's assistant to collect a piece of meat for her.

The teacher's assistant answered, "You can do that yourself."

The girl looked very shy, and the assistant asked "Don't you dare to ask? Why is that?"

"Because he is a hearing person. . . ."

"Well, he won't bite you and will kindly give you a piece of meat if you kindly ask him."

"But he's not able to sign. . . ."

"You can point or do some simple gesturing, like for sausage [demonstrates a way to gesture]."

With an uncertain expression, the pupil slowly slinked off to the man tending the barbecue and returned with the piece of meat she had requested.

"You see, it wasn't that difficult, huh?"

Here, the deaf assistant encouraged the deaf pupil to communicate with "sign-impaired" hearing people, and offered strategies for how to communicate with them.

Deaf teachers also help deaf children realize how they can educate hearing people who are ignorant about deafness. For example, a group of hearing pupils frequently harassed a couple of deaf peers on a deaf–hearing mixed playground. In class, they talked about this with the deaf teacher, and together they concluded that the hearing children lacked knowledge about sign language and about being deaf. The deaf pupils then gave an awareness-raising presentation for an audience of hearing peers about sign language and about what it means to be deaf. The harassment subsequently stopped. Such problem-solving skills are often organized and encouraged by deaf teachers, because teachers know that throughout their lives, deaf children repeatedly will be confronted with incomprehension and ignorance on the part of hearing people.

Information about Deaf Clubs, Events, and Networks

Deaf teachers feel responsible for informing their pupils about deaf events such as World Deaf Day and Deaflympics, activities and camps, deaf clubs, the Flemish deaf association and its work, and well-known deaf role models in Flanders and around the world. In this way, deaf teachers contribute to the (future) social capital of deaf children:

> I want to try to give them the opportunity to meet each other. [...] Then they know that it exists [the deaf community, deaf clubs] and then they can go over there in the future, if they want to.

> I know some deaf people who disappeared. They do not come [to the deaf community]. What do they do? Are they bored? With family, at work, maybe they feel alone, lonely. No, it should not be like this. [I say to them:] Come! Come to the deaf club, to the deaf community. Friends, a network, that's important.

Deaf teachers also transmit cultural capital, such as teaching students about Deaf history, Deaf art, and other deaf-related topics. A teacher said: "I feel I need to give that information, because it's a part of the child, of its life."

Being Deaf as a Way of Life

Deaf teachers want to pass on pride about being deaf and explain the difference between deaf and hearing persons in a positive, rather than a problematic, way. One teacher explained that it is important to have deaf people on earth and that deaf people contribute to the world in particular ways, with their language and culture: "Many hearing people negatively stereotype being deaf. I don't. I want to give them [the deaf pupils] another perspective." This perspective of "being deaf as a way of life" (thus recognizing deaf ontologies) is an important approach for deaf teachers, which they believe should be the dominant approach in deaf schools. One teacher explained that they taught about differences between deaf and hearing people, that both have strengths and weaknesses, and that hearing people are not necessarily better than deaf people.

This perspective is implied in Ladd's Deafhood tenets, wherein sign languages are regarded as a gift for hearing persons, and deaf people are described as global citizens who are models for the rest of society and are present on earth with the intention to manifest these valuable qualities (Ladd 2003). Similarly, Ladd suggests in his cultural holism model that deaf teachers tell their pupils that the biological difference between deaf and hearing can be seen from a positive perspective (i.e., the strength of the visual and tactile senses) (Ladd & Gonçalves 2012). Those ideas also underlie the concept of Deaf Gain (Bauman & Murray 2009).

CONCLUSION

In analyzing intergenerational responsibility of deaf teachers toward deaf children, I am inspired by Hannah Arendt. According to Arendt (1994), the purpose of education is to care for the younger generations and to prepare them for public life and society. Central to this pedagogical relationship is that it is a relationship *between different generations*. According to Arendt, educators have a dual responsibility: They are responsible for the living conditions and the development of the child *and* for the continued existence (and transformation) of the world. This means that the child, a newcomer, should be protected against the world, by being given opportunities to learn to speak and act. It also means that the world should be protected against the child, a stranger: Educators need to represent the world and educate the child about the appropriate way of being in the world.

Deaf teachers do protect the world against the child through the transmission of social and cultural capital and educating them about their visual–tactile strengths and the positive aspects of being deaf. Deaf teachers want the deaf community to continue to exist, particularly for deaf children, corroborating with Tijsseling's (2006) important statement that "Deaf children should not be used for the continuation of the deaf community, but the deaf community should continue to exist for deaf children" (99). At the same time, the teacher protects the child against the world, by attempts to change deaf education and to dismantle barriers and oppressive mechanisms, and by preparing the child to participate in public life as a deaf person. Deaf teachers feel loyalty toward the younger generation, more specifically the *deaf* younger generation. Those feelings of loyalty and responsibility are rooted in shared ontological experiences of being deaf.

If the need to change deaf education were less urgent than it currently is, deaf teachers would have to invest less time in advocacy and in challenging current practices and policies. Consequently, they would be able to invest more time and energy on the transmission of ideas of being deaf and further explore and develop deaf ways of teaching, indeed, develop and nurture deaf pedagogies (Ladd & Gonçalves 2012). The former teachers explained that their oppressive working environment gave them the feeling they could not focus on developing their deaf-specific pedagogical and didactic skills. Even years later, those negative experiences in deaf education still had a personal impact on them: during the retrospective in-depth interviews, lots of frustrations came to the surface.

As a deaf researcher, I feel it is very important to recognize and validate deaf ontologies in pedagogical practice, and thus I feel an urgency to disseminate the research results. I have presented this research in Flanders and in international conferences, for deaf audiences, mixed audiences, and one hearing audience. Mixed audiences of hearing and deaf people actually became deaf-led spaces, where deaf people commented or participated in discussions about the research, and hearing people were merely spectators, even when the majority of the audience was hearing. Typically, after a presentation, deaf teachers, former teachers, teacher's assistants, dormitory supervisors, students on work placements, parents, and deaf professionals who work on deaf/sign language topics in areas other than education, approached me to tell me they recognized the issues at stake. This confirms that the experiences of the five deaf teachers in this research were recognizable beyond their particular contexts. Some deaf people shared their experiences, sought recognition of the work they are doing, or asked my advice about potential research themes.

Furthermore, I am committed to connect my research with activism: I want to contribute to strengthening the network of deaf teachers, teacher's assistants, dormitory supervisors, and other deaf professionals in the field of deaf education, in Flanders and worldwide, for them to share experiences, to feel empowered, and to identify, recognize, and understand their deaf educative practices. I am currently working for the cell advocacy of Fevlado (the Flemish Deaf Association) and focusing on the possible future establishment of a new sign-bilingual school in Flanders. This advocacy, this research, and the dissemination of my research are my ways of contributing to the quality of deaf education and the recognition of deaf ontologies and intergenerational responsibilities in deaf education.

Thus, shared ontologies led to intergenerational responsibility, which appeared to be the incentive of both the active and the former deaf teachers not only to teach, but also to participate in the research, and for myself as the researcher to conduct this research.

REFERENCES

Andrews, J., & Franklin, T. (1996/1997). Why hire deaf teachers? *Texas Journal of Audiology and Speech Pathology, 12*(1), 120–131.

Antoons, I. (2012). Bilinguaal-bicultureel dovenonderwijs in Vlaanderen. In G. De Clerck & R. Pinxten (Eds.), *Gebarentaal zegt alles* (pp. 71–87). Leuven: Acco.

Arendt, H. (1961/1994). De crisis van de opvoeding. In *Tussen verleden en toekomst*. (J. Masschelein & P. Peeters, Trans.). Leuven: Garant.

Baarda, D.B., de Goede, M.P.M., & van der Meer-Middelburg, A.G.E. (1996). *Open interviewen: praktische handleiding voor het voorbereiden en afnemen van open interviews*. Groningen: Stenfert Kroese.

Bauman, D., & Murray, J. (2009). Reframing: From hearing loss to Deaf-Gain. *Deaf Studies Digital Journal, 1* (1).

Baynton, D. (1996). *Forbidden signs: American culture and the campaign against sign language*. Chicago, IL: The University of Chicago Press.

Bourdieu, P. (1997). The forms of capital. In A. H. Halsey, H. Lauder, P. Brown, & A. S. Wells (Eds.), *Education: Culture, economy and society* (pp. 46–58). Oxford, UK: Oxford University Press.

Buyens, M. (2005). *De dove persoon, zijn gebarentaal en het dovenonderwijs.* Antwerpen/Apeldoorn: Garant.

De Meulder, M., Smessaert, I., & Vermeerbergen, M. (2008). Onderwijs aan dove en slechthorende kinderen, jongeren en volwassenen. Onderwijs van Vlaamse Gebarentaal en Dovencultuur. In M. Vermeerbergen & M. Van Herreweghe (Eds.), *Wat (geweest/gewenst) is. Organisaties van en voor doven in Vlaanderen bevraagd over 10 thema's* (pp. 73–140). Gent: Academia Press.

Gonçalves, J. (2010). *The role of Gaucho culture and Deaf pedagogy in rethinking Deaf Education* (Unpublished doctoral dissertation). University of Bristol, Centre for Deaf Studies.

Kusters, A., & Friedner, M. (2015). Introduction: DEAF-SAME and difference in international deaf spaces and encounters. In A. Kusters & M. Friedner (Eds.), *It's a small world: International deaf spaces and encounters.* (pp. ix–xxx) Washington, DC: Gallaudet University Press.

Ladd, P. (2003). *Understanding deaf culture: In search of Deafhood.* Buffalo, NY: Multilingual Matters.

Ladd, P. (2013). A final frontier—Can Deafhood pedagogies revolutionize deaf education? [film].

Ladd, P. (forthcoming). *Seeing through new eyes—Deaf pedagogies and the unrecognised curriculum.*

Ladd, P., & Gonçalves, J.C. (2012). A final frontier? How deaf cultures and deaf pedagogies can revolutionize deaf education. In L. Leeson & M. Vermeerbergen (Eds.), *Working with the deaf community: Deaf education, mental health & interpreting.* Dublin: Interesource Group Ireland.

Mindess, A. (1999). *Reading between the signs: Intercultural communication for sign language interpreters.* Yarmouth: Intercultural Press.

Nespor, J. (2000). Anonymity and place in qualitative inquiry. *Qualitative Inquiry, 6*(4), 546–569.

O'Brien, D., & Emery, S.D. (2014). The role of the intellectual in minority group studies: Reflections on Deaf Studies in social and political contexts. *Qualitative Inquiry, 20*(1), 27–36.

Rogers, K., & Young, A. (2011). Being a deaf role model: Deaf people's experiences of working with families and deaf young people. *Deafness & Education International, 13*(1): 2–16.

Scheiris, I., & Raemdonck, L. (2007). *Ongehoord verleden: dove frontvorming in België aan het begin van de 20ste eeuw.* Gent: Fevlado Diversus vzw.

Smith, D.H., & Ramsey, C. (2004). Classroom discourse practices of a deaf teacher using American Sign Language. *Sign Language Studies, 5*(1), 39–62.

Tijsseling, C. (2006). *Anders doof zijn: een nieuw perspectief op dove kinderen.* Twello: Van Tricht.

Van Herreweghe, M., De Meulder, M., & Vermeerbergen, M. (2015). From erasure to recognition (and back again?): The case of Flemish Sign Language. In M. Marschark & P. E. Spencer (Eds.), *The Oxford handbook of Deaf Studies in language research, policy and practice* (pp. 45–61). Oxford: Oxford University Press.

Van Herreweghe, M., & Vermeerbergen, M. (1998). *Thuishoren in een wereld van gebaren.* Gent: Academia Press.

West, D. (2008). *Deaf children's wisdom (Seeing through new eyes)* (Unpublished work). Centre for Deaf Studies, University of Bristol.

West, D. (2011). "We're the same, I'm deaf, you're deaf, huh!" In G. Mathur & D.J. Napoli (Ed.), *Deaf around the world: The impact of language* (pp. 367–371). West Yorkshire: Oxford University Press.

Wilkens, C.P., & Hehir, T.P. (2008). Deaf education and bridging social capital: A theoretical approach. *American Annals of the Deaf, 153*(3), 275–284.

SECTION III

Ethnographic Methodologies

11

Visual Methods in Deaf Studies: Using Photography and Filmmaking in Research with Deaf People

Dai O'Brien and Annelies Kusters

Deaf people have long claimed a unique corporeality in their experience of the world and one very important example is that many deaf people have a strong visual orientation, which in this chapter we call visucentrism, in opposition to audiocentrism, which refers to the wider society's focus on hearing and speaking (Eckert & Rowley 2013). We argue that, as a result, visual research methods carry a lot of potential for exploring deaf ways of being in the world.

Before we go on, we want to stress that we are aware, and want the reader to be aware, that not all deaf people are visually oriented to an equal or similar extent, or in the same ways. Deafblind people are an important example, including deaf people with Usher Syndrome (which causes reduced peripheral vision and nightblindness), who have other experiences of visuality.[1] In addition to, or instead of the visual orientation, many deaf people are strongly tactically oriented, whether they are sighted or blind (Edwards 2015, Barnett 2015, Napoli 2014). Bahan (2014) summarizes deaf people's corporeality as "visual-tactile orientation." In this chapter, we focus on visual methods rather than methods that engage both the visual and tactile, or only the tactile. We also show how the use of visual methods can be significant in research with deafblind people. We hope that Deaf Studies researchers will experiment more with methodologies that explore how deaf people experience the world through different senses.

---

[1] In her PhD study, Barnett (2015) who is deafblind herself, has used research methods that were designed for, or adapted to, doing research with deafblind people who use hands-on signing (i.e., the deafblind person touches the hands of the signing person) or a reduced visual frame (i.e., signing within certain spatial boundaries so that a deaf person with reduced peripheral vision can perceive what one is signing). Barnett organized "speed dating dyads," in which deaf and deafblind people had 10-minute conversations in pairs.

Originally, within the field of Deaf Studies, visucentrism was thought to be a *sociocultural* feature, which united members of the community and fit into the primacy and value bestowed on sign languages by deaf people. In addition to using *visual languages,* most deaf people are able to use vision when *interpreting* the world by taking note of the behaviors of other people, or animals such as dogs, in order to understand and observe the environment. For example, if a deaf person observes people or dogs looking in a specific direction, he or she can surmise that something is happening in that particular location; or if people suddenly disappear from a train platform a deaf person can surmise, without needing to hear a public address (PA) announcement, that the train is cancelled or will arrive at a different platform. Most deaf people also make use of visual strategies to *engage with* the world: looking back before leaving a room (to make sure nobody needs them, given that they might not hear when they are called by means of voice/noise); informing each other of obstacles in their path when having a signed language conversation while in motion, in which their vision is focused more on each other than on the physical environment; making sure the sightline is clear when sitting at a table (such as removing vases and bottles); and sitting or standing in circles or ovals in order to ensure all conversation partners are in their field of vision (Bahan 2004, Mindess 2006, Sirvage 2009, Hauser et al. 2010).

Recent research into cognition has suggested that deaf people's visucentric way of engaging with the world is *biological* as well as sociocultural, and that deaf people do process visual information in a qualitatively different way to hearing people, with this difference being influenced both by the use of sign languages and the effect of hearing loss (Capek et al. 2010, Cardin et al. 2013). Examples are the development and use of peripheral vision and spatial processing, or the way in which deaf people understand and organize visual information. Bauman and Murray (2014) argued that this unique visuality is an important example of Deaf Gain. Thus, the visucentrism of deaf people is not simply another version of the postmodern visual culture of contemporary Western life (Rose 2012:2–3) but something unique to deaf peoples' corporeal experience of the world.

Researchers in the field of architecture are working to explore and utilize this visual nature and visual experience (e.g., the DeafSpace project in Gallaudet) and make use of features of the deaf experience to inform and influence more mainstream architectural practices to make them more accessible and open to everyone (Bauman 2014, Edwards & Harold 2014). As such, it is long overdue that Deaf Studies researchers try to tap into this visucentric experience of the participants in their research methodologies. Despite the seemingly perfect fit between visual research methods and the deaf experience of the world, remarkably little work has actually utilized these methods (see Thoutenhoofd

2009 and Sutherland & Rogers 2014 for exceptions). This may be because researchers think that, for example, conducting interviews in sign language or analyzing signed poetry is visual per se, and so specific attention to "visual methods" is unnecessary.

Visual research methods are those that use "various kinds of images as ways of answering research questions" (Rose 2012:10), through the production of images by means of photography, drawing, cartography, filmmaking, and so on. These images could be used as stand-alone texts to be analyzed in the research project, or be used to elicit responses from research participants. They could be researcher-produced or participant-produced. Visual research methods have been part of various research disciplines for many years. The field of anthropology, in particular, has a rich history of using photography and video in capturing the lives and customs of its research participants (De Brigard 2003). The use of visual methods (Banks & Zeitlyn 2015), also called visual methodologies (Rose 2012) and visual ethnography (Pink 2013), have enjoyed a surge in popularity in fields such as sociology and cultural studies in recent years, although even in those fields visual research methods have been in use for many decades.

In contemporary Deaf Studies, within the wider influence of what is now considered to be the "contemporary visual culture" or, the way in which "looking practices are engaged in symbolic and communicative activities" in current Western society (Sturken & Cartwright 2009), the time is right (and long overdue) for Deaf Studies to explore further the potential of these methods. This chapter explores and considers what kind of research findings can be gathered when visual methods are used in the field of Deaf Studies and concludes that there should be a greater exploration of such methods in Deaf Studies. We first discuss traditional methods in Deaf Studies, visual methods in other disciplines, and visual methods in Deaf Studies. We then discuss and evaluate two examples of our own research in which we explored the use of visual methods. The first example is O'Brien's use of auto-driven photo-elicitation interviews with young deaf people to explore their experiences of transition from childhood to adulthood in England. The second example is Kusters's use of filmmaking when doing linguistic ethnography in Mumbai. This discussion also considers the question of what happens if Deaf Studies researchers who use visual methods are deaf themselves and thus employ their own visual orientation in their research practice.

"TRADITIONAL" METHODS IN DEAF STUDIES

Traditionally, Deaf Studies has employed methods, principles, and practices that were previously in use in many different fields including education, psychology, and linguistics. The most commonly used methods are both qualitative and/or quantitative: interviews, focus groups, (participant) observation, questionnaires, surveys, and other methods. Methods have been adapted to a greater or lesser extent to try and provide *access* to signing deaf people, such as using written English to supplement spoken English in interviews (Dee 2006) or using sign language interpreters in interviews (Valentine & Skelton 2007). Other researchers have held interviews and focus groups *directly* in sign languages, that is, without the involvement of sign language interpreters.

There are a number of common patterns here. First, because sign languages do not have widely used written versions, for the most part qualitative data gathered in/through sign language ultimately is translated to the written version of a spoken language. Thus, many Deaf Studies scholars record the visual (interviews, poetry, performances, dialogue, etc.) until the point of analysis and/or dissemination: the end product is typically a text in the written version of a spoken language (usually English) with or without accompanying stills and/or DVDs. It is, however, increasingly possible to annotate and analyze pictures and videos directly in qualitative data analysis programs, so sign language data can be annotated and analyzed in such programs without first being translated into a written language. Some notable exceptions to dissemination in written languages have originally been published in, or been translated into, a signed language (see, for example, *Deaf Studies Digital Journal* and *ASLize*, along with Emery 2011), venues of publishing that unfortunately are seen as less prestigious (see Kusters et al, this volume, for a further discussion on this issue).

Second, most research projects in Deaf Studies prioritize *the use of language* in its various modalities: spoken, written, or signed, directly or in translation. A critical concern linked to these methods is that of linguistic competence. In order to express oneself in any language, and/ or understand others, one must possess a degree of linguistic competence in that language. Without this ability for participants to express themselves, any research method that tries to engage with participants through "talk," spoken or signed, is limited. This is particularly important for deaf people. In the United Kingdom and United States (where a lot of Deaf Studies research is undertaken), deaf people lag behind their peers in their comprehension and production of English in both spoken and written forms (Lederberg 2013). Similarly, due (at least in part) to the policy of mainstreaming and cochlear implantation, which discourages the use of sign languages in childhood, many deaf children do not achieve fluency in sign languages at an early age. This means that they lack linguistic competence not only in the spoken/written form of their national languages, but also in the sign languages used by the deaf community. Importantly, this is compounded in countries where deaf people do not have access to formal education or a shared signed language. Also, of course, researchers themselves might have limited linguistic competence in a particular language (e.g., when doing research in another country or with immigrants). This lack can lead to problems in research, where participation relies on the researchers' ability to express their questions and comments clearly; the participants' ability to understand the researchers' questions (in whatever form or modality they are presented); and the participants' ability to articulate their own feelings and opinions. As such, lack of linguistic competence can lead to problems for researchers and participants to understand each other.

Third, as discussed in the introduction to this chapter, traditional Deaf Studies methodologies do not tap into deaf people's visucentrism. We argue in this chapter that neglecting this essential feature of deaf people's ontologies is a failing that should be addressed. Addressing this creates potential for more emancipatory research.

VISUAL RESEARCH METHODS

There is a long history of engagement with photography and video in humanities and social science research. Anthropologists, for example, have used photographs and video since the late 19th century to record particular environments, rituals, and practices for analysis afterward or for display in classrooms (De Brigard 2003, MacDougall 2011). Around the turn of the 21st century, large numbers of social science researchers began to (re)engage with, and develop, visual research methods, viewing them as a vital way to engage with the burgeoning visual culture of the day (Rose 2014).

As mentioned earlier, visual research methods use images (which could be photos, film, artwork, or advertisements, among others) as research resources. These images could be collected or created in many different ways. Pre-made images can be collected and analyzed for research. Such research can include analysis of advertising images, artwork, postcards, television programs, and so on. These images would not be created specifically for the research project in question, but would be collected and sampled for analysis. Other research uses images that the researchers themselves create for the purpose of the project. Images are thus used as prompts to elicit responses from research participants, as ways to record the research process itself, or as ways of recording researchers' own impressions or feelings about the research process. When used as prompts, images can be used to supplement researcher's questions, or they may replace the questions altogether, as when the interviewer simply presents a photograph and asks the participant to "tell me about this image."

The reason for using images in interviews is to build "communication bridges" (Collier & Collier 1986:99) between the interviewer and participant and to ease communication by displacing the focus of the interview from the participant to the photograph in question. In such contexts, the images are thus not analyzed separately (although they could be if required), but used as a "jumping-off point" for the interview to begin. This is not to say that the images themselves are unimportant. They can be used as a window into the worlds of the research participants, to provide an insider's view on their lives. This means that images are not simply used as interview prompts and then put aside, but rather, they play an active part in steering the subsequent interview and the researcher's interpretations of the participants' views. Use of images allows the participants to take control over the interview (Clark 1999:41) and impose their own frames of reference on the researcher (Samuels 2007) in ways that would be very difficult in an interview conducted solely through questions produced by the researcher.

Many such elicitation interviews thus use images that have been made, taken, or selected by the researcher for the purposes of the research. Although this can be an advantage in that the standardization of images acts in the same way as standardization of interview schedules, for example, in that the stimulus is a constant from which varied responses can be compared, this runs a risk of not really getting to the root of the participants' world views. Researchers may capture "visually arresting images," images they find unique or beautiful (Clark-Ibáñez 2007:171), which, while resonating with the researchers themselves, may have no bearing on the lives of the participants. Good examples of this are the many uses of sign languages in television advertisements, music videos, or theater productions. Non-signing people may find the use of sign languages in these contexts to be fascinating and comment-worthy, even reverential, although for many deaf people the perception that this gives is the opposite, one of tokenism or even insult, if the director or writer of the piece has no understanding of deaf cultural practices. On the other hand, of course, such reactions offer insight into deaf people's worldviews.

A third way to use images when eliciting data, one which side-steps this problem, is to engage with participants by letting them create visual material themselves as part of the research process. In these cases, researchers will provide participants with the means to take photographs, produce videos, or create artworks, and they either will provide a script or will give the participants free rein to make/take images of whatever they like. The script could be very detailed, requesting a certain number of images on specific themes, or much less detailed, providing rough guidelines or themes for the participants to follow. The interviews then focus on these images in such a way that both the researchers' and participants' initial interpretations of the images presented can be subject to renegotiation of meaning. The first subjective response of both the participant and researcher goes through a process of co-construction, in which meanings are discussed and shared to come to a fuller understanding of the image being presented.

The latter method has been a very popular approach, because it encourages collaboration between researcher and participant. It often is claimed that this method, in which participants create the images themselves, reduces the power imbalance inherent in the researcher–participant relationship (Rose 2012:306). This sort of collaboration, it is argued, also empowers the participant, which makes it a very popular method in research with oppressed groups. By asking the participant to create something, such as photographs, artworks, or a piece of film footage, the interrogation shifts its focus from the participants themselves to the artifact that they have produced. This change in focus has been argued to have a number of benefits for the research project, not least of which is that the focus on the visual artefact enables the participants themselves to see things through "new eyes." This process allows deaf research participants to impose their own visucentric frames on the research (see Thoutenhoofd 1999). The distancing effect of interrogating a produced object, rather than the participants themselves, can remove barriers of defensiveness, or of reluctance to engage, and can almost "depersonalize" the research to such an extent that a previously defensive participant fully engages and contributes to research. Images also can play an important part in the dissemination of data: rather than (or in addition to) providing written quotes, photographs, artworks, or videos can be published in research reports.

A major advantage of some (but not all) visual research methods is that by focusing on the visual, emphasis is taken away from self-expression through language. Instead, the meanings and information one might want to express are focused in the visual artefacts. Of course, this still assumes that participant and researcher have access, however basic, to a shared language, but having a common frame of reference in the artefact, adds to the common basis the researcher and participant have for creating understanding. This can sidestep, or at least moderate, some of the issues linked to linguistic competence discussed earlier, and makes creative visual methods a favorite in research projects with children and young people, immigrants, and other groups who either might lack linguistic competence or not have a language in common with the researcher (see Clark-Ibáñez 2008, and Clark 1999, for examples).

VISUAL RESEARCH METHODS IN DEAF STUDIES

As mentioned earlier, there have been very few engagements with visual research methods in the field of Deaf Studies. Ironically, Harold (2013) writes in her article on access of deaf people in cities that acknowledging the visual in Deaf Studies research and in deaf ontologies is very important, but this is not reflected in her research methodology, which consisted of audio-recorded interviews and focus groups conducted through an interpreter. Similarly, in the first textbook on methodology in Deaf Studies, Young and Temple (2014) write that recognizing the visual and deaf ontologies is crucial, but they do not explore visual methods in their book. Many Deaf Studies researchers have made abundant use of photography and/or video-recording, (such as Baynton, Gannon & Bergey 2007, in a project on deaf history, and Sutton-Spence's poetry projects [2005]) however they did this predominantly with the aim of analysis of data, documentation, and dissemination rather than elicitation of data.

The earliest example of the use of visual methods in Deaf Studies known to us is Thoutenhoofd's (1996) Sociology and Social Policy PhD study (published as *See Deaf* in 1999) in which he explored what he called the "ocularcentrism" (what we call visucentrism) of the deaf experience. This project used a combination of both researcher-created images (photographs taken by Thoutenhoofd during visits to a Deaf Club) and participant-created images using autophotography to explore the "potential use of photographs in uncovering elements of the particular visual perception shared collectively by Deaf people" (1996:267). Through the use of the researcher-created images, Thoutenhoofd hoped to explore what he termed the "scopic spaces" of the Deaf Club (1999:217), that is, how the collective visual experience of deaf people organizes and structures their use of space. The autophotography element of the project focused on the photographs taken by a group of young deaf people specifically for the project, depicting everyday life experiences for this group. Again, the intention was to explore whether there was an identifiable collective approach to the visual nature of the task by deaf young people. Thoutenhoofd (1998) states that photographs capture some of the visual symbolism in deaf community life: young people asserted their pride of being deaf and sign language. Thus, the use of photography can lead to greater understanding of "the deaf way."

Another, more recent, study to use visual research methods was Sutherland and Roger's study (2014) of the experiences of deaf children. This study took a mixed-methods approach to the research, including use of drawing, video diaries, and photography to explore deaf children's experiences of sign-bilingual education. These visual artefacts were used to stimulate further discussion with the young people and to explore further their feelings and views of their educational experience. They stated that "Research paradigms need to be decentred and visually oriented, to gain a greater understanding of Deaf Gain. (...) in order to capture Deaf people's perspectives and linguistic and cultural characteristics in a positive way" (280).

Both of these studies sought to place the visuality of deaf people in a preeminent position in the research and to prioritize and explore the visual nature of the participants' lives. These studies not only utilized the deaf visucentric experience of the world, but also explored how it affected the ontology and epistemology of deaf people involved in the study.

A few researchers have used video as a participatory research method or within focus groups. For example, in the frame of a small research project, De Clerck created a film ("Wereld doof") with young people who attended a school for the deaf, in which the world was deaf and hearing people were a minority (De Clerck 2009). In a cross-comparative sociological/anthropological project on the acculturation of deaf children in preschools in the United States, Japan, and France, Tobin and Hsueh (2007) used what they called "video-cued multivocal comparative ethnography": using video "neither as data nor as description but instead as rich nonverbal cues designed to stimulate critical reflection" (77–78). The project focused on pedagogy, curriculum, and goals of early childhood education. They video-recorded a day at each preschool, edited it down to 20 minutes, and used this video for reflection in focus groups within the same preschool, other preschools in the country, and preschools in the two other countries in the project. They found that the videos helped them challenge taken-for-granted approaches (Che, Hayashi & Tobin 2007). The videos were afterward produced as an ethnographic film. We will now turn to exploring and evaluating our own experiments with visual methods.

CASE 1: AUTO-DRIVEN PHOTO-ELICITATION IN ENGLAND (DAI O'BRIEN)

This research was undertaken to explore the transitional experiences of young deaf people from childhood to adulthood in England. In undertaking this research, I had a dual focus, looking at both the policy of transition planning created by the UK government, and the impact of this policy on the young people and professionals affected by the policy (O'Brien 2012, 2013, 2015). In order to explore the experiences of the young people who participated in this research, a combination of semistructured interviews and auto-driven photo-elicitation methods were used. The semistructured interviews were used as a way to elicit basic background information about educational experiences, family background, and experiences of transition planning in order to obtain baseline data, which could be compared among the eight participants. The auto-driven photo-elicitation interviews, on the other hand, were used in order to get a more personal and in-depth perspective on their lives, to understand what they felt was important to their transition to adulthood and beyond.

In this project, all the photographs used in the interviews were taken by the participants themselves. The photographs were not only discussed in terms of what the image showed, but also the motivation behind the image and the way it was captured. Along with the information gleaned from the semistructured interview, this discussion of the site of production (Rose 2012) of the image allowed a deeper insight into the participants' intentions and the meanings behind the photograph taken.

Each participant was given instructions about what they should focus on when taking photographs. I left these instructions deliberately vague, asking only that participants take photographs of things and places that were important to them. For reasons of confidentiality, they were asked not to take photographs of people, but some found interesting and creative approaches to challenge this instruction. Of the eight participants who agreed to take part in the photo-elicitation stage of the research, only four actually returned photographs in time for the photo-elicitation interview to be conducted. The reasons for this were varied, from work pressures, to photographs getting lost in the mail. At the time of the fieldwork of the research (2010–2011) smartphones and digital cameras were still considered to be prohibitively expensive for young people. A decision was made to hand out disposable cameras to the participants because it could not be assumed that they would have access to a digital camera, or, indeed, access to the Internet in order to submit their photographs. Some reflections on the importance of the chosen method are presented here.

The Visual Nature of the Research Task

Many of the participants reflected that they were better able to express themselves through the photographs rather than through responses to interview questions. This suggests that they did have a visucentric worldview, that they felt better able to understand and explain the world through their use of photographs than through signed or spoken explanations.

Participants in this research project had a range of linguistic competence in sign language, from basic sign language ability to fluency. The range of ability in spoken English was similarly spread between basic and fluent. Participants generally preferred to express themselves in the language in which they were most fluent, although I found that this did not always guarantee they were easy to understand. For example, some participants chose to speak, even when their speech was not clear. Lip-reading, never an easy task, was thus made even more difficult for me, and equally, those participants sometimes found it difficult to understand my speech. This made some elements of the semistructured interviews quite difficult to conduct, when the meanings of questions and answers were distorted or misinterpreted simply through mutual incomprehension between us, even though I am deaf and consider myself to be fluent in both British Sign Language (BSL) and English. In the photo-elicitation interviews, however, the visual nature of the interviews bypassed this difficulty, with the photographs acting as "clear, tangible prompts" (Clark-Ibáñez 2004:1512) that made communication much easier and clearer between us. This was particularly the case in one interview, which had been markedly difficult at the semistructured interview stage, with continual communication breakdowns and incomprehension on both our parts. The limitations of the semistructured interview had obviously frustrated the participant, and he took the most photographs of any of the participants, resulting in a rich and informative interview. By using the photographs as reference points to provide us each with a shared understanding of the topic under discussion, we were able to communicate much more effectively.

The nature of the photographs taken was also suggestive of a particularly visual worldview. Some of the photographs were of visual decor, such as mosaics of personal photographs on the walls of university dormitory bedrooms, to evoke feelings of home. These deaf young people created these feelings of home by displaying visual mementos such as photographs and postcards that reflected various aspects of their lives. These mosaics constructed visual records to reflect aspects of life important to these young people. Emotional and affective states also were tied into photographs that were taken. One participant took photographs of a sunny day to reflect the feelings of happiness that she felt at a certain stage of her life when she was growing up. Other participants took photographs of magazines and posters. When asked about this, they replied that the photographs represented interest in the visual nature of the media shown in the pictures. This showed their interest in working in graphic design, TV production, and other visual media in the future. It could be argued that, particularly in the contemporary visual culture in which these young people grew up, hearing young people could have taken similar photographs. This is, of course, the case, but the reflections of the research participants show that these young people believed themselves to have a visucentric nature, suggesting more than a simple reflection of mainstream visual culture (Hauser et al. 2010, Bahan 2004, Lane et al. 1996) (Figure 11.1).

Importance of Deaf Identity in Photographs

In many of the photographs that were taken, there was very clear reference to the participants' identification as deaf people. Sometimes this was deliberate, and the participant explained to me that the photographs were intended as a statement of identity. At other times the participants' deaf identity came through in the photographs in an unintended way, revealing itself to us as viewers of the photograph when we interpreted it anew from a different perspective, rather than the

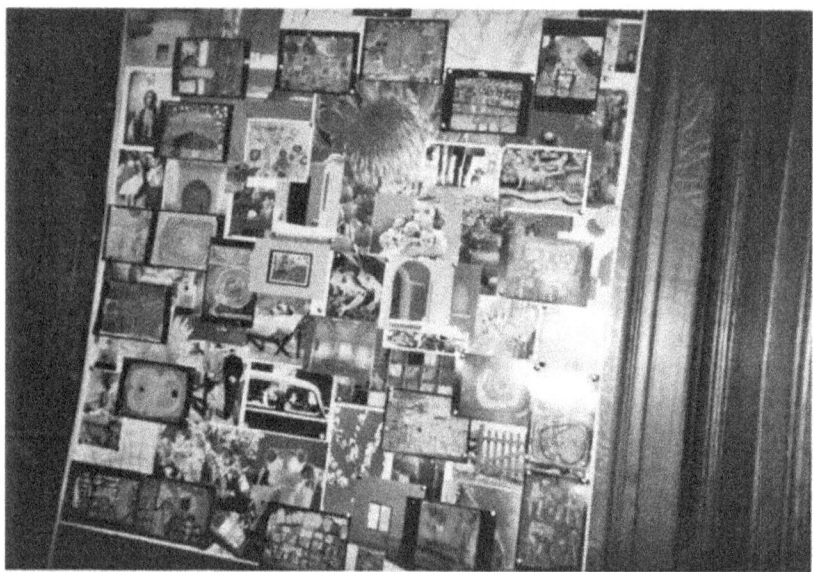

Figure 11.1 *"...a lot of the things that I took are visual things, like photographs and drawings and ... like photos. There's some research saying about deaf people are more visually aware, and I thought that's obvious..."*

meaning the photographer intended when the photograph was taken. One participant took photographs of her BSL interpreter (represented by her shoes in picture two), her English support tutor, and her deaf mentor, all representative of services that were offered to her in university. For her, these were vital parts of her identity as a deaf person. It was interesting that she chose to portray support services, given that these could be interpreted through a deficit view of deafness and that she "needed" these services in university. She was adamant, however, that these pictures showed her pride in her deaf identity as a signing deaf person, resisting the pressures from the hearing world to conform to the spoken monolingual norm. This presentation of meaning, which felt paradoxical to me at the time of the interview, shows the importance of discussion about the meanings of images. My initial response to the photographs was to assume that they showed feelings of barriers, of exclusion from her university course (influenced, no doubt, by my own experience at university). Instead, she explained that having this support was a positive statement of identity; it showed her pride in using BSL in university rather than English. Although the intentions of photographers are often thought to be of little importance in the meaning of the image they capture (Rose 2014:31), the experience I describe shows the risk of misinterpreting these images, especially if meanings are not explicit in the image captured (Figure 11.2).

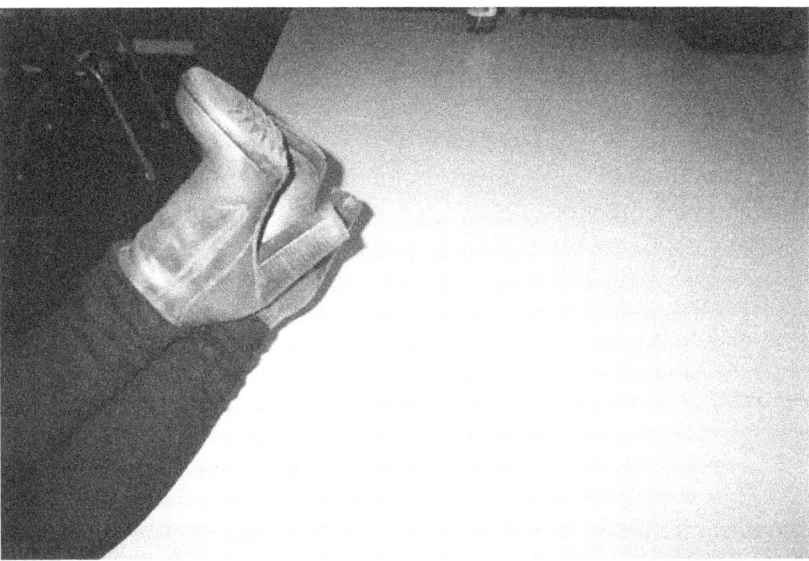

Figure 11.2 *"Maybe this 'support' could be seen as being linked to disability, but actually it's not. . . Deaf people have to be involved in the real world, and it's a hearing world. So how can we be hands-on and positive about that? So that's why I have an interpreter, they provide full access in real time."*

Other images captured almost incidental statements of identity, which only came to the fore during discussion in the interview. One participant took a photograph of her disability bus pass, intended as a comment on her independence and ability to travel by herself without needing her parents to drive her around (she was too young to drive herself). However, she also discussed this photograph in light of the question of whether she considered herself to be disabled. Traditionally, Deaf Studies scholars would reject the disability model (see Ladd 2003, for example), and, instead, refer to barriers linked to language or culture. Her conclusion was that she felt disabled by the hearing world's inability to communicate with her, which could be seen as similar to the social model of disability (Oliver 1996). However, rather than taking a proactive stance like the previous participant in assuming a signing deaf identity, she preferred to avoid confrontation with the hearing world. She used the bus pass because it meant that she would not have to try to communicate with the driver about her destination or the price of the ticket, she simply presented her pass to the ticket machine as she boarded the bus. This single image was thus able to articulate a very complex statement about identity and everyday life strategies. The same participant presented what would be considered to be a "visually arresting image" (Clark-Ibáñez 2007:171) of her cochlear implant connected to an MP3 player. When I asked about this photograph, whether it was intended to be a statement of identity, she replied that this was simply to show her love of music. Finding a visual way to illustrate what is not visual at all was a challenge that this participant negotiated effortlessly (Figure 11.3).

Both of these examples show that deaf participants were able to capture complex, nuanced meanings about their identity as deaf people within the photographs they took. They negotiated the overlap and conflict between the imposition of deafness as a disability and the ontology of being deaf in their everyday lives, and found ways of presenting that negotiation of identity in their photographs. These examples also show the importance of considering the interpretations that the audience brings to the photographs, and the potential of auto-driven photo-elicitation interviews to stimulate deep discussion of what a participant may consider to be a clear and unproblematic image (Meo 2010:161). The image that an amateur photographer captures may not express the meaning the photographer intended. In other words, the process of encoding and decoding (Hall et al. 1980) must be itself interrogated, to ensure that symmetry/asymmetry of the encoding/decoding relationship is established and the meanings of the image clarified, thus producing a "collaborative representation" (Banks 1995) of what the participant wished to portray.

The Composition of Images

Having emphasized the importance of intentionality and encoding/decoding, it is also very important to consider any meanings in the

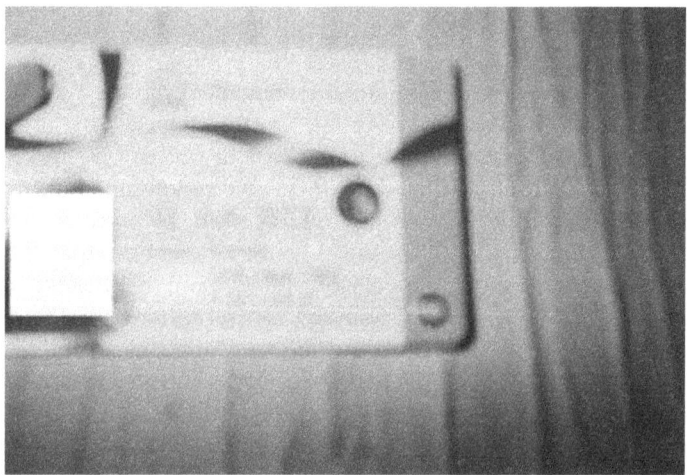

Figure 11.3 *"This is a bus pass, because I always use a bus pass 'cause I always go on the bus to town all the time because it's very easy..."*

photographs that may have crept in unintentionally. This can be illustrated by looking at the composition of the photographs taken by two different young people in the project. The first was a young woman who took all of her photographs from inside her bedroom, including a view out of the window of her bedroom. The limited location of the photographs gave the impression of a relatively isolated young woman, something that was belied in the photo-elicitation interview. The other set of photographs were taken by a young man, in several different locations, including from a moving car. These were taken to show the various places in the young man's locality that he felt were important to him, including the gym and youth club he frequented and his friends' houses. The photographs from the car, however, showed that his apparent mobility and independence also could be interpreted as an illusion. All the photographs were taken from the passenger side, and when asked, he revealed that he could not drive (although he was of driving age) and that a family member had given him lifts around to take the photographs.

This shows that it is important to analyze the site of production in the photographs (Rose 2012). It is not enough simply to consider what is portrayed in the images; consider, too, how the images were produced, where they were shot, what sort of unintended meanings are revealed in the way in which the images have been produced. Some ways of analyzing visual images take these elements into account (see Rose 2012 for examples), but many of these approaches are intended for analyzing professionally produced images, such as advertising, television programs, paintings, and so on. These methods must be used with caution if they are to be used with images produced by unskilled amateur photographers, who might not have put much thought or planning into the images they captured. These methods, however, can reveal certain elements that would otherwise not have been revealed without analyzing the images themselves.

Negotiating the "No People" Rule in Visually Creative Ways

Interestingly, some of the participants found inventive, visual ways to negotiate my request not to show people in the photographs they took. This was intended as a way of simplifying the ethical issues of the project and to avoid the need to gain informed consent from people captured in the photographs. Some of the participants were able to exploit the "gaze" of the photographs to capture people in their images without identifying them. One such was a photograph taken of the crowd at a sporting event, meant to signify the participants' love of her father and the sport to which he introduced her. The photograph captures thousands of people, but they are all facing away from the camera, homogenous in a mass of undifferentiated sports fans. The participant successfully utilized the power of the camera's

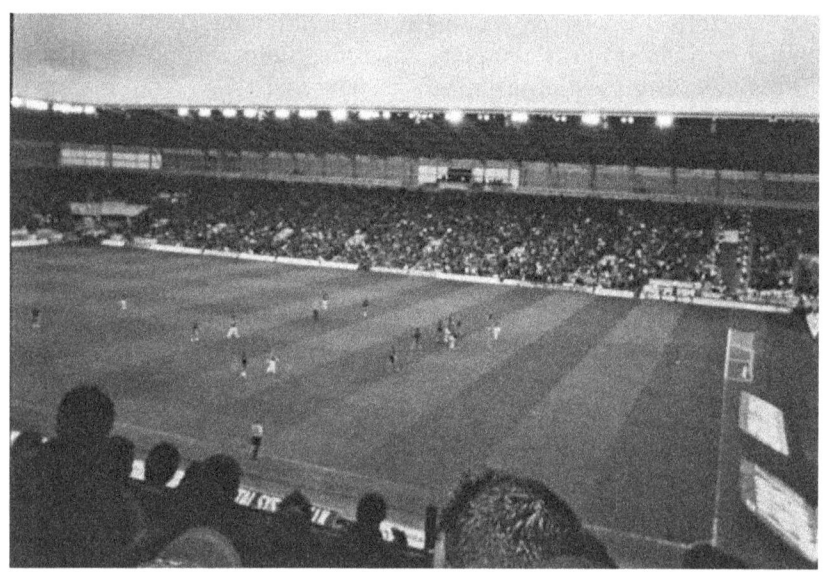

Figure 11.4 *"That's at the football game, because [team name] I'm a really big supporter ... But unfortunately that game was a really bad game and we lost."*

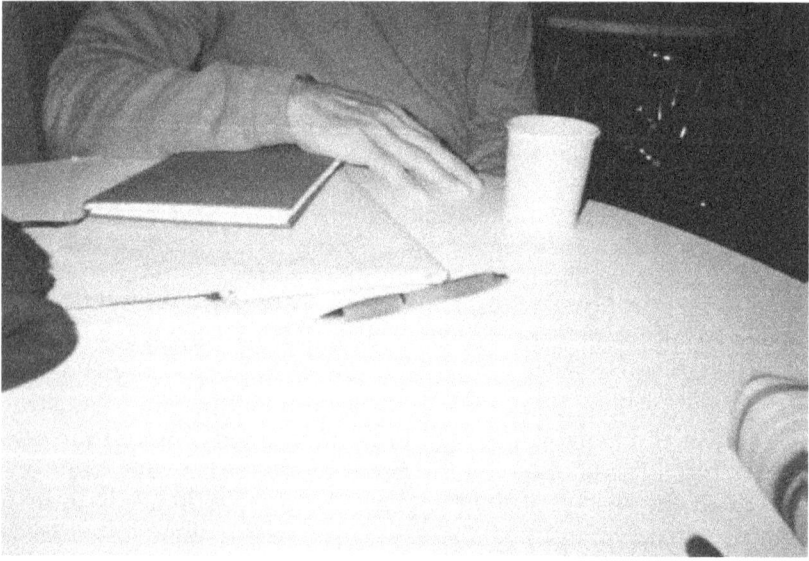

Figure 11.5 *"This is my mentor. He's like, someone I meet up with to discuss my emotions, how I feel about what's going on. He's a good mentor, and I feel like he's an important person to me because he's got a lot of knowledge about deaf culture."*

gaze to capture an image that contains thousands of individuals but also represents one. In contrast, another participant exploited the ability to focus so closely on a single aspect of a person that they became unidentifiable, differentiated into a component part, for example, through a close up of an earring, a hand making notes on a page, somebody's shoes. These creative ways of subverting the "no people" rule show visual imaginations at work, young people well versed in thinking about the world in visual ways (Figure 11.4 and Figure 11.5).

CASE 2: FILMMAKING IN MUMBAI (ANNELIES KUSTERS)

This research project documented communicative strategies during customer interactions and small talk between fluent deaf signers and hearing non-signers in Mumbai. When people from these different linguistic backgrounds meet, they typically use both conventional and spontaneous gestures to communicate with each other, often combined with mouthing and/or writing in different languages. Because this way of communication is mostly visual, video-recording was deemed essential within the project methodology. Linguistic ethnography was undertaken in public and parochial spaces such as markets, shops, food joints, and public transport in Mumbai. Six deaf research participants (including one deafblind person) were selected, and 300 interactions between them and hearing strangers and acquaintances were video-recorded, when they were buying or ordering, selling or serving, or chatting.

The focus of the research was not limited to language strategies: We (the research team) also explored how such communicative situations were experienced, as well as discourses and ideologies on the use of gesture, its potential and limits, and discourses on how it differed from Indian Sign Language. To that end, semistructured interviews with the six deaf participants, and 130 impromptu mini-interviews were conducted with both deaf and hearing people immediately after recorded gesture-based interactions. In addition, three exploratory discussions were organized in deaf clubs. Furthermore, recorded gesture-based interactions and interviews were used to create an ethnographic film called *Ishaare: Gestures and Signs in Mumbai. Ishaare* is an anthropological film, "representing ethnographic knowledge about an event and how it is experienced" (Pink 2013:105).

Filmmaking allows researchers to capture individuals' agency and experience, as well as interactions between people and their relationship with physical environments. Researchers have argued that "viewing a film is closer in character to the visual and auditory experience of the anthropologist in the field than to reading an anthropological text, where much of the detail must be reconstructed in the reader's imagination" (MacDougall 2011:100). The expectation is often that ethnographic (or anthropological) films are both neutral and comprehensive: They present a variety of perspectives and elaborate as much as needed to produce a relatively representative picture. Some anthropological filmmakers believe that the film will explain itself, while others believe that metacommentaries are necessary for guidance. While films are specific and case-based, written texts, on the other hand, are important for making general (scientific) statements and drawing overall conclusions (MacDougall 2011). Films, however, are more than dissemination tools: "Filmmaking is a way of looking, sometimes motivated by intellectual objectives and sometimes anticipating thought" (MacDougall 2011:101). Filmmaking is another way of exploring themes (Figure 11.6).

The production of *Ishaare* was a cooperative effort between myself (Annelies Kusters, the deaf researcher), a deaf Indian research assistant (Sujit Sahasrabudhe), a hearing Indian research assistant cum sign language interpreter (Amaresh Gopalakrishnan), an agency of trained deaf filmmakers (Visual Box), and three deaf Mumbaikars who took turns working as cameramen. This contrasts with documentaries on deaf people that are made by hearing filmmakers and often experienced as not entirely in correspondence to lived deaf experiences. Indeed, there is a need for deaf-led sign language media (Rijckaert 2012).

My role was to coordinate the whole project, direct the film, and analyse the data. Sujit's role was to lead discussion groups, conduct interviews, and translate interviews to written English. Amaresh's role was to interpret during interviews with hearing people, to translate/transcribe interviews with hearing participants, and to annotate gesture-based interactions. Visual Box's role was to train the cameramen and to edit *Ishaare*. Part of this five-day training was creating a pilot film (eight and a half minutes in duration). This way the team (researcher, two assistants, and a cameraman) could practice working together, and the cameramen could receive feedback on their materials and insight on what would/could be done with their recordings in the editing stage.

The first stage of the project consisted of field work in Mumbai (five months in 2014), including exploratory discussions in deaf clubs, the selection of the six participants, the training of the cameramen by Visual Box, and the recording of gesture-based interactions and interviews. The second stage of the project consisted of transcriptions, translations, analysis, the creation of a storyboard, and the creation of *Ishaare*. In stage three (2015), seven film discussion groups were organized in Mumbai. In addition to *Ishaare* and the pilot video, two more videos were created to document the research and the process of creating *Ishaare*: one eight-minute video on the cameramen's training and one

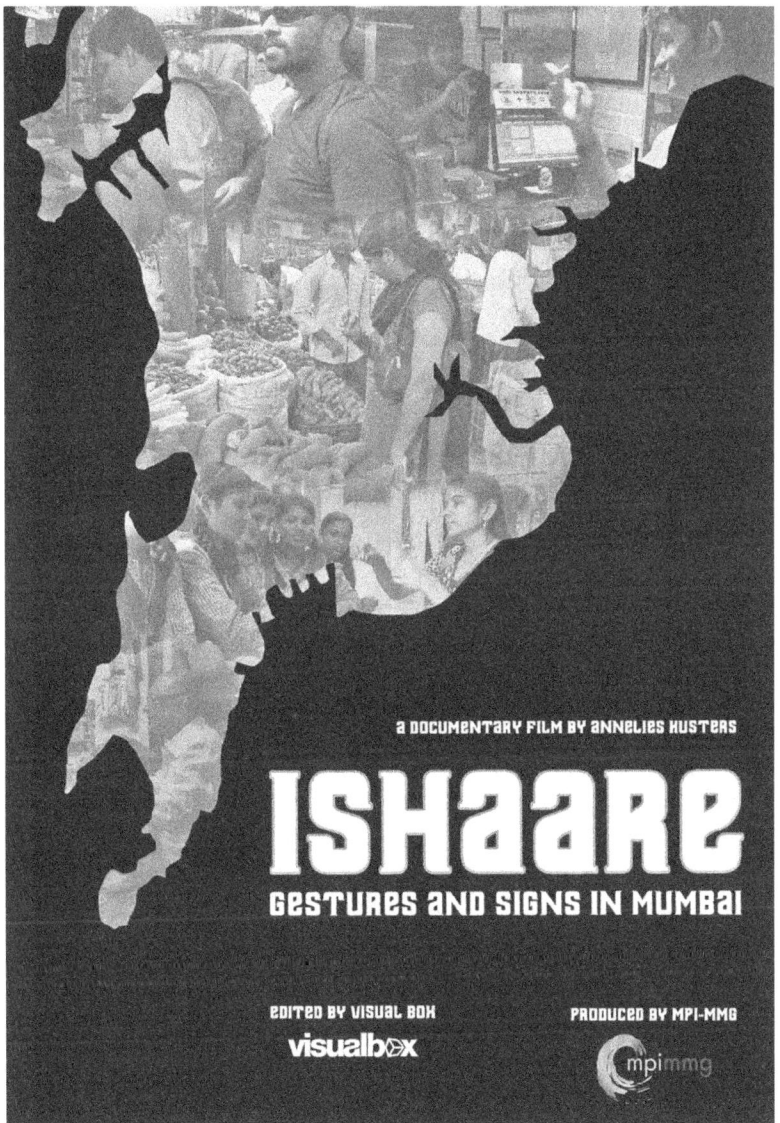

Figure 11.6: Film poster for *Ishaare*.

20-minute video on the making of *Ishaare*. All videos can be watched on the project's website.[2]

The use of video was thus inherent in all steps of the research proc-ess: from data production to triangulation (which means using different

---

[2] http://www.mmg.mpg.de/de/forschung/alle-projekte/deaf-hearing-gestural-interaction-in-mumbai-an-ethnography-of-communication/

methods to check research results; in this case the film was used to triangulate findings in discussion groups) and dissemination, to optimize
reflexivity and feedback. The gesture-based interactions and interviews were video-recorded with five aims: (1) extraction, (2) reflection,
(3) projection and provocation, (4) articulation, and (5) dissemination.
Here, I summarize each aim, and further in the text, I describe and evaluate them in greater depth.

(1) *Extraction* means "using video to record a specific interaction so that it can be studied in more depth by the researcher"
(Haw & Hadfield 2011:2). Gesture-based interactions were
recorded with the aim of further close-up observation: playing and replaying the videos, annotating them, and making
extensive notes on the interactions in the videos. In the case
of interviews, videos were translated to written English. After
analysis of data, *Ishaare's* storyboard was created. The choice
of sequences that are included in *Ishaare* was thus based on the
data analysis.

(2) *Reflection* means "using video to support participants to reflect
upon their actions, understandings and constructions" (Haw
& Hadfield 2011:2). *Ishaare* was shown to deaf audiences to
elicit further thoughts on gesture-based interactions and reflect
on the recorded utterances and practices. Previously to the
research, Sujit and I got the impression that communication
through gesture is often regarded as "low" (in contrast to communication in fully fledged signed or spoken languages) or is
something to be ashamed of. We expected that *Ishaare* would
trigger conversation on the issue.

(3) *Projection and provocation:* "using video to provoke participants
to critically examine and challenge existing norms, traditions
and power structures" (Haw & Hadfield 2011:2). To this aim,
Ishaare was shown to, and discussed with, four hearing audiences (8–15 people): hearing parents of deaf children, hearing
teachers of deaf children, and two hearing lay audiences. "Lay"
is understood to mean people with no background of work-
ing/living with deaf people (although during the discussion
groups, it turned out that some of them did have such experiences). Particularly because deaf education policies often seek
to prevent the use of signed language (or gesture), we (Sujit and
I) thought *Ishaare* could be thought-provoking for hearing parents and teachers of deaf children. In the case of lay audiences,
the aim was to elicit and compare perspectives before and after
showing *Ishaare*. The expectation was that *Ishaare* would allow
a deeper and more informed discussion than when no film had
been shown.

(4) *Articulation* means "using video to help participants voice their opinions and communicate these to others" (Haw & Hadfield 2011:2), which we found important in the process of giving deaf people a platform to express their experiences of communicating in the city, as well as important in the process of dissemination.

(5) *Dissemination*: Firstly, because we were recording visual communication, more particularly Indian Sign Language and gesture-based interactions, we wanted to maintain the original data source in the process of dissemination. Secondly, we regarded producing an ethnographic film as a method of dissemination wherein the research participants (rather than the researcher) are the leading voices and faces of the project. Thirdly, because of the visual nature of sign languages, we believe that documentaries are accessible to a wider variety of audiences than, for example, written academic texts, including those for deaf audiences (see, however, further discussion later in this chapter).

We will now share some insights from this process of using video and creating *Ishaare*, but see Kusters, Sahasrabudhe, and Gopalakrishnan (2016) for a more elaborate description and discussion of the research methodology.

Visual Methods within the Frame of a Wider Research Methodology

As explained earlier, this linguistic ethnography entailed more than the six case studies. The combination of these case studies with three exploratory discussions in deaf clubs, seven film discussions, the production of field notes on our own gesture-based interactions, as well as Sujit's ability to wear multiple hats in the project, was important in helping us identify gaps in the recorded data and interviews, and in further informing and complementing data from the case studies. Thus, in this context, it was fruitful to integrate visual methodologies in a broader methodology wherein the visual methods were not the only methods in use.

Exploratory Discussions

Because Sujit (the deaf research assistant) is a native Mumbaikar, and I (Annelies, the deaf research leader) had lived and researched in Mumbai before and compiled field notes on the theme since 2006, the theme and location were not new for us. Still, before starting the recordings of gesture-based interactions in the frame of the six case studies, we organized and video-recorded discussions in three deaf clubs: one club for women (Bombay Foundation of Deaf Women,

BFDW for short), one for youth (Yuva Association of the Deaf, YAD for short), and one for a more general membership (India Deaf Society, IDS for short). The number of attendees varied between 30 and 100. Sujit started off with an explanation about the project and what would be done with the recordings, and then directed questions toward the audience, giving the stage to whomever was interested in sharing their thoughts and experiences. Questions included, for example: In which situations do you use gesture? What is the potential and limitation of communication in gesture? What is the difference between gesture and Indian Sign Language?

A wide range of people took the stage. Deaf people shared examples and experiences, added to examples shared by others, and challenged one another's perspectives. Sujit managed the discussions, offering new questions in the process, often prompted by me. The discussions (one and a half to two hours in duration) were video-recorded and afterward analyzed according to the premises of grounded theory. These discussions were very fruitful in initiating the research, in that we were able to gather a wide range of perspectives and experiences, which helped to further inform and specify the questions asked during the six case studies. Also, because the research focused on six main participants, it was important that these exploratory deaf club discussions (in combination with the after-film discussions; see remarks later in this chapter) include varied perspectives. Furthermore, and importantly, this information and these insights were not only made available for and shared with the researchers but also were shared with others who were present in the audience. It was clear that many people were personally engaged by these discussions. The theme, as such, was introduced into Mumbai deaf community discourse. After these discussions, we selected participants, undertaking pilots (without camera) with some of them.

Field Notes and Positionality

The kinds of (customer) interactions under investigation in this project were those that we (Sujit and I) engaged in ourselves on a daily basis. Our own gesture-based interactions (and reflections upon those) were laid down in field notes. While Sujit is a native Mumbaikar, I lived in Mumbai for three years (after marrying Sujit) and did my daily grocery shopping in the street markets of Mulund (the suburb of Mumbai where we lived). It was trial and error, especially in the beginning: I had to learn gesturing conventions and marketing scripts. I had to learn the usual price for fruits and vegetables and how to communicate about them. For example, when buying tomatoes, pointing at the tomatoes and gesturing "one" means you want "one kilo of tomatoes" (rather than "one tomato"); when the seller then gestures "one" it means you have to pay ten rupees (and not one rupee or one hundred rupees). I learned in which situations bargaining is expected and acceptable and in which situations it is not. Furthermore, I experienced the importance of building up communicative acquaintance with sellers. Thus, my position as a deaf foreigner who lived for three years in the same neighborhood, led to insights that I found very useful in the process of research. Indeed, a deaf Indian or a hearing foreigner would not have gone through this same learning process.

Sujit's Multiple Hats

As can be seen in the list of case studies, Sujit was included as one of them. Sujit's gesture-based interactions very much informed the project and it was decided not to limit the (self-)observation of his interactions to field notes. During the project, Sujit shared a lot of metalinguistic reflection on gesture. Furthermore, because he was my husband, discussions about gestures and *Ishaare* were part of everyday life discussions not only during work time but also at home. Sujit and I decided that such metalinguistic reflection, in combination with an analysis of his own practices of gesturing, should be part of the research and part of *Ishaare,* particularly because there was no plan to include a separate "guide" in the film. Thus, in the film, Sujit appears during interviews with research participants, but also when he engages in gesture-based interactions himself and when he reflects upon these language practices. The decision to include Sujit as a research participant provided him with a range of different perspectives: engaging in gesture-based interactions with or without the presence of a camera; being the observer of gesture-based interactions of the other participants; and being their interviewer. In addition, he led the exploratory discussions in deaf clubs and the after-film discussions in Stage Three of the project. This combination of perspectives led to the deeper level of metalinguistic reflection that he showcases in the film.

Using *Ishaare* for Eliciting Reflection, Projection, and Provocation

As explained earlier, using *Ishaare* to elicit perspectives on gesture was an inherent part of the project methodology. The idea was thus not merely to organize "feedback sessions" or "film discussions," but also to further reflect on gesture-based communication, using the movie as a tool to illustrate what is meant or to refer to during discussion. This was an experimental and innovative aspect of the methodology, because audience reception of ethnographic films is an under-researched method and theme (Rutten & Verstappen 2015). As Rutten and Verstappen (2015) document, an anthropological documentary can be received very differently by different audiences, and for filmmakers, screenings can lead to unexpected surprises about people's reactions. Having screened an ethnographic film on Indian migrants in London, Rutten and Verstappen document a variety of reactions by various audiences with different backgrounds (regarding class, nationality, age, ethnic group, urban vs. rural life, etc.). Audience reactions included recognition and identification, curiosity, feeling estranged, feeling certain parts were controversial or comical. Rutten and Verstappen (2015:416) state that "visual anthropology has much to gain from taking audiences seriously, not only as students that may learn something through our films, but also as teachers, who may have something important to say." Only a limited number of authors have written about film elicitation, however, which is much less frequently used than photo elicitation. Film elicitation includes showing archival film footage or ethnographic documentaries as visual prompts to elicit discussion (Banks & Zeitlyn 2015).

We first organized a screening for the deaf community in Mumbai, in a hall that could seat 1,000 people (to make the film accessible to as broad an audience as possible). We distributed tickets (funded by the Max Planck Institute for the Study of Religious and Ethnic Diversity, which also funded the research as a whole and the creation of *Ishaare*) through several deaf clubs and organizations. The hall was full, and almost all the people present were deaf. The screening consisted of three parts: first a 15-minute presentation in which the aim of the research and the creation of the film were explained, then, *Ishaare* was shown, and, finally, the *Making of Ishaare*. The day after, Sujit and I visited BFDW, and the next weekend we visited IDS and YAD for discussions lasting between one and one and a half hours. The number of attendees again varied between 30 and 100. Again, Sujit moderated most of the discussions, but I also participated by asking a few questions. Questions included: What were you thinking when you watched the film? What have you learned? What did you think of the interviews with hearing people?

Some people started telling about their experiences of gesture-based interactions, but that was not really what we were looking for, given that we already had gathered such data in the exploratory discussions that were held in the clubs before the recordings. Yet, the film led to some further discussion of the difference between sign and gesture. It also appeared that the film had led to increased awareness about the importance of acquaintance and cooperation between interactants for the success of gesture-based interactions; since several deaf people contrasted the film with negative experiences in daily life. Many people also came with suggestions for situations that also should be recorded to create a more complete picture: such as communication in banks (which they said is much more difficult than buying vegetables), at the doctor's office, in villages, and in families. A few people expressed that after watching *Ishaare,* they had a better understanding of emic perspectives on the difference between gesture and sign. People sometimes referred to specific excerpts in *Ishaare* when giving examples, and in this way having watched the film aided discussion. For example, there were a few comments on hearing perspectives that were portrayed in the film; expressing skepticism regarding some hearing people's positive utterances about deaf people.

Interestingly, and against our expectations, most deaf people seemed to find it difficult to reflect on the film, especially in BFDW and IDS. Although many of them enjoyed and applauded the film (such as in "Very good," "The best!"), it seemed that many people could not explain what they found good or even what the movie was about. Sujit and I had expected that the film would, in fact, be most accessible for Indian deaf signers because they were the only ones who would not need to read the subtitles (because deaf interviews were in ISL, gesture-based interactions featured deaf people, and hearing people's quotes were translated into ISL by the in-screen interpreter). Although perhaps the language itself was accessible, a number of deaf Mumbaikars reported that they found it hard to identify the connecting thread in *Ishaare*; asking "What is the message?" "Where is the politics?" or saying that the point did not "hit" them.

There is a tradition of documentary filmmaking in India; Discovery Channel sessions are screened on television in India and many fiction films are subtitled in English on the TV (though because of generally limited English literacy rates among deaf people in Mumbai, subtitles only provide fragmentary access). A few news sessions do have an in-vision Indian Sign Language interpreter. Still, although deaf people do watch serials, documentaries, films, and news on the TV, they might not have the experience of fully accessing and critically watching (ethnographic) documentary films. *Ishaare* is not a film in which a lot of guidance is given: Viewers have to look for the lead/structure themselves. Films produced by Indian deaf people either contain fiction and/or a very clear moral message such as "study well," "save trees," "don't hit women," "work hard," "don't cheat in exams," "don't cheat on your partner" "don't throw rubbish on the street," and so on. *Ishaare* in contrast was much more nuanced, and also much longer in duration.

The primary purpose of *Ishaare* was to portray under-researched communication strategies. "Spreading a message," per se, was not the first priority, though *Ishaare* could be (and has been) used in that way, such as to demonstrate that it is possible to communicate in gesture, and that speech is not necessary in everyday interactions. Indeed, customer interactions and travel are the classic examples that (ignorant) hearing people use when arguing that deaf people should be able to (or be taught to) speak. Only a very small minority of deaf people seemed to understand that the film could be used to illustrate this, not only to hearing parents, teachers, and lay people, but also to deaf people who were not confident using gestures rather than speech when communicating with shopkeepers, for example.

In the end, I got the impression that the movie did not accomplish one of its intended purposes to a satisfactory extent, namely, letting research results flow back into the community by means of an accessible means of dissemination. This made us aware that it is necessary to organize presentations and workshops, engaging directly with the audience, rather than (only) making them the passive audience of a film. Preceding the film with a 15-minute presentation was not enough to make the majority understand how the film was embedded within the research project. Another way to engage with this audience could be to produce a different style of film, with clearer guidance.

In this context it is very important to mention that in Mumbai, the concept of "gesture" is still quite new (in stark contrast with the perspectives of many international viewers for whom "gesture versus sign" was an established way of looking at deaf–hearing and deaf–deaf communication). Indeed, while the *use* of gesture is widespread in India, the concept of gesture is less well-known: In emic discourses, hearing people's gesturing often was referred to as "signing." In Hindi, the word for gestures/signs is one and the same: *Ishaare* (hence the title of the film). Often, rather than separating "gestures" and "signs" into different concepts, deaf and hearing people's *Ishaare* were distinguished by explaining that hearing's *Ishaare* is often slower, bigger, more context-dependent and less specific. That being said, the concept of "gesture" was by no means absent in India and in the Mumbai deaf community, yet it was definitely less established than in Western deaf communities or in sign language research, for example.

Also, deaf people in Mumbai longed for comparisons. They were aware that the project was motivated by my fascination with the contrast between the West and India, because I found that successful gesture-based interactions are much more common in India (and other countries in the global South) than in Europe. Some Indian deaf people said that it would have been enlightening if the film also had included a depiction of gesture in Europe, rather than only providing a "mirror."

Thus, many Indian deaf people did not instinctively understand the researcher's intention behind creating *Ishaare*, perhaps because such reflection on documentaries is not part of their everyday epistemologies and/or because of the non-Indian frames of reference that impacted the film, namely, its non-Indian director and editors.

Yet during the after-film discussions it also appeared that a film made in the context of a research project can positively impact a community in ways unexpected or unpredicted by the researchers: Deaf people in Mumbai valued *Ishaare* for certain aspects other than those the researchers regarded as central to the project. The most important impact or intervention for Mumbai deaf people was seeing Pradip, the deafblind participant, who made a lasting impression on many viewers: The movie has led to an enormous boost in deafblind awareness. Pradip is well known in the Mumbai deaf community, but viewers expressed that even though they regularly had conversed with Pradip, and knew how to communicate using hands-on signing (during which the deafblind person touches the hands of the signing person), they had no idea about how he communicated with hearing people when he was on his own.

The second most significant impact was that many deaf people were happy with the portrayal/recognition/attention accorded to three deaf businesses. Many deaf people who took the stage in the deaf clubs told of other deaf-led businesses (*pan*-makers, sandwich stalls, a deaf rickshaw driver) they knew, and reported that these deaf people communicated in ways similar to those portrayed in *Ishaare*.

After the deaf club discussion groups, we organized four film screenings and discussions with hearing people: In each case, we first organized a pre-film discussion, then screened *Ishaare*, and then organized a post-film discussion. In contrast to deaf audiences, hearing audiences in India seemed to better "get" the film, perhaps because the film portrayed interactions by "others" and offered new insights, or because as hearing people they had better access to films and were more exposed to them in general, as compared with deaf people. Two of the discussions were with teachers and parents of deaf children, respectively. Based upon Sujit's personal experiences, teachers and parents of the deaf often believe very much in the need for deaf people to *speak* to be able to go to shops or to gain employment, and model their educational practices to this, to the extent of prohibiting the use of sign and gesture. The aim of targeting those groups was to demonstrate (with the film) how deaf people navigate society if they do not speak and are not accompanied by hearing people who speak for them. The educational policy of the school that was selected is not straightforwardly in favor of or against one particular way of communication; instead, it favored combining gesture, sign language, speech, and so on. The school was chosen because it is one of the bigger and better-known schools for the deaf in Mumbai.

In the pre-film discussions, Sujit gathered perspectives on how the participants (eight parents and eight teachers) thought deaf people communicate in the city, and on the difference between gesture and sign. Although parents did not have a clear idea about this difference, most teachers did. The conversation with teachers was enlightening because they had very specific experiences with, and detailed insights into, the use of gesture versus sign language. For example, they expressed that gestures are important for communicating with deaf children who use gestures at home and do not know Indian Sign Language yet; and that they use gestures rather than Indian

Sign Language in informal conversation, while using Indian Sign Language when teaching particular concepts. The (constructed) difference between gesture and sign language became clearer to them after viewing the movie, even though they already had preconceived ideas on the difference. In this aspect, seeing the movie aided and triggered further discussion. As for the parents, most of them did not seem to recognize a difference between gesture and sign language in advance of the screening; after the screening, however, they said they had a better understanding of this. Parents experienced the screening as hugely eye-opening, and parents of younger children said the film made them confident about their children going out to shops, for example. Yet, in terms of research this screening did not yield a lot of new data. Both groups were very impressed by Pradip, so among hearing people the film also led to deafblind awareness.

The two other film discussions were organized with lay people: a class of 15 students in a postgraduate course on community media, and a group of 11 neighbors, friends, and relatives of a neighbor of Sujit's parents. Both groups found the movie very educational and said their pity for deaf people was replaced by respect. Some expressed a desire to learn sign language. The discussion with the media students was enlightening, given that several of them gave informed and detailed perspectives on gesture-based communication. They were especially critical of perspectives in the interviews recorded with a range of customers at Café Coffee Day, a coffee house with deaf staff. According to the students, the hearing interviewees were idealizing their interactions with the deaf staff, so much so that it seemed theatrical.

Thus, the screenings and discussions were central in starting the process of dissemination in Mumbai. Different groups regarded different aspects of the film as eye-opening, and their reception of the film was, in turn, eye-opening for the research team. The film discussions found to be most fruitful for eliciting research data were those with the deaf audiences, the hearing teachers, and the media students.

CONCLUSION

The case studies presented here offer support for the use of visual methods and the ability of deaf participants and researchers to exploit these methods to the fullest, presenting complex, rich data. A number of challenges and precautions as to how to interpret and use these images also were discussed. In both cases, visual methods were used within the frame of a wider project methodology, and in both cases there were some surprising results: For Dai this included the ease with which participants were able to negotiate the "no people" rule through visually creative ways of photography; for Annelies this included the reception of *Ishaare* by deaf audiences in Mumbai. Our being deaf informed the research project in several respects: Annelies made field notes on her own gesture-based interactions, and the project of creating *Ishaare* was deaf-led; indeed, it was led by a deaf foreigner rather than an Indian, but in the film, Sujit and the other research participants are the main faces of *Ishaare*. Dai was able to use his own experience of growing up deaf in a mainstream environment to interpret and unlock some of the more complex meanings shown in the photographs taken for the project.

Many have claimed that deaf culture is a visual culture, but we do not see the corresponding utilization of visual methods in research involving deaf people and deaf communities. Rose (2014) talks about the difference between "visual culture" and "visual methods." Rose's point is that the relationship between visual research methods and visual culture, wherein visual culture refers to the new multimodal ways of communication that focus more on image rather than on writing (Kress 2004), which are emerging from "new digital technologies and neoliberal globalisation" (Rose 2014:37), is not as straightforward as it appears. Rose posits that although many believe that visual research methods are a way of representing the visuality of the new visual culture, they are, in fact, a way of *performing* a contemporary visual culture (Rose 2014:39). In other words, visual culture is expressed in the very act of using visual research methods. If we, as deaf scholars, truly want to represent our own deaf ontologies and visucentric nature in our work, the use of such visual methods is a fundamental part of this expression. We then could see this increased engagement not simply as a pragmatic choice of research method to better communicate with research participants, but as a radical departure from the hegemonic methodology of the academy in order to fully express, and experiment with, the researchers' and their participants' visual ontologies.

REFERENCES

Bahan, B. (2004). Memoir upon the formation of a visual variety of the human race. In B. K. Eldredge, D. Stringham, & M. M. Wilding-Diaz (Eds.), *Deaf studies today: A kaleidoscope of knowledge, learning and understanding: 2004 conference proceedings*. Orem: Utah Valley State College.

Bahan, B. (2014). Senses and culture: Exploring sensory orientations. In: H. Bauman & J. Murray (Eds.), *Deaf Gain: Raising the stakes for human diversity* (pp. 233–255). Minneapolis: University of Minnesota Press.

Banks, M. (1995). Visual research methods. Social Research Update 11. Retrieved from http://sru.soc.surrey.ac.uk/sru11/sru11.html.

Banks, M., & Zeitlyn, D. (2015). *Visual methods in social research* (2nd ed.). London: Sage Publications.

Barnett, S. (2015). *Being equal—A deafblind community of one* (Unpublished doctoral dissertation). University of Bristol.

Bauman, H. (2014). DeafSpace: An architecture toward a more livable and sustainable world." In H. Bauman & J. Murray (Eds.), *Deaf Gain: Raising the stakes for human diversity* (pp. 375–401). Minneapolis: University of Minnesota Press.

Bauman, H., & Murray, J. (2014). Deaf Gain: An introduction." In H. Bauman & J. Murray (Eds.), *Deaf Gain: Raising the stakes for human diversity* (pp. xv–xlii). Minneapolis: University of Minnesota Press.

Baynton, D., Gannon, J. R., & Bergey, J. L. (2007). *Through deaf eyes: A photographic history of an American community.* Washington, DC: Gallaudet University Press.

Cardin, V., Orfanidou, E., Rönnberg, J., Capek, C. M., Rudner, M., & Woll, B. (2013). Dissociating cognitive and sensory neural plasticity in human superior temporal cortex. *Nature Communications, 4,* 1473.

Capek, C., Woll, B., MacSweeney, M., Waters, D., & McGuire, P. K. (2010). Superior temporal activation as a function of linguistic knowledge: Insights from deaf native signers who speechread, *Brain & Language, 112,* 129–134.

Che, Y., Hayashi, A., & Tobin, J. (2007). Lessons from China and Japan for preschool practice in the United States. *Educational Perspectives, 40*(1), 7–12.

Clark, C. D. (1999). The autodriven interview: A photographic viewfinder into children's experience. *Visual Sociology, 14,* 39–50.

Clark-Ibáñez, M. (2004). Framing the social world with photo-elicitation interviews. *American Behavioural Scientist, 47*(12), 1507–1527.

Clark-Ibáñez, M. (2007). Inner-city children in sharper focus: Sociology of childhood and photo elicitation interviews. In G. C. Stanczak (Ed.), *Visual research methods: Image, society and representation.* Los Angeles, CA: SAGE.

Clark-Ibáñez, M. (2008). Gender and being 'bad': inner-city students' photographs. In P. Thomson (Ed.), *Doing visual research with children and young people.* London and New York: Routledge.

Collier, J. Jr., & Collier, M. (1986). *Visual anthropology: Photography as a research method.* Albuquerque: University of New Mexico Press.

De Brigard, E. (2003). The history of ethnographic film. In P. Hockings (Ed.), *Principles of visual anthropology* (3rd edition). Berlin: Mouton de Gruyter.

De Clerck, G. A. M. (2009). Tussen droom en werkelijkheid: Dove jongeren als filmmakers. In R. Pinxten (Ed.), *Mensen: Een inleiding in de culturele antropologie* (pp. 234–239). Tielt: Uitgeverij Lannoo.

Dee, L. (2006). *Improving transition planning for young people with special educational needs.* Maidenhead, Berkshire: Open University Press.

Eckert, R. C., & Rowley, A. J. (2013). Audism: A theory and practice of audiocentric privilege. *Humanity and Society, 37*(2), 101–130.

Edwards, C., & Harold, G. (2014). DeafSpace and the principles of universal design. *Disability and Rehabilitation, 36*(16), 1350–1359.

Edwards, T. (2015). Bridging the gap between DeafBlind minds: Interactional and social foundations of intention attribution in the Seattle DeafBlind community. *Frontiers in Psychology, 9,* 1–13.

Emery, S. D. (2011). *Citizenship and the deaf community.* Nijmegen, the Netherlands: Ishara Press.

Hall, S., Hobson, D., Lowe, A., & Willis, P. (1980). *Culture, media, language: Working papers in cultural studies, 1972-79.* London: Routledge.

Harold, G. (2013). Reconsidering sound and the city: Asserting the right to the Deaf-friendly city. *Environment and Planning D: Society and Space, 31*(5), 846–862.

Haw, K., & Hadfield, M. (2011). *Video in social science research: Functions and forms.* London: Routledge.

Hauser, P. C., O'Hearn, A., & McKee, M. (2010). Deaf epistemology: Deafhood and deafness. *American Annals of the Deaf, 154*(5), 486–492.

Kress, G. (2004). Gains and losses: New forms of texts, knowledge and learning. *Computers and Composition, 22,* 5–22.

Kusters, A., Sahasrabudhe, S., & Gopalakrishnan, A. (2016). A reflexive report on the use of video and the production of Ishaare when doing linguistic ethnography in Mumbai. MMG Working Paper 16-04. http://www.mmg.mpg.de/fileadmin/user_upload/documents/wp/WP_16-04_Kusters-Sahasrabudhe-Gopalakrishnan_Filmmaking.pdf

Ladd, P. (2003). *Understanding Deaf culture: in search of Deafhood.* Clevedon: Multilingual Matters Ltd.

Lane, H., Hoffmeister, R., & Bahan, B. (1996). *A journey into the DEAF-WORLD.* San Diego: DawnSign Press.

Lederberg, A. R., Schick, B., & Spencer, P. E. (2013). Language and literacy development of deaf and hard-of-hearing children: Successes and challenges. *Developmental Psychology, 49*(1), 15–30.

MacDougall, D. (2011). Anthropological filmmaking: An empirical art. In E. Margolis & L. Pauwels (Eds.), *The Sage handbook of visual research methods* (pp. 99–114). London: Sage.

Meo, A. I. (2010). Picturing students' habitus: The advantage and limitation of photo-elicitation interviewing in a qualitative study in the city of Buenos Aires. *International Journal of Qualitative Methods, 9*(2), 149–171.

Mindess, A. (2006). *Reading between the signs: Intercultural communication for sign language interpreters* (2nd edition). Yarmouth, ME: Intercultural Press.

Napoli, D. J. (2014). A magic touch: Deaf Gain and the benefits of tactile sensation. In H. Bauman & J. Murray (Eds.), *Deaf Gain: Raising the stakes for human diversity* (pp. 211–233). Minneapolis: University of Minnesota Press.

O'Brien, D. (2015). Transition planning for d/Deaf young people from mainstream schools: professionals' views on the implementation of policy. *Disability and Society, 30*(2), 227–240.

O'Brien, D. (2013). Visual research with young d/Deaf people – an investigation of the transitional experiences of d/Deaf young people from mainstream schools using auto-driven photo-elicitation interviews. *Graduate Journal of Social Science, 10*(2), 152–175.

O'Brien, D. (2012). *d/Deaf Young People's Experiences of Transition Planning in England: Using Auto-driven Photo-elicitation Interviews and Critical Discourse Analysis to Explore Experiences of Policy and Practice.* Unpublished PhD Thesis. University of Bristol.

Oliver, M. (1996). *Understanding disability: from theory to practice.* Basingstoke: Palgrave.

Pink, S. (2013). *Doing visual ethnography* (3rd ed.). London: Sage Publications.

Rijckaert, J. (2012). Op weg naar erkenning van Deaf Cinema? In G. De Clerck & R. Pinxten (Eds.), *Gebarentaal zegt alles. Bijdragen rond diversiteit en gebarentaal vanuit emancipatorisch perspectief* (pp. 103–116). Leuven: Acco.

Rose, G. (2014). On the relation between "visual research methods" and contemporary visual culture. *The Sociological Review, 62,* 24–d46.

Rose, G. (2012). *Visual methodologies* (3rd ed.). London: Sage Publications.

Rutten, M., & Verstappen, S. (2015). Reflections on migration through film: Screening of an anthropological documentary on Indian youth in London. *Visual Anthropology, 28*, 398–421.

Samuels, J. (2007). When words are not enough: Eliciting children's experiences of Buddhist monastic life through photographs. In G. C. Stanczak (Ed.), *Visual research methods: Image, society and representation* (pp. 1528–1550). Los Angeles: Sage.

Sirvage, R. (2009). The deaf walk: Proximics, space and the collectivist way of being. Retrieved from http://video.mit.edu/watch/speakers-and-signers-robert-sirvage-the-deaf-walk-proximics-space-and-the-collectivist-way-of-b-4311/.

Sturken, M., & Cartwright, L. (2009). *Practices of looking: An introduction to visual culture* (2nd ed.). Oxford: Oxford University Press.

Sutherland, H., & Rogers, K. D. (2014). The hidden gain: a new lens of research with d/Deaf children and adults. In H.-D. L. Bauman (Ed.), *Deaf gain: raising the stakes for human diversity* (pp. 269–282). Minneapolis: University of Minnesota Press.

Thoutenhoofd, E. D. (1999). See deaf: on sight in deafness. https://www.academia.edu/527261/See_deaf_On_sight_in_deafness

Thoutenhoofd, E. (1996). *Occularcentrism and deaf people: a social photography project*. Unpublished PhD dissertation: Durham University.

Thoutenhoofd, E. D. (1998). Method in a photographic enquiry of being deaf. *Sociological Research Online, 3*(2). Retrieved from http://www.socresonline.org.uk/3/2/2.html.

Tobin, J., & Hsueh, Y. (2007). The poetics and pleasures of video ethnography of education. In R. Goldman (Ed.), *Video research in the learning sciences* (pp. 77–92). New York: Lawrence Erlbaum Associates.

Valentine, G., & Skelton, T. (2007). Re-defining 'norms': D/deaf young people's transition to independence. *The Sociological Review, 55*(1), 104–123.

Young, A., & Temple, B. (2014). *Approaches to social research: The case of Deaf Studies*. Oxford: Oxford University Press.

12

Writing the Deaf Self in Autoethnography

Noel O'Connell

PROLOGUE

The idea for this chapter grew out of my doctoral work after I successfully graduated with a PhD in Education in 2013. As a deaf scholar with over 10 years of experience in qualitative research, I am intimately acquainted with academic life. My work intersects autoethnography with storytelling, deaf education with sociology, and Deaf Studies with Communication Studies. I am also an autoethnographer, Deaf Studies researcher, academic writer, and one amongst a "minority of Deaf intellectuals" working in the field of Deaf Studies (O'Brien & Emery 2013). Deaf narratives and deaf people's life stories form the core of my research projects. My life experience can be described as Deafhood, defined as "deaf people's own ontologies" or "ways of being in the world" (Kusters & De Meulder 2013:428). Deafhood, for me, encompasses all aspects of the lived ontological deaf experience. In my line of work, I write stories, not only about life in residential schools for deaf children, but also about my experience of oralism, an educational ideology that prohibits the use of sign language and promotes spoken language communication through articulation and pronunciation drills and lip-reading exercises (O'Connell & Deegan 2014).

This chapter begins by critically and reflexively exploring my experience of writing autoethnography into my PhD thesis, titled, *A critical (auto) ethnographic study of deaf people's experiences of education and culture in Ireland*. My doctoral project involved a study of 20 deaf participants and the researcher in a critical (auto) ethnographic study of deaf education. I found autoethnography a useful form of inquiry for the doctoral research. The method involves doing "research, writing, story, and method that connect the autobiographical and personal to the cultural, social, and political" (Ellis 2004:xix). In many ways autoethnography helped create space for a counternarrative to the dominant deaf education research paradigm, which describes deaf people without including them as research participants and giving "voice" to their stories (e.g., Mathews 2011). When hearing researchers write about deaf people's experiences of education, they cannot help but represent these experiences through their own lenses as people who are biologically and culturally hearing. When Deaf Studies and autoethnography intersect, deaf autoethnographies are created in ways that make fertile ground for sharing experiences of education with the world.

This chapter seeks to answer the following questions: How does one represent the lived Deafhood experience through autoethnography? What are the challenges and resolutions for doing autoethnography? How does one address criticism, ethical issues, and narrative truth? To answer these questions, I show examples of doing autoethnography by layering in five "present-tense vignettes" (Humphries 2005:840) extracted from my autoethnographic stories. These vignettes are utilized as bracketed phenomena linked with the text to illustrate how autoethnography is constructed, evaluated, and produced.

BEGINNINGS

Vignette 1: Discovering Autoethnography
Autumn in Ireland, a doctoral supervisor meeting almost four years ago to the day I start writing this chapter on autoethnography. I glance at the clock on the wall behind "Professor John,"[1] my doctoral supervisor. It is 2.45 pm. "Lucy," my sign language interpreter is sitting beside Professor John translating my comments in Irish Sign Language (ISL) into spoken English. I tell my supervisor about the autobiographical journal writing that I have written as a separate project from the doctoral research.

"How do you feel about including your story in your thesis?" the professor asks. "I would suggest writing an autoethnography into your research as a way to respond to the challenge of subjective research."

"Autoethnography?" I make a mental note to do some research on the subject. "What does that involve?"

"Don't worry about that for now. Your questions will soon be answered after you do some reading on autoethnography. You can decide what to do later. Have you ever heard of Carolyn Ellis?"

"No. I can't say I have."

"She is an American sociologist working in the field of Communication Studies. She has published widely on the subject."

"I don't think I have come across her work." I point out. "I am thinking of the viva voce. How will an autoethnography stand up to scrutiny?"

---

[1] This is a pseudonym. The etymological root of the term *auto,* as derived from the Greek αὐτο, denotes the idea of "self," "one's own," and "by oneself"; ethnography is literally the writing of culture.

"Let's wait until you have read her book, The Ethnographic I: A meth-odological novel about autoethnography. *The book is written in the form of a novel that weaves together personal stories, theory, and narrative about her teaching a fictional university graduate course. Ellis uses characterization, plot, scene-setting, dialogue, and action to show the reader autoethnography's methodological meanings and form."*

"I must get a copy of the book."

"Good idea. You might also like to read the work of Art Bochner and Norman Denzin. They've published papers on autoethnography. We can discuss Ellis's book at our meeting next month and you can decide what you want to do for your thesis writing."

So began my entry into autoethnography. As this vignette shows, my own route to autoethnography was via autobiography. The impetus for doing autoethnography grew out of a willingness to understand how theory and reflexive engagement could help elicit meaning from my autobiographical stories. After reading Ellis's book and the work of Ellis and Bochner (2000), I made the decision to introduce a series of autoethnographic vignettes into the research alongside the study of 20 deaf participants for the doctoral thesis. My first initiative in "creating autoethnography" (Muncey 2010) was to combine tenets of my autobiographical writing with ethnography (Ellis 2004). Before taking on the task, the first step was to learn about the distinction between autoethnography and autobiography.

According to Alexander (1999:309), auto*biography* is "a process of recreating, re-viewing and making sense of the biographic past." The autobiographer uses retrospection to write about his or her life in order to capture all the fundamentals of that life remembered (Ellis, Adams & Bochner 2011). Autobiography may include stories about "epiphanies," or remembered moments that cause the writer to reflect on lived experience after which life does not seem quite the same. Interviews, journals, photographs, and newspaper articles also are used as sources to help the autobiographers with their memories of certain events described in their writing. Autobiographers sometimes write by "showing"—a form of writing that uses the literary conventions of characterization, scene-setting, plot development, and dialogue intended to "bring readers into the thoughts, feelings, emotions and actions" in the story (Ellis et al. 2011:4). In the mode of "telling the tale," the autobiographer attempts to put some distance between writer and text in order to describe an event in a more abstract way. When both "telling" and "showing" are employed, they help elucidate an understanding of what is happening in a story.

Auto*ethnography*, on the other hand, is "an autobiographical genre of writing and research that displays multiple layers of con-sciousness" (Ellis & Bochner 2000:739). Autoethnographers also write about "epiphanies" (Denzin 2014) and may use journals, photographs, letters, and newspaper articles (Muncey 2010). Similarly, they employ the literary technique of "showing" to give readers a sense of "being there" (Spry 2001) with the author going through an experience. They also employ the technique of "telling" to describe an experience in a less intimate way. By contrast, autoethnographers write (graphy) about personal experience (auto) that arises from being part of a culture (ethno) and show how they acquire a specific cultural identity. Unlike autobiography, autoethnography connects the personal with the cultural and political and uses ethnographic methods to analyse personal experience reflexively in order to elicit meaning from the stories (Ellis 2004). Ethnography entails the use of "thick description" to make cultural experience familiar to readers (Ellis et al. 2011). Thus, the hybridity of *auto* and *ethnography* means researchers make cultural and personal experience accessible and meaningful by using a systematic approach to analyzing and interpreting sociocultural understandings of self (1). This systematic approach sets autoethnography apart from other self-narratives such as autobiography.

A number of Deaf-authored autoethnographic texts have emerged in recent times. McIlroy and Storbeck's (2011) study, for example, is written as an output of McIlroy's master's thesis assignment on deaf identities. The idea of including two authors—McIlroy, the Deaf author experiencing the autoethnography and working in collaboration with the hearing author Storbeck—raises questions around the meaning of "auto" in this ethnographic study. Valente's (2011) book is based on the author's experience as a young child attending mainstream school and as an adult looking back on his attempt to find a place in society. The author blends autobiographical stories with elements of ethnographic writing and critical theory. Though Valente's most recent article on autoethnography (2014) explores a number of topics covered in the book, he also includes details omitted from the narrative—details that prompted a reconsideration of the way he shaped his stories. As Valente looks back in time, he finds himself adding details about his father. In a moving telling of the father–son relationship Valente adopts the metaphor of the Incredible Hulk to analyze the emotions generated by the effects of his father's alcoholism. As Valente writes autoethnographically, he is very much aware of his feelings and conflicting thoughts as a young deaf boy and of the hidden depths of his anger. There is courage displayed in writing the narrative about issues that are of a sensitive nature. The stories are powerful enough to evoke in me an emotional reaction that causes me to reflect on my relationship with my father, which I detail later in this chapter.

Embedded in West's (2012) narrative inquiry concerning the life stories of deaf and hearing bilingual families is a series of autoethnographic vignettes about the hearing author who has no corporeal experience of deafness. Both McIllroy and Valente take insights gained from a particular position as deaf people and use these as vantage points to write about their identity, culture, and language. Ruiz-Williams, Burke, Chong, and Chainarong (2015) claim that their work is based on autoethnography. However, I found little evidence of a reflexive engagement, an important feature of autoethnography, wherein the autoethnographer stands back from the stories and begins to ask questions to help reflect on the stories and the writing experience (Ellis 2004).

Though a number of Deaf-authored autobiographical writings, including Laborit (1999) and Bragg (2002) have been published, it is perhaps surprising given the history of deaf people's experience of marginalization and discrimination, that relatively few Deaf-authored autoethnographies are available to us. A number of possible explanations for this neglect can be offered. First, researchers may be reluctant to break away from long-held beliefs about objective research. Second, researchers may have avoided taking this approach due to a general lack of awareness or understanding of what constitutes autoethnography in terms of how it is defined and how it should be written, constructed, and produced.

History of Autoethnography

Historically, certain writers from the anthropology tradition paved the way for autoethnography. Jomo Kenyatta's (1966) *Facing Mount Kenya* is said to be the first published autoethnography, although it received heavy criticism for being too subjective (Hayano 1979). Although Karl Heider (1975:3–17) used autoethnographic method in a study of the Dani people, Hayano (1979) is credited as the originator of the term after he championed a form of "insider ethnography" (Ellis 2004). Hayano published *Poker Face* (1982) based on a study of semiprofessional poker players and argues that researchers' "insider status" should be made transparent in research.

The early 1980s saw a paradigm shift in the way qualitative research was conducted. In that period, postmodernist thought began challenging the legitimacy of the "objective observer" position of the researcher. Throughout the 1990s and the early 21st century, scholars placed great value in personal stories within various social science research disciplines including sports science (Sparkes 2000), nursing (Muncey 2010), health care (Ellis 1995), and education (Hayler 2010). Subsequently, autoethnographic stories emerged on a wide range of subjects, including loss and trauma (O'Connell 2016a), stigma (O'Connell 2016b), and communication (Ellis & Bochner 2006) and have been written using a variety of literary genres from poetry and fiction to novels, photographic essays, journals, and prose poetry (Muncey 2010).

Defining Autoethnography

There are subtle variations in the way autoethnography is defined because various uses of the term and their associated meanings can differ depending on the relationship between the researcher's personal experience and the phenomenon under investigation (e.g., education, health, sports). Reed-Danahay (1997:2) suggests that its meaning contains "a double sense—referring either to the ethnography of one's own group or to autobiographical writing that has ethnographic interest." This is true to the extent that autoethnography may be described as "a self–(auto–) ethnography or an autobiographical (auto –) ethnography."

Sparkes (2000:21) defines autoethnography as "highly personalized accounts that draw upon the experience of the author/researcher for the purposes of extending sociological understanding." Writing about performance autoethnography, Spry (2001:710) proposes a form of "self-narrative that critiques the situatedness of self with others in social contexts." Maréchal (2010:43) describes autoethnography as a "method of research that involves self-observation and reflexive investigation in the context of ethnographic field work and writing."

Ellis et al. (2011) offer a catalogued list of autoethnographic "cousins" in the form of "layered accounts," using vignettes, reflexivity, multiple voices, and introspection. Another form of autoethnographic writing listed in the catalogue are the "indigenous ethnographies" produced by native and indigenous authors in response to colonized systems, power relations, and the outsider-researcher's right and authority to study their people. In "narrative ethnographies," the ethnographer produces narrative text detailing his or her personal experiences of doing ethnography. The researcher's perceptions around doing research and interacting with participants while doing field work are revealed in "reflexive ethnography."

The one register that closely identifies with my doctoral thesis writing is *indigenous ethnography*:

> Indigenous ethnographies are written by researchers who share a history of colonialism or economic subordination, including subjugation by ethnographers who have made them subjects of their work. You could write as a bicultural insider/outsider and construct your own cultural story to depict a way of life. (Ellis 2004:46)

Given that indigenous ethnography attempts to make "characteristics of a culture familiar to outsiders and insiders" (Ellis et al. 2011), I took the liberty to write my "own cultural story" in order to "depict a way of life" and reveal the extent of my experience of oralism around the subjugation of sign language. These stories were written as evocative accounts detailing some painful memories of the past. They are called evocative stories because they are powerful enough to evoke an emotional response in the reader. They are stories not only of oppression and marginalization but also of steadfast determination and positive life transformations. Just like the stories presented in this chapter, they were written as evocative autoethnography.

EVOCATIVE AUTOETHNOGRAPHY

Vignette 2: Lost in Translation

My teacher, Miss Carey, is a commanding presence in class. Today, she is talking to us as if we are hearing children. I have no idea what she telling us to do. All she does is point her index finger to the floor.

" . . . . do it now!"

I notice her lips quivering and wavering in frustration. She seems powerless to help us understand her instructions. I wonder what she wants us to do. I am 12 years old and everything seems hazy in this semi-dark classroom. We are seated in darkness save for the light of the overhead projector shining onto the silver screen behind her. I try to read the figures displayed on screen, but they are blurred. In a show of impatience, Miss Carey turns swiftly around and stares at the screen through a maze of wavy shoulder-length hair that partly covers her face and mouth. Then she quickly pushes the projector to the other side of her desk and adjusts the head to make the screen display clear. It is then that I can start counting numbers and figures.

Miss Carey does not sign because she does not know how to sign. Reading her lips strains my eyes. I know she is telling us to do something, but the words from her mouth are elusive; they are like quicksand. She keeps saying, "Do it . . ." and continually adjusts the microphone around her neck. She rolls her eyes heavenward, showing frustrated annoyance.

"Can you . . ."

When her eyebrows are raised, I can see she is asking questions. Only a few of us nod in reply.

"What are we to do?" I ask her. Something in my throat forces me to swallow hard. Miss Carey does not hear me. Instead, she looks at the screen and back at us. Pointing to the floor, she says,

"There . . . stop that . . . now do it . . ."

I take a deep breath, a sense of anger rising inside me. Tim taps me on the arm and leans sideways. Crouching under the table, he makes discrete signs.

"Is that a question?"

"I don't know."

Miss Carey says, "Stop . . . now . . . get ..."

For a second, I place my hands on my face not knowing whether to like or hate her. I see her through the gap between my fingers. She is writing something on the projector. Taking my hands down, I study her notes. The writing is round and slanted like a scribble. We start writing notes onto our notepads. No wants to ask questions. We think she will respond in the same exasperated way. And she still talks to us like we are hearing children. I know she is talking but not what she is telling us to do.

" ... No ... make it ..."

One of our classmates, Bob, is partially deaf. He can hear with a hearing aid. Bob does not sign to us because he is terrified of getting punished. When Miss Carey moves across the room, we ask for repeat instructions, but she ignores us. Instead, she tells us to "... Stop ... look...." She is irritated at our show of indifference and throws her hand up in desperation. My teacher is about to lose control of herself. As if sensing that we are watching, she moves into the shadow and becomes submerged in the semi-darkness. My classmates start writing on paper, trying to guess the question. What does she want us to do? Once more frustration squeezes my heart. I take deep breathes. Before long, Kevin taps my elbow.

"What did she say?"

There are two particular genres of writing produced by autoethnographers: "evocative" and "analytical" autoethnography. While the first appreciates the emotional context in stories, the second is analytical and does not deal with the emotions of the characters or people in autoethnographic stories (Anderson 2006). Evocative autoethnography has been criticized by Anderson (2006) for using emotion in qualitative research. In his view, autoethnographers should avoid engaging in "emotionalism" and, instead, adopt a more analytical approach using systematic ethnographic methods to find answers to questions about social life. In analytic autoethnography, the researcher is (1) self-identified as a full member of the cultural group or community under study; (2) visible as a member in the researcher's published text; and (3) committed to an analytical approach to enhancing theoretical understandings of social phenomena and "objective" writing and analysis of a social or cultural group under study. Based on his personal experience of family, work, and sports skydiving, Anderson (2006) analytic autoethnography examines personal experience against the broader social phenomenon involving stories of other skydivers. Similarly, Hayler (2010) constructed personal stories were shared with six other teacher educators as a means of gaining new understandings of experiences, beliefs, and practices. Haylor's analytical approach is based on comparing and sharing stories with other participants in order to increase his understanding of an experience. Ellis and Bochner (2006:433) accuse analytical autoethnography of encouraging the reader to "become a detached spectator" with little emotional context available in the narrative to engage them. According to the authors, the analytical approach to autoethnography is a genre of realist ethnography that excludes the emotions, thoughts, and feelings of the researcher (Ellis & Bochner 2006).

As Vignette 2 illustrates, this chapter is framed as evocative autoeth-nography because it shows emotional contexts of experience based on my memories of the events that took place in the classroom sometime in the late 1970s. The story is purposefully written in the present tense in order to summon rich and contextualized information about the experience of oralism. The aim was to cause readers to feel and think about their lives in relation to my life. The chaos in the story is bound together in a systematic way to give coherence to the narrative using dialogue, scene-setting, plot, characterization, and description (Ellis 2004). Thus, the vignette is an exemplar of how emotion can be used to elicit a response from readers and help "generate conversation" (Ellis 2004). The vignette is written in the present tense to create a sense of verisimilitude and to make the experience lifelike and real on the page. Dialogue, for example, is constructed so as to capture the subjective experience of the lip-reader. The reader may experience the author's feelings of anguish, discomfort, and frustration in the experience of being lost in translation.

NARRATIVE TRUTH

Vignette 3: A Walk in the Woods
"Where are we going?" I ask Patrick.

It is a mild October Saturday morning. The sky is overcast with occasional sunshine bursting through clouds. The air is cold and crisp. We are standing in the middle of the queue, hidden out of sight of the authorities. I am probably seven or eight years of age. All of us are children of similar age dressed casually in jumpers and overcoats with a small rucksacks sitting snugly on our backs. Standing in line, two abreast, we wait for the signal to move forward. Patrick glances nervously over his shoulder looking to see if anyone is watching us. Then he signs.

"We will walk near the trees," he says, "and pick nuts from the ground and throw them into the field."

"Yes," I say. "We can play with the leaves on the ground."

"We can run around and hide and play catch."

"Yes!"

My eyes widen with excitement. Suddenly Patrick turns his head and looks toward the end of the queue. All heads turn round, and I stand on my toes peering over shoulders. Beyond the queue is a towering figure looming over a red-haired boy. The woman is holding his hand. She has a large tree branch in the other hand. The sight of the boy receiving three lashes on the palm of his hand causes me to recoil in shock. I gasp with fright and stagger backward. After steadying myself, I turn and stand on my toes and see the distress on the boy's face. The woman's eyes glare with anger, lips tightly shut, almost slanted at the corner. I cannot take my eyes off her face, the pulse surging through my body. My heart quickens apace. The boy picks himself up off the ground and holds his hand under his armpit, tears streaming down his face. Unable to watch any longer, I turn round quickly and face Patrick. Patrick signs with deliberate ease, making sure not to stir his shoulder.

"She saw Joe signing," he says.

I push my hands down and scuffle backward trying to find my footing. I am back in the row again staring at Patrick's pale face, searching for answers. But there is nothing more to be said. Time to move on. My teacher steps forward walking past us down toward the end of the queue. I look on anxiously and, when the queue starts moving again, I follow the line ahead of me. Soon the wooden gate appears in sight, a hundred yards ahead. At the gateway, we step into the clearing and walk on grass. I feel the crunch of copper leaves under my shoes until we come to a pathway. From there, we move to an opening where dark pine trees hover above us.

After writing this vignette, I found myself reflecting on standards of truth or verisimilitude in the story. Given that I was somewhere between seven and eight years old at the time the events took place, the issue uppermost in my mind was the question of narrative truth. What is truth? How can we know it? As Denzin (2014) states, there are different types of truths: *facts* and *facticities*. Facts relate to events that are believed to have occurred, while facticities describe how facts were lived and experienced by people interacting with one another. Truth refers to "statements that are in agreement with facts and faculties as they are known and understood" (Denzin 2014:13) and narrative truth "is based on how a story is used, understood and responded to" (70). In this particular vignette, I present my own version of truth by narrating a story about a deeply disturbing incident that occurred when I was a young boy. I had not managed to write about this incident until recently because memory can be fallible. People may either tell different stories of the same event or describe the same event differently (Denzin 2014). I tried various ways to write this eye-witness account but, because it happened over 40 years ago, I was not sure whether this was my story at all. I wondered if the victim should be the one to tell it himself, because I was merely a bystander in the drama that unfolded before my eyes. I wrote the story knowing that the boy was the one who experienced pain and suffering. Although I did not experience his pain, I was overcome with shock and fear given that I also used sign language and the violence inflicted on the boy easily could have befallen me.

To portray accurately the experience of witnessing the violence, I felt it was important to test my memory of the event. While looking back on the past, I reached the conclusion that the walk in the woods did actually happen because this was a frequent event in childhood. Though I remember witnessing the violence inflicted on the boy it was difficult to know whether this happened on the day we went out for a walk. I asked myself whether the incident occurred on the same day and whether this was my version of the truth. My response was that regardless of whether this was true or not, my truth lay in the painful experience of witnessing and the joys of going out to play in the woodlands. In the interest of description and to make the narrative work, I wrote about the incident as though it happened on the same day. The dialogue was constructed to the best of my recollection. Although I can remember the scenes played out in my mind, I cannot remember details of conversation.

According to Ellis (2011:10), autoethnographers rely on narrative truth, on "what a story of experience does—how it is used, understood, and responded to for and by us and others as writers, participants, audiences and humans." Although it is impossible for anyone to recall events in language that represents how they were lived, autoethnographers reflexively ask whether the event has been remembered and described correctly in the story. Is the report "fact" or "facticities"? Such questions around narrative truth and the narrator's credibility as a writer, performer, and observer often are raised by autoethnographers (Denzin 2014). Where validity is maintained, the story must have verisimilitude in that the author's actual experience is portrayed in a way that is lifelike, "true, coherent, believable, and connects the reader to the writer's world" (Denzin 2014:70).

SELF-INDULGENCE OR SOMETHING MORE?

Vignette 4: Stars of the Silver Screen
It is seven o'clock, an hour after Saturday evening supper. We are back in the play hall and there is a minute or two before the film begins showing. We are seated in cast-iron chairs all lined up in rows at the end of the play hall. Six rows of ten chairs, five on each side of the walkway, all lined up in eager anticipation of the start of "Butch Cassidy and the Sundance Kid." The play hall is pitched in total darkness and the silver screen before us flickers with light from the film projector behind us. On our right is the theater stage, where curtains are drawn and a wall poster informs us that "Jack and the Beanstalk" will be showing in the spring.

The man in charge of the film showing, Brother Johnson, is inserting rolls of film into the projector reel. Earlier, he had warned us about signing, telling us that anyone caught would be sent upstairs to bed. Halfway through the film there would be a break to allow him time to change the reels. He would take off the reel and replace it with the next roll of film. That night, I arrive in the hall just before the start of the film, and I see Paul's hand waving in the air. Paul waves me over to an empty chair beside him. By the time I reach my seat, I am greeted by back slaps and thumbs up from the lads seated behind me. Paul's face lights up with a bemused smile, and I turn round to face Patrick, Colm, and Kevin, friends I have known for eight years, ever since I started residential school at the age of five.

"Do you know what tonight's film is called?" Paul asks, excitement written all over his face.

I finger spell words: "B-u-t-c-h C-a-s-s-i-d-y..."

"The S-u-n-d-a-n-c-e K-i-d!" Patrick interjects "Robert Redford and Paul Newman are in the film!"

"I don't know," I respond. "I have never seen the film. Is it a cowboy film?"

"Yes. Plenty of action!"

"We should be allowed to choose films we want to watch," Patrick says glancing over his shoulder at the projector. "Is he watching us?"

Colm lowers his hands and makes discrete signs. "I have seen many boring films. All talk and no action."

"I know," I say. "Last week's film was good."

"Yes. That was True Grit."

"J-o-h-n W-a-y-n-e."

"I like cowboy films," Paul signs, lowering his hands. "In cowboy films we see action. If there is too much talking, I get bored. So hard to follow the film."

"I think tonight's film is full of action," Colm signs. "James is sitting near the projector. He has just read the name."

As Paul nudges my left elbow, I turn around several degrees and follow the direction of his hand to the projector at the far end of the room. "Brother Johnson is like a sheriff in a cowboy film. Always watching us."

"Yes, I know. He can be cruel. If he catches us signing, he will send us to bed."

"I would hate to miss the film," Patrick says glancing over his shoulder. "Did you know Brendan was sent to bed last week? He missed the show. It was terrible for him. I think he was caught signing to another boy."

"Did you see it happen?" Colm wants to know.

"Yes I saw it happen...."

Suddenly lights are turned off, and we turn in our chairs to face the silver screen. It flickers on and on. Fifteen minutes into the show, we start asking questions among ourselves trying to figure out the heroes and villains in the film. The film is about two outlaws who are on the run from the sheriff and a group of lawmen. We decide the outlaws are our heroes. We love the all-action film. There are anxious moments because the outlaws cannot escape. They are still being followed. Tensions rise near the end of the film as the group of lawmen closes in on them. Then Butch and Sundance end up in some strange country, hidden inside a hut, and surrounded by soldiers with guns aimed at them. There is no hope. They cannot make a getaway. My heart is racing and I am unable to bear the tension. Their fates already sealed, I hold my breath and wait in hope, not wanting to believe they are about to die. The scene before my eyes is now tinged with tragedy. A short time later, the two men run out of the hut, guns in hand. Then the screen goes still.

There is frantic tapping on my shoulder. I turn around.

"Is this the end?"

"I don't know."

"Are the reels being changed?"

"But the lights are not turned on!"

I turn around, crouch low, and wave at John. John says he heard shots being fired in the background.

"You mean they are dead?"

"Yes, I heard shots," he says, holding an imaginary gun in his hands and making a show of firing shots.

"Fire! Fire!"

"Are you sure shots were fired?"

"Yes, this is the end of the film. Our heroes are dead."

This vignette is condensed from my personal narrative based on a version of my childhood lived in residential school and focusing on my experience doing weekend activities. It is a highly subjective account of an event that occurred during the latter half of the 1970s when I was 13 or 14 years old and at a time when subtitling facilities were unavailable. Like all vignettes presented here, this story was written from inside the head of a young boy using an adult's sentiment and outlook. I wrote it from my imagination, using my own sense of reality based on my subjective experience. I emphasize the word "subjective" in the context of autoethnography's focus on the self in relation to others. Because of its strong emphasis on self, autoethnography's status as proper research has been called into question by scholars committed to "objective" social science research (Sparkes 2000). Delamont (2002), for example, argues that self-narratives are "too personal" (Sparkes 2000), highly subjective, too individualized, and self-absorbed. Ellis (2009) notes that critics describe autoethnographers as "navel-gazing, self-absorbed narcissists who don't fulfil scholarly obligation to hypothesize, analyze, contextualize, and theorize." Such criticism emerged subsequent to Ellis and Bochner's (2000:745) statement that autoethnography "is always a story about the past and not the past itself." Sparkes (2002) argues that there must be something more to the way scholars reject personal narratives, that perhaps therein lies a deep mistrust in valuing self and experience. Ellis and Bochner (2000) argue that the personal is always present in ethnography and, therefore, personal narrative should be utilized "to allow another person's world of experience to inspire critical reflection on your own" (22). In that sense, I wrote the vignette because not only did personal narrative help to understand the experience of oralism better, but it also invoked in readers a feeling for the experience and could inspire critical reflection of that particular experience. Despite criticism leveled at autoethnography, I believe it is my duty as a Deaf scholar and member of a sign language community to create space in which to share my experience through stories and make these stories accessible to readers (Bochner & Ellis 2000).

ETHICAL DILEMMAS

Vignette 5: Homeward Bound

At nine years of age, I am sitting in the front passenger seat of my father's car. On my right, my father is staring straight ahead, his hands gripping the steering wheel. We turn out of the school gateway onto the street under dark clouds. Behind me, in the back seat, are my school friends. It is a Friday evening in February, and we are heading home from school for the weekend. As part of the car pool arrangement, my father is driving the boys to meet their parents in another town. The drive is three hours long. So far, rain has turned light, but dark clouds hover above us. Soon rain starts to fall heavily, pouring needles of water onto the windscreen. My father turns on the windscreen wipers and rests his hands on the steering wheel. He squints his eyes at the road ahead as rain comes down in torrents. At this point, he seems unaware of the boys signing to each other in the back seat behind him. When one of the lads taps me on the shoulder, I turn half a circle and rest my knees on the seat. I lay my arms on top of the seat and watch the boys sign stories about school.

"Did you see the Virginians today?" Paul signs excitedly, imitating the man in a black leather waist-coat.

"I saw it," I reply, half-conscious of my father's disapproval. He has been throwing glances my way since I turned around. For some time, I have been aware of his hostility toward sign language. Still, I cannot find a way to stop signing. The last time he collected us from school, I incurred his wrath.

"Why can't you speak to them?" he had demanded.

I did not wish to argue with him, so I simply ignored his warning and allowed it pass without protest. When I turned around, Stephen wanted to know what my father said to me. So, I told him and the other boys looked at each other in disbelief. I remember feeling ashamed then. I vowed that this time I was not going to let him dictate how I communicated with my friends.

By now buckets of rain are pouring out of the sky. We continue through narrow winding country roads. While we share football stories, my father gives me a persistent tap on the leg, and I turn around to face him.

"Will you stop!" he mouths angrily.

I look at him and turn back to the boys, ignoring his furtive warnings. Paul looks at me enquiringly.

"What is wrong?"

I sign: "He said stop signing."

Before long, my father pulls up to the side road. I quickly turn around to face the windscreen. My father turns toward me looking furious and I recoil in shock. He says something about, "What in the name of Jesus..." Could I not

*stop signing? I attempt a meek apology, mouthing sorry, but he does not see
or hear me. As rain lashes against the windscreen, tension fills the air. Time
stands still. I make up my mind not to sign for the rest of the journey. It is as
good as guaranteed. So, we drive on through winding country roads. With
my back turned to the boys, I look straight ahead feeling submerged in misery.*

This vignette raises important questions around ethical responsibilities
toward intimate others who are implicated in the stories (Ellis 2009).
The question of whether or not to obtain consent from people included
in the narrative must be considered (Wall 2008). Due to the sensitive
nature of this evocative story, special considerations were taken into
account. Ellis (2007) adds "relational ethics" as a new dimension to
ethics in autoethnography, which refers to ethics involved in writing
personal narratives wherein intimate others, such as family members,
friends, partners, and colleagues are described. Ellis (2007) maintains
that no definitive rules or universal principles are available to guide
autoethnographers on how to address ethics. Besides following the
generic rule of "do no harm," autoethnographers must strive to be ethical and honest about the events described as well as to be true to the
comments made by all those involved in the stories.

While writing the story about my father, I considered the question of
consent and, as a consequence, experienced a persistent sense of anxiety over whether or not to contact the participants in the story. Because
my father was deceased, I sought consent from my family, including
my mother, because I was concerned about implications for their reputation. Following Ellis's (2007) suggestion, I shared extracts of my stories with the participants and my family members and subsequently
obtained their consent. In order to add some perspective to my father's
actions, I added details about his upbringing as part of my reflections
on the vignettes. To help give credence to the stories, I described the
school's influence on shaping his beliefs about the value of sign language. Writing the story allowed me to look inward into my thoughts,
feelings, and experiences and outward into my relationship with others
(Ellis 2004). In that sense, autoethnography proved a useful method not
only in my research but also in my search for self-understanding and
understanding of others. It has given new meaning to the experience
I explored in the vignette in that I am able to put some distance between
myself and the past.

EPILOGUE

This chapter explored how I engaged in creative expression by combining autobiography with ethnography and reflexivity. I have demonstrated ways in which autoethnography could be constructed
and produced within and across Deaf Studies research. The process

involved writing autobiographical stories from the heart, revealing my thoughts and feelings "uncensored" (Ellis 2009) on the pages. This was followed by a process of deleting parts that I did not want to reveal. When I returned to the text later, I adopted the ethnographer's critical eye to analyze and reflect on the stories in order to find meaning attached to emotional experience. While engaging in reflexivity, I became self-questioning about stories to gain meaning. Meaning was derived from stories through writing. Meaning was discerned through the use of plot, action, dialogue, scene-setting, and characterization. Meaning stemmed from "showing" rather than "telling." Meaning became accessible when evocative stories were produced and subjected to interpretation and reflexive engagement. I engaged in the ethnographer's task of writing, reading, re-reading, thinking, questioning, consulting with people, communicating almost every day about history, society, sign-language-community issues, identity politics, and sign language, all of which I incorporated into my stories and my analysis of the stories. In doing so, I was able to produce an "evocative autoethnography," one that was not "presented" but rather "communicated" to readers in such a way that they would feel those experiences as if they were part of the story.

Although there are no specific criteria for doing autoethnography, I have managed to raise questions about how exactly it could be constructed and produced. What I have presented here is an argument for its possibilities as a new, innovative, and unconventional research method in Deaf Studies. I have shown how autoethnography provides us with an avenue to address unanswered questions around deaf people's social, educational, cultural, political, and economic lives. Autoethnography offers the possibility for a critique of power systems and for including new ideas and methodologies in Deaf Studies. Autoethnography gives "voice" to deaf scholars whose story historically has been silenced by dominant hearing narratives that attempt to explain away their experiences without due regard for their worldviews. I hope that the discussion I have presented here about the challenges I faced and how I dealt with them will help inform future Deaf scholars and inspire them to share their autoethnographies with the world.

Postscript

In what seems to be late morning, I wake up and look at the clock on the bedside table. It is already 8.30 am on a Thursday in October 2013, one month since I passed the viva voce examination. I yearn to get back to sleep and instead of turning over, I lie on my back, thinking about the class I am about to teach later in the day. No rest today, I think to myself. Then I leap out of bed and get myself ready to drive to university. Dressed in casual clothes, I head down-stairs to the kitchen for breakfast. On my way, I pass the front door and catch a glimpse of a large brown envelope lying on the doormat. Seeing the university stamp marked on the envelope, I think back to a conversation I had with my supervisor about my viva voce examination report. When I enquired about it, he told me the report was in the post.

Before I submitted my doctoral thesis the previous July, I asked Professor John what he thought my chances were at the examination. I had in mind my concern about autoethnography. "Will it pass?" I asked him. "The thesis is in good shape," he replied, "and I am confident it will." I trusted his judgment and felt sure it was a strong piece of work.

On this dark and dreamless morning, I pick up the envelope and hurry inside the kitchen. Seating myself at the breakfast table, I open the envelope with eager anticipation. Slightly tired but anxious to know the examiners' views on my work, I start reading the report. This is what they wrote:

> *Well framed, systematic, elegantly written and courageous, the thesis author combined the narrative sensibilities of a novelist and the analytical skills of a social scientist. It is a bold, critical and self-critical study which deliberately blurs the boundaries between the researcher and the research in an attempt to acknowledge the hybrid identity of the researcher and the complexity of the bi-cultural identity of deaf people as presented in the research topic and data. Drawing from extensive autobiographical writing, edited and carefully selected for the thesis, the doctoral candidate presented a series of vignettes throughout the thesis that allowed him to then pause and reframe them through the lens of a range of social science theorists especially Foucault in explicating identity, knowledge and power in the life experiences of the Deaf community in Ireland over the last fifty years. In doing so, the thesis unfolds a story about education, religious-run schools for the deaf and the state that is powerful, at times disturbing, engaging and speaks to how we understand the complexities of inclusive practices in education today. Each chapter in the thesis was crafted in a way that brings another layer to a complex critical autoethnography. Both examiners agreed it was a privilege to read and undertake a viva for such a new ground break-ing thesis.*

I sit back in my chair feeling relaxed and at peace. If I cannot feel the hap-piness of getting the doctorate, then I have known the joy of producing an autoethnography. I think I am a different person from the one who started this journey over five years ago. This does not mean I am not myself. On the contrary, I remain the same, only my perspectives have changed for the better. I cannot offer conclusions here because the writing journey must go on, and I will continue writing evocative stories and producing autoethnographies. That is my destiny. I hope it is yours, too.

ACKNOWLEDGMENTS

The author wishes to thank Professor Jim Deegan, Mary Immaculate College, as well as Rachel Sanchez and the book editors for their constructive comments on earlier drafts of this chapter.

FUNDING: The author received the following financial support for the research, writing, and/or publication of this chapter: This research was supported by the Irish Research Council Postdoctoral Fellowship GOIPD/2015/73 awarded to Noel P. O'Connell.

REFERENCES

Alexander, B. K. (1999). Performing culture in the classroom: An instructional (auto) ethnography. *Text and Performance Quarterly, 19*(4), 307–331.

Anderson, L. (2006). Analytic autoethnography. *Journal of Contemporary Ethnography, 35*(4), 373–395.

Bragg, B. (2002). *Lessons in laughter: An autobiography of a deaf actor*. Washington, DC: Gallaudet University Press.

Delamont, S. (2002). *Fieldwork*. London: Falmer.

Denzin, N. K. (2014). *Interpretive autoethnography*. New York: Sage.

Ellis, C. (1995). *Final negotiations: A story of love, loss and chronic illness*. Philadelphia PA: Temple University Press.

Ellis, C. (2004). *The ethnographic I: A methodological novel about autoethnography*. Walnut Creek, CA: Alta Mira Press.

Ellis, C. (2007). Telling secrets, revealing lives: Relational ethics in research with intimate others. *Qualitative Inquiry, 13*(1), 3–29.

Ellis, C. (2009). Fighting back or moving on: An autoethnographic response to critics. *International Review of Qualitative Research, 2*(3), 371–378.

Ellis, C., Adams, T. E., & Bochner, A. P. (2011). Autoethnography: An overview. *Forum Qualitative Sozialforschung/Forum: Qualitative Social Research, 12*(1), 10. http://nbnresolving.de/urn:nbn:de:0114-fqs1101108.

Ellis, C., & Bochner, A. (2006). Analyzing analytic autoethnography: An autopsy. *Journal of Contemporary Ethnography, 35*(4), 429–449.

Ellis, C., & Bochner, A. (2000). Autoethnography, personal narrative, reflexivity: Researcher as subject. In N. Denzin and Y. Lincoln (Eds.), *The handbook of qualitative research* (pp. 733–768). Thousand Oaks, CA: Sage.

Hayano, D. (1979). Autoethnography: Paradigms, problems and prospects. *Human Organisation, 38*(1), 99–104.

Hayler, M. (2010). *Autoethnography, Self-Narrative and Teacher Education*. The Netherlands: Sense Publishers.

Humphries, M. (2005). Getting Personal: Reflexivity and Autoethnographic Vignettes. *Qualitative Inquiry, 11*(6), 840–860.

Ladd, P. (2003). *Understanding deaf culture: In search of Deafhood*. Clevedon: Multilingual Matters.

Mathews, E. S. (2011). *Mainstreaming of deaf education in the Republic of Ireland: Language, power, resistance* (Unpublished doctoral dissertation). National University of Ireland, Maynooth.

Ruiz-Williams, E., Burke, M., Chong, V Y., & Chainarong, N. (2015). "My deaf is not your deaf": Realizing intersectional realities at Gallaudet University. In M. Friedner & A. Kusters (Eds.), *It's a small world: International deaf spaces and encounters*. Washington, DC: Gallaudet University Press.

Heider, K. G. (1975). What do people do? Dani auto-ethnography. *Journal of Anthropological Research, 31*(1), 3–17.

Kenyatta, J. (1966). *Facing Mount Kenya*. New York: Vintage Books.

Kusters, A., & De Meulder, M. (2013). Understanding Deafhood: In search of its meanings. *American Annals of the Deaf, 158*(5), 428–438.

Laborit, E. (1999). *The cry of the gull*. Washington, DC: Gallaudet University Press.

Maréchal, G. (2010). Autoethnography. In A. J. Mills, G. Durepos, & E. Wiebe (Eds.), *Encyclopedia of case study research* (pp. 43–45). Thousand Oaks, CA: Sage Publications.

McILroy, G., & Storbeck, C. (2011). Development of deaf identity: An ethnographic study. *Journal of Deaf Studies and Deaf Education, 16*, 4.

Muncey, T. (2010). *Creating autoethnographies*. New York and London: Sage.

O'Brien, D., & Emery, S. (2013). The role of the intellectual in minority group studies: Reflections on Deaf Studies in social and political contexts. *Qualitative Inquiry, 20*(1), 27–36.

O'Connell, N. P. (2016a). Childhood interrupted: A story of loss, separation and reconciliation. *Journal of Loss and Trauma: International Perspectives on Stress and Coping, 21*(3), 225–234. doi: 10.1080/15325024.2015.1048151.

O'Connell, N. P. (2016b). "Passing as normal": Living and coping with the stigma of deafness. *Qualitative Inquiry, 22*(8), 651–661. doi: 10.1177/1077800416634729.

O'Connell, N. P., & Deegan, J. (2014). "Behind the teacher's back": An ethnographic study of deaf people's schooling experiences in the Republic of Ireland. *Irish Educational Studies, 33*(3), 229–247. doi: 10.1080/03323315.2014.940683.

Reed-Danahay, D. E. (1997). *Auto/ethnography: Rewriting the self and the social*. Oxford: Berg.

Sparkes, A. C. (2002). Autoethnography: Self-indulgent or something more? In A. P. Bochner & C. Ellis (Eds.), *Ethnographically speaking: Auto-ethnography, literature, and aesthetics* (pp. 209–232). Walnut Creek, CA: Alta Mira Press.

Sparkes, A. C. (2000). Autoethnography and narratives of self: Reflections on criteria in action. *Sociology of Sport Journal, 17*, 21–43.

Spry, T. (2001). Performing autoethnography: An embodied methodological praxis. *Qualitative Inquiry, 7*(6), 706–732.

Valente, J. M. (2011). *d/Deaf and d/Dub: A portrait of a deaf kid as a superhero*. New York: Peter Lang Publishers.

Valente, J. M. (2014). Monster's analysis: Vulnerable anthropology and deaf superhero-becomings. In M. Sasaki (Ed.), *Literacies of the minorities: Constructing a truly inclusive society* (pp. 10–36). Tokyo: Kuroshio Publishing Company.

Wall, S. (2008). Easier said than done: Writing an autoethnography. *International Journal of Qualitative Methods, 7*, 38–53.

West, D. (2012). *Signs of hope: Deafhearing family life*. Newcastle upon Tyne: Cambridge Scholars Publishing.

13

When Inclusion Excludes. Deaf, Researcher—Either, None, or Both

Hilde Haualand

A core concept in the social reforms that have been launched in the past decades to improve the lives of people with disabilities is *inclusion*. Inclusion is (among other things) a policy or ideology used by governments and other policymakers to change or improve schools, workplaces, housing, or other community institutions so as to adjust them to meet human diversity, and in particular, to embrace people who experience exclusion. The concept is, however, multifaceted and contentious, and has multiple meanings.[1] Inclusion also may describe a state in which everyone participates in the same areas; a process to increase participation (of groups who are not already participating); or a means to meet an end (e.g., legislation that enhances workplace access for people with disabilities so that they also can earn a living). It is often not clear which of these meanings of inclusion are meant in various situations (Powers 2002); nor is it always evident who or what inclusion and inclusive measures target: society as a whole, policymakers, or people with disabilities. To a deaf social anthropologist and researcher who repeatedly and overtly has been marked and sometimes questioned on the basis of what sometimes is perceived as an identity, sometimes as a disability, and sometimes as a physical impairment that supposedly limits access to certain data (bluntly ignoring that being deaf may give access to data that could be overlooked by one who hears), the various ideas of inclusion and their targets do not only represent epistemological challenges, but also manifest themselves as tangible and ambiguous experiences.[2]

---

[1] Inclusion is especially contested when used in discussions on deaf education and the rights of deaf signers (Kusters, De Meulder, Friedner & Emery 2015, Powers 2002), but this debate will not be pursued here.

[2] In this article, "deaf" is not only considered as an identity or as a linguistic minority. Being deaf also is discussed and viewed as a disability that arises as a consequence of discrimination and lack of access to society. This use of "deaf" is also a consequence of the services that were studied in the research process that will be described. In all three countries, the establishment of and right to use a video interpreting service is regulated in disability legislation, and deaf

In this chapter, the multisited fieldwork I conducted in the United States, Sweden, and Norway between 2006 and 2010 serves as a case study to show how the concept of inclusion became a source of epistemological and ontological crisis during the research project, and how a reflexive approach to this discomfort and ambiguity became an asset for analysis. This work formed the basis for my PhD project, and I studied the development and organization of the novel and quickly evolving video interpreting services[3] in these countries. First, I will present the project and some of the underlying ideas about inclusion, technology, and disability in the project and the field. Next, I will discuss my multiple roles and positions, and how they caused an ontological crisis, through presenting excerpts from the fieldwork. These positions were not only relevant when doing fieldwork, but also in the political and research communities where the questions and assumptions related to the video interpreting services were discussed. In the last section of the chapter, I more explicitly reveal how my reflexivity, or self-appraisal (Berger 2015), as a deaf researcher made it possible to recognize and take responsibility for both my own (multiple) positions as well as the outcomes of the research.[4]

Writing and talking about positionality in social science research is about acknowledging the researcher as a person with a gender, certain abilities (and other personal traits), a personality, and lived experiences. It also recognizes the fieldwork as a dialogical process, wherein the researcher both influences the informants and is positioned and influenced by them (England 1994). For the sake of simplicity, the discussion in this chapter is confined to situations where being deaf and/or being a researcher influenced the relationship with the field and the research project. Other aspects that influenced my positionality and relationship to the field and the informants, such as gender, socioeconomic resources, and ethnicity are mostly left out, although these certainly also have an impact on the research process. This simplification is not to say that my experiences of being or positioned as "deaf" are universal,

---

people are entitled to receive or use these services by virtue of hearing loss, regardless of their linguistic or cultural identity or background.

[3] International discourse related to these services often uses Video Relay Service with the abbreviation VRS as a common name for the services provided in a growing number of countries worldwide. I have, however, chosen to use "video interpreting" or "video interpreting services" as a common name, unless it has been important to emphasize that a particular national system is discussed. The reason for this is the prevailing position VRS has in the United States, and its specific reference to a telecommunication service. The telecommunication aspect is, however, only one of several possible definitions or ways to organize the service; therefore, the more encompassing concept "video interpreting" is used as a general term.

[4] Parts of the text in this chapter are from the methods chapter in my PhD dissertation (Haualand 2012).

that a "researcher" is a simple category, or as the chapter shows, that it is possible to separate these roles for someone who is both.

DISABILITY RESEARCH AS DISABILITY POLITICS

The multisited fieldwork (and my PhD project) was part of a project funded by a Norwegian research council program on disability and disabling barriers. The project aimed to study how new information technology influenced the employment situation of disabled people, with an emphasis on systems for technology provision and access, and less emphasis on how individuals actually used these technologies. The research program was in line with a long tradition in Norway, where research on disability to a large extent has been about "applied welfare research intended to provide policy makers with the knowledge on which to act in order to bring about social reform" (Moser 2003:10). Following the social model of disability (see Oliver [1990] and an explanation below), the research program funded research projects on disabling structures, and disabled people were not the sole research subjects. In addition to disabled people, employers, teachers, social workers, public administration workers, and politicians (regardless of whether they were related to or worked with disabled people) were research subjects in several of the projects (Norges forskningsråd 2008). Rather than viewing disability as a consequence of impairments and an (unfortunate) fate of individuals, the social model of disability views disability as a consequence of discrimination and inaccessible social and material constructions (Oliver 1990). According to this view, those social and material conditions need to change, not the individuals with various impairments. The social model of disability has been supported by research that has documented disabling social and material structures (Oliver 1990, Shakespeare 2006, Söder 2009, Tøssebro 2004) and has guided disability politics and motivated social reforms (Moser 2003, Tøssebro 2009). A few examples of legal documents that adopt a social model of disability to protect against discrimination, impose accessibility requirements, and encourage inclusive practices are the Americans with Disabilities Act (1990), the Norwegian Discrimination and Accessibility Act (2009), and the United Nations Convention on the Rights of People with Disabilities (2008), which is being ratified by an increasing number of countries.

Exclusion as the Counterpart of Inclusion

All of the aforementioned legal documents, as well as the research project my PhD was part of, emphasized inclusion as an overarching ideal and underlined the equal right to participate in all areas for everyone. In the context of governmental disability policies (of which my research project also was part), inclusion has in many ways replaced "integration." Integration was about allowing disabled people into ordinary public schools and other arenas of society, without necessarily changing these arenas to make them accessible to all. The concept of integration succeeded a politics of segregation, which meant offering and planning specific and often isolated services for disabled people. Inclusion (as a government policy) is thus historically contingent on both integration and the previous segregation of disabled people in separate schools and institutions (Foucault 1967, 1971, Hacking 1999). The politics of inclusion differs from the politics of segregation, and partly also from integration, in its view on disability, and it has by and large adopted a social view on disability. The continued focus on disability and disabled people in legal documents, as well as various actions to promote inclusion, indicate, however, that people with disabilities, rather than society as such, have continued to be the target of many so-called inclusive measures. Critical voices have emphasized how inclusion as a government policy is discussed as something disabled people "need," or eventually should have the right to, and hence, reconfirms the exclusion it aims to remove (Buckmaster 2009, Goodin 1996, Haualand 2012, 2014, Kusters et al. 2015, Moser 2003). There is an ambiguity embedded in the concept that on the one hand emphasizes inclusion as "active or coercive on the part of the state and, on the other hand, as passive where it comes to those people who are being included" (Buckmaster 2009). The way the inclusion concept guides politics not only confirms that exclusion exists, it also defines disabled people *as* excluded and reproduces categories such as included/excluded and disabled/nondisabled.

One arena in which these categories are reproduced is discussions on technology and disability. Although there has been a gradual move toward defining disability as a consequence of inaccessible social and material structures, the fact that everyone is thoroughly dependent on technologies in everyday life (Latour 1993, Miller 2005) is rarely discussed. Few common definitions of assistive technology recognize that services and products that enable independence for nondisabled people are assistive, too; "Since all useful technology is assistive, it is peculiar that we stipulate that some devices are assistive, while others need no qualification" (Ott, Serlin & Mihm, 2002:21). In my PhD research project, I did not want to uncritically reproduce a conceptual distinction between technologies primarily used by disabled people and other, more generic technologies. Rather than accepting the asymmetric relationship between deaf and hearing people, or between those who are included and those who are not, as given facts, I wanted to analyze and describe the technological dependence that permeates any society, without isolating disabled people's dependence on technology as special or exotic. Technology and institutions are continuously reproduced and "do not exist by themselves. They are being *crafted*, assembled as part of a hinterland" (Law 2004:54). This crafting is not something that belongs to a historical phase of construction or establishment, but exists as a continuous process, in which the objects are reproduced—or enacted—in numerous ways (Mol 2002). Just like the concept of inclusion may reproduce exclusion, the idea that some technologies are assistive while others are not continues to define people through the technologies they use.

As a Norwegian deaf researcher with a scholarship from a disability research program, which was initiated and funded by the government in order to identify and consequentially remove disabling barriers, the ambiguity of inclusion did not only represent a theoretical challenge or curiosity. The experience of being an active agent of inclusion policies while at the same time being a target of various inclusion measures, lent a personal touch to the question of how these more or less given categories of included/excluded, deaf/hearing, disabled/nondisabled were constructed in the first place. I could not avoid observing how I was constructed as a deaf person, as a researcher and a foreigner, to name a few positions, when I interacted with my research subjects. It was difficult to see myself as a passive target of inclusive measures, especially because I was in a quite privileged position as a permanently employed researcher at a renowned labor and welfare research institute in Norway. This institute did (and still does) research that provided the Norwegian government with an evidence base for their disability politics and the goal to enhance inclusion of all, with a special focus on inclusion of disabled people in employment. When talking with deaf people about access to videophones, interpreting services, and, in particular, about their limited access to the labor market, my privileged position as a doctoral researcher often came to the fore. Being a deaf person communicating in Norwegian Sign Language, I was also part of the target group of the video interpreting services—and, hence, belonged to a predefined group of "excluded" or less privileged people who potentially would benefit from the services. When interacting with fellow (hearing) researchers at the disability research program of which I was a part, my lack of access to information and communication that my colleagues could take for granted often put me in an inferior and partially excluded position. I will return later to the ontological crisis I experienced during the research process and will now present the field: videophones and video interpreting in the United States, Norway, and Sweden.

VIDEOPHONES AND VIDEO INTERPRETING AS SOCIAL CONSTRUCTIONS

The different definitions of videophones in Norway and the United States offer an example of how technology and technology provision reproduce social categories and hierarchies. The different definitions of videophones are related closely to the general disability politics in the two countries. As welfare states of the universal type (Esping-Andersen 1990), the Nordic governments (Norway, Sweden, Denmark, Finland, and partially Iceland) cover a broad range of assistive technologies for disabled people. In order to keep the state budget under control, a medical diagnosis indicating some kind of impairment functions as gatekeeper to distinguish those qualified for support (Solvang 2000). Those who qualify have an individual right to the technology they need in order to function in everyday life and at work. Deaf and deafblind people in Norway, are entitled to sign language interpreter services through the same system. Dedicated videophones or software that give access to the video interpreting service are defined as "equipment for video interpreting" in public documents and were listed in the database for assistive technology provided by the government.

In the United States, provision of assistive technologies to individuals is not considered a public responsibility, but a liability of both private and public institutions, or for disabled people's employers. In the United States, the Americans with Disabilities Act (ADA) has required public institutions to make their products and services accessible to all citizens for more than 25 years. According to Berven and Blanck (1999), the Americans with Disabilities Act fosters innovation and activity in the consumer market (especially related to assistive technology) and has expanded the market for goods that improve accessibility. One argument is that universal technological solutions that can be used by as many as possible reduce the need and expenses related to provision and development of special technologies for a few. Videophones are conceived as more generic technologies in the United States. They can be dedicated videophones provided by video-interpreting service providers, computer software, or cell phones with an integrated camera that can be purchased by anyone, and all these solutions provide access to video interpreting services.

Simply assuming that videophones were "assistive technology" or generic technology, or taking the existing hierarchies (of disabled and nondisabled, included and excluded) as facts, limits insights into what technologies do in their interaction with social entities such as political regulations and various private and public institutions. Because videophones and video interpreting had been defined as assistive technology in Norway and Sweden, the United States provided an interesting case for seeing how a different system of technology and service provision functioned.[5] By contrasting different systems of video interpreting, it

---

[5] The three countries have quite similar populations of deaf people with almost equal employment and educational rates, and all countries rank high on the scale of Internet penetration within the overall population.

also was anticipated that it would be easier to detect the particularities of each system, and to see how systems of videophone and video interpreting service provision (which primarily targeted deaf people) re- or deconstructed social categories like those already mentioned.

Although there might be similarities among the video interpreting services in the three countries, the moment they are in use by consumers, they are the result of different policies to achieve the aim of inclusion and participation of all in society. The video interpreting services (like other complex public services) are the result of an assemblage of various pieces of legislation, financial arrangements, ideological aims, and technologies, not to mention the efforts of numerous people, all of which have to intersect in order to make the service "work" (Haualand 2011, 2014). These entities differ in each of the three countries, which also was reflected in the discussion, definition, and organization of the services. Although the particularities of each system are not the focus of this chapter, it is hoped the description will serve to clarify some fundamental differences among the video interpreting services in the three countries.

In the United States, there is a sharp demarcation between *video relay service* and *video remote interpreting,* which respectively refer to interpreting telephone calls between a signer/deaf person and a non-signer/hearing person, and interpreting in situations where the communicating parties are located at the same site, and the interpreter provides the service via a videophone. This distinction is barely visible in Sweden and Norway. At the time of fieldwork, the bulk of American discussion, financing, and regulations were related to video relay services (VRS), and video remote interpreting was diminutive compared to it. VRS is confined to concerns regarding the right to functionally equivalent telecommunication services (as stipulated in the Americans with Disabilities Act and the Telecommunication Act). This means that the features, functions, and capabilities of the video (and text) relay services must mirror the experience of using voice telephone services as closely as possible (Strauss 2009). VRS is regulated by the Federal Communication Commission, the sign language interpreters at the call centers are called *operators* or *call assistants,* and the deaf (and hearing people) who use the service are regarded as *consumers,* or sometimes as *clients.*

In Norway, the name *bildetolktjeneste* (literal translation; *video interpreter service*) indicates an emphasis on a service, which interpreters provide by way of video. In public documents, the service is defined as an extension of the nationwide sign language interpreting service. This also is reflected in the name, which emphasizes the interpreters, and also indicates the medium (video) of the interpreting service. The national social insurance agency provides both the videophones and the video interpreting services. The service is rarely discussed as a telecommunication service (as it is defined in the United States), even though 75% of the assignments are what Americans would define as video relay service (NAV 2010). In Norway, video interpreting is organized entirely as a means to provide (and receive) interpreter services by way of videophones.

In Sweden, regional public rehabilitation service offices distribute the videophones, and the Post and Telecommunication Agency funds the service. The Swedish name *förmedlingstjänst via bildtelefoni* (literal translation; *relay (or liaison) services via videophones*) indicates a separation between the service and the technology not seen in the other two countries. Just like in the United States, the public telecommunication authorities regulate the service, but a sign language interpreting company provides the service. The video interpreting service also can be reached by way of generic cell phones with video software. The word *förmedlingstjänst* emphasizes a service focused on passing on communication or information, and it is not restricted to phone calls. The sign language interpreters work alternately in a studio and in situations where they are present in person, and under the same working title; sign language interpreter *(teckenspråkstolk)*.

THE FIELDWORK

The fieldwork (2006–2010) took place during a period when video interpreting services were evolving quickly in the three countries, and government agencies, various nongovernmental organizations, and product developers did extensive work to establish and develop a service enabled by a new technology. The "field" was hence not a definite place or a specific group of people, but rather a bundle of technologies, disability issues and politics, and the fieldwork reflected this definition of the field. When I engaged in participant observation and conducted interviews with those who used and/or worked with the video interpreting services (whether these were signers/deaf people, designers, service providers, interpreters, or other stakeholders), I wanted to see how they related the service to themselves and to others, and how they viewed their own roles and responsibilities in a system of videophone and video interpreting service organization and provision. By tracing the relationships among the various pieces of legislation, public and private institutions, people, and technologies, I aimed to understand how the "specific ways in which the phenomenon studied exists in the world, about the ways in which it is entangled" (Sørensen 2010:44). Defining the field as bundles of technologies and politics had two profound impacts on the fieldwork. First, defining the field as a bundle, directed the glance toward a search for connections and assemblages in and between these bundles. The fieldwork could itself be regarded as an assemblage, or a "process of bundling, of assembling, or better of self-assembling in which the elements put together are not fixed in shape, do not belong to a larger pre-given list but are constructed at least in part as they are entangled together" (Law 2004:42). Second, when the focus is on a system, rather than a predefined group of people, the fieldwork is bound to be multisited, which in "more practical terms (. . .) involves following processes in motion, rather than units in situ. It also involves a reconsideration of the politics of ethnography, away from an investigation of "subaltern" peoples, seen in the context of an exploitative world system, towards an investigation of the system itself". By focusing on *systems* of video interpreting, I hoped to escape a view that defined the deaf consumers or users of these services as excluded per se (cf. critique of inclusion by Buckmaster [2009]). Rather, I wanted to analyze how the anticipated roles of deaf people were constructed within these systems.

Taking Communication for Granted

The United States not only provided an interesting contrast to the Nordic systems for technology provision, but also provided opportunity for a unique case study in Gallaudet University, given that a majority of its employees and students know and use sign language every day.[6] Residing and working at Gallaudet would provide an opportunity not only to study how deaf people use a particular technology in everyday work life, but also would provide a milieu that would serve as a contrast with work settings where deaf people using videophones were alone or a minority. Located in the middle of America's capital city, the geographical and mental distances were also very short to the political and legal institutions and organizations that not only had first-hand knowledge and expertise on video interpreting services, but also worked actively to either change or implement these services.

Being a visiting researcher at Gallaudet University from late 2005 until July 2006, I also was provided with a comfortable position from which to study life on a campus where sign language was ubiquitous. Because I already knew American Sign Language from the time I had been an exchange student at a high school in the United States, I could quickly take part in the everyday routines of faculty and staff. I also was given access to all their technological resources and could use them the way they did. The fieldwork included visits to federal departments, nongovernmental organizations (NGOs), and other institutions involved in developing video interpreting services. In most of these places, people who knew ASL, whether they were deaf or hearing,

---

[6] Many of the readers of this book should be familiar with Gallaudet University (Washington, DC), which is the world's only liberal arts university for the deaf, where the lectures, instructions, and tutoring by and large are in American Sign Language.

welcomed me, or they already had arranged for an interpreter to talk with me. With permission from the Internal Review Board at Gallaudet University, I conducted several interviews with both colleagues at the university and deaf people in the Washington, DC area about their use of technology to communicate at their workplaces. The topic of videophones came up early in these interviews, and one informant demonstrated how the sign for videophones (fingerspelled "VP") was no longer only a noun to describe a videophone, but also was used as a verb, as in, "We'll VP tonight?" or "VP later, OK?" There was a glut of commercial material and gatherings by video relay service providers around the campus. People could still recall what it was like not to have this technology around and one could inevitably observe an intense diffusion period of a new communication technology.

The prevalence of sign language at Gallaudet and its surroundings quite soon gave me a sense of being ordinary, a feeling of being "at home among strangers" (cf. the book with the same title [Schein 1989]). It would, however, misleadingly simplify the experience(s) of being deaf if I claimed I was totally "at home" when living in a foreign deaf community. Deaf people are always deaf in the context of a region, a nation state, or the social or cultural group within which they reside. The experience of being deaf in the United States is different from the experience of being deaf in Norway or any other part of the world (Friedner & Kusters 2015). When I claim I felt at home at Gallaudet, I am foremost referring to a shared mode of visual communication and partially to similar (but not identical) experiences with hearing, non-signing people.

As a Norwegian who normally resided in a rural suburb outside Oslo, I was, indeed, also an outsider in downtown Washington, DC. I struggled to adjust to the pace of life in the capital city and at the university, and to understand formal procedures related to receiving a social security number or opening a bank account. I spent hours in the huge local grocery store only to leave with a bottle of juice, a few apples, yogurt, and muesli. Another trivial, yet vital task was to decode the East Coast social codes in order to blend in, and to keep track of a rhythm of life I experienced as speedier than what I was used to from Norway. With all the practical mysteries I had to solve and the quest to understand the dynamics of life in the political heart of the United States, I was also a continuous outsider who never really blended in with life in Washington. This did not, however, prevent me from soon sharing the thoughts of a woman who had been working at Gallaudet for more than 20 years. She and I discussed the difference between her work situation at Gallaudet and the struggles of her deaf husband, who worked in downtown Washington, DC. He was frustrated with the process of convincing his boss to allow a videophone at his desk, and she commented, "One reason I am still working here is that I don't tolerate those frustrations." After only a few months at Gallaudet, my tolerance and patience with communication barriers decreased. I was beginning to take the ease of access to communication technologies and other people for granted, just like most hearing people do every day without ever giving this access a second thought.

Being an Excluded Token of Inclusion in the Research Group

When I went home to Norway, my conception of myself as a deaf person had changed through a process of "looping," described by Hacking (1999) as a process in which someone classified gets new knowledge related to this classification, and this knowledge consequently "loops back to force changes in the classification and knowledge that exist about them" (105). At Gallaudet, I gradually learned to take access to communication for granted, and rarely had to give the struggle for participation a second thought. The inclusion I sensed (and very soon took for granted) was not the kind of inclusion discussed in public documents, but was more like a state of being wherein my access, right, or possibility to participate were rarely challenged. My behavior and understanding of others and myself changed in the interaction with the community in and around Gallaudet University. The intense focus on videophones and VRS in the United States had provided me with many new questions to explore in the continued fieldwork in Norway, and later also in Sweden. These were a result of the empirical observations made in and around Gallaudet, but the very tangible reality I had lived in at this same place also changed my experience of being a communicating human being.

From taking communication for granted, the re-encounter with an audiocentric world in Oslo, Norway was harsh. From previous experience, I knew that I would use interpreters more often in Oslo than at Gallaudet, but I was not prepared for all the work I had to do merely to be able to participate in the research community. After nine months at Gallaudet, I had become accustomed to participating in a broad range of arenas and expected to continue this participation at home, but the work required to organize interpreters for this became a part-time job.[7] The daily e-mails to and from the regional interpreter service and other people I needed to consult in order to get the right interpreters in place at the right time added up to about 500 e-mails every semester, not to mention the numerous text messages I also had to handle.

The practical work was cumbersome, but what was really annoying was that co-researchers in the field of disability studies, whom I thought would be sensitive to the issues of inclusion and communication,

---

[7] In Norway, access to sign language interpreters is considered an individual right of deaf and deaf blind people. There are no limits on the amount of interpreter services, other than the limits on available interpreters/resources.

turned out to be completely oblivious to these issues. I had been working with some of these researchers for years, and many also had a long
record of disability research. They did not see handling interpreters
as a mutual responsibility, and many had a difficult time seeing that
the interpreter not only worked "for" the deaf person but was there to
facilitate communication between at least two parties. Further, the presence of interpreters at meetings often was viewed as sufficient to secure
equal participation and access for all participants. They did not see that
communication and inclusion of all was about much more than just
having an interpreter present at a meeting. The disability research community discussed research on inclusion in schools, workplaces, and
other locations where the idea of inclusion was "implemented," as if
inclusion were something to be practiced in the schools and workplaces
we researched. Inclusion once again became a government policy and
a goal to implement, by someone else, but not something to consider
right here and now among us. Due to the struggle I faced to participate and to organize the interpreters we needed in the research group,
I kept asking myself if my co-researchers really wanted me there. As a
deaf researcher, I felt like a condensation of the tangible consequences
of exclusion and a fantasy of what inclusion policies make possible.
I defended the ethical imperative of inclusion while I also questioned it,
because it failed me over and over again. I could not take the position of
the active and coercive part/agent, because I repeatedly found myself
left out as a deaf person among hearing researchers. I could not take
the position of a passive receiver, because I also was a product of the
politics of inclusion and had been empowered with tools to take action.
The feeling of being an excluded token of inclusion was growing.

Legitimacy as a Deaf Researcher

It was, however, not only the work to "include" myself that made me
question my position as a researcher. As one of the first deaf PhD students in Norway, I also belonged to a quite novel group of academics in
the Norwegian research community. Some of the comments I received
questioned my ability to treat my data with the desired analytical distance. Because I sometimes also used or tested the video interpreting
services, which were then emerging in Norway, a few co-researchers
warned me against the danger of becoming "my own informant," and
suggested that I would not be able to stay objective because I was "too
deaf." By virtue of my difference or deviance (as a deaf person), they
then claimed I could be no different than all other people embodying
the same difference, irrespective of all other potentially different backgrounds, such as education, employment, or personal interests.

From discussions with fellow deaf academics and from anecdotal
examples shared through social media, I knew I was not alone in facing
a somewhat outdated, yet prevailing objective/subjective-divide when

more or less implicitly being accused of not being as "objective" as hearing research fellows (in particular if the research material or questions involved other deaf people). These accusations are rarely seen in print, and in my case, they often were disguised as questions or comments at conferences or in discussions with lay persons or other (hearing) academics. Braided as they were with the struggle to participate at both formal and informal meetings, these comments nevertheless effectively undercut my sense of legitimacy as a deaf researcher.

My fieldwork in the United States, and my observations of the different ways videophones were discussed in public in Norway and the United States, had confirmed the assumption that the divide between technologies used primarily by disabled people and other (and more generic) technologies, was socially and politically constructed. I was becoming increasingly aware of how everyone was and is thoroughly dependent on communication technologies, but only disabled people were discussed and identified as "dependent" on "special" or "assistive" technology, and as vulnerable in times of technological change. The significance of the existing material infrastructure to everyone, not only disabled people, was concealed in discussions on the significance of technology to include disabled people in the labor market. It was not possible to identify videophones or other technologies as "assistive" by studying their appearance or function. Rather, their function was the result of political processes in which the users of the same technology could, on one hand, be defined, for example, as "disabled," or having a "special need" for "assistive technologies" to carry out everyday tasks, and, on the other hand, be defined as consumers in a competitive, commercial market. My study of videophones and video interpreting services was nevertheless reduced to a project wherein "a deaf anthropologist studies how other deaf people use technologies for deaf people." The implicit divide between those whose stated aims are to include and the excluded targets of inclusive action (cf. Buckmaster 2009) was persistently prevailing.

HARAWAY'S CYBORG AND VISION METAPHORS

After returning from the United States, I encountered a research community that could not or would not recognize their own responsibility for making it possible for everyone to participate; comments that questioned my legitimacy as a researcher; and a general ignorance toward how government policies and the disability research program contributed to reinforcing the conceptual divides they aimed to reduce. The sum of all this made me lose my faith in the possibility of being a deaf researcher in this field without being a walking reconfirmation of the very divides I wanted to deconstruct. As a result, I escaped academia for about a year and a half and found a project job in a deaf media company, where I did not have to work continually to find interpreters to "include" myself, to wonder whether I was eligible to do the job I was doing, or to wonder who I was.

I did not, however, abandon academia totally; I continued to read books and articles, especially texts that in some way or another focused on minority researchers, research positions, and reflexivity. One author who in particular echoed my sense of being multiple, of being both included and excluded, of being both a deaf person struggling to participate in a hearing work community and a privileged researcher, was Donna Haraway. Although she was primarily problematizing the essentialism of gender, her description of the cyborg (1991) echoed the feeling of being a hybrid (a mix or blend of being deaf and being a researcher, as if it were possible to extricate these categories from each other). A cyborg is one and many at the same time; it can juggle identities and positions. In the quest to keep the various perspectives apart, while also trying to grasp a whole, the cyborg metaphor was inspirational; the cyborg demands a double gaze—to see simultaneously what is unitary and what is different, what is specific and what is general. Haraway also revealed to me how I as a deaf researcher also was an imagination of a politics of inclusion (through access to interpreters and various technologies), who continually also risked exclusion by the shortcomings of the same mechanisms. Rather than being paralyzed by a double, and sometimes self-contradictory position, the cyborg metaphor revealed the productive possibilities that could be provided by an active consciousness and attention to being "double." There was no need to be either included or excluded—I could be both. As a deaf social scientist within a disability research community, I could never leave totally behind the questions I researched, given that in many ways they directly affected my everyday life. This did not, however, deprive me of the ability to observe, or to possess a vision.

Vision is the other concept from Haraway I contemplated when I wondered whether I should re-enter academia. Vision is not a research method, but it is a tool to reflect on our own position and where we are situated as researchers. There are no researchers who do not have a vision, and no two researchers share the same vision. This does not ultimately disqualify any of them, but makes us all equally responsible for what we see, and for confessing that our vision is always partial. This insight is fundamental to taking responsibility for the research—and the possibility of being objective in a way, in the sense that we are aware of how we see and why we observe what we see. Knowledge is always partial—and it is the partial and situated perspective for which we can account. This is, as Haraway presents it, an "argument for situated and embodied knowledges and against various forms of unlocatable, and so irresponsible, knowledge claims" (Haraway 1991:191). As an embodied proficiency, vision enables us to go beyond fixed appearances. We can use vision to go behind the surface, behind phenomena as they first appear. It allows us to explore. As such—in the metaphor of vision— "we find means for appreciating simultaneously *both* the concrete, 'real' aspect and the aspect of semiosis and production in what we call scientific knowledge" (Haraway 1991:195). Just like the people who are our informants, we social scientists also are influenced by the people we meet and interact with (cf. Hacking's looping concept), and we are never completely naive or innocent when engaging in participant observation. The key to taking responsibility for our knowledge is to be aware of this process and the continuous multiplicity of experiences when doing fieldwork and analyzing field notes.

Haraway's cyborg and vision metaphors, as well as conversations with other deaf academics and a few allied hearing researchers, (re) established a sense of equality and symmetry vis-à-vis the research community I had left. What was more, my double position as both deaf and a researcher within the field of communication technology, disability, and employment may have made me able to direct the focus toward categories and perceptions I, as well as my colleagues, perhaps more or less took for granted.

RESUMING THE FIELDWORK: THREE WORKSHOPS ON VIDEO INTERPRETING

About a year after resuming the research project, I attended three workshops on video interpreting services in three countries, and these will serve to illustrate how a fluid research position provided access to information and insight that were significant for the final analysis of the material. The workshops took place just as I had started to analyze the material from prior fieldwork, which certainly also influenced what I saw and looked for this time. I already had started to discuss deaf and hearing peoples' dependence on technologies and services as two sides of the same coin, and what needed explanation was why public policies and documents used different terms to define this dependence. Further, I was starting to get quite a firm grip on the particularities of each system for provision of video interpreting services. In many ways, attending the workshops confirmed what I had already observed earlier. They are described here to illustrate how my positions as a deaf person and as a researcher were relevant in different ways, and how this influenced the relationship with the informants.

In September 2009, I received an invitation to attend a workshop at the Federal Communications Commission (FCC) premises in southwestern Washington, DC. Most of the approximately 40 participants were from various service providers and consumer and lobby associations in the United States. Of these, about one quarter to one third were deaf, representing both service providers, federal agencies, and lobbying NGOs. The event was an open discussion between parties that expressed slightly different interests, but simultaneously shared a common basic understanding of what video relay service was about. They were discussing a newly introduced measure, which required that consumers take action to register their addresses. The participants had a common interest in developing a best practice to make the consumers register. I was introduced as a "researcher from Norway," and one of my informants, who was also present, invited me to lunch. Some of the other people around the lunch table were people whose names I recognized from historical accounts of how video interpreting was established in the United States. It felt like a "scoop" to be able to talk directly with them about the work they had done.

At the workshop and lunch, I was, like most of the informants I actually talked to, deaf. We shared a few other traits, such as knowing ASL, and we probably came from similar socioeconomic and educational backgrounds. At the same time, this workshop was an occasion where my role as an outsider was quite clear. They were a group of American people who knew each other and their respective roles quite well, and I was a researcher from Norway asking potentially ignorant questions and using odd words to try to grasp what I saw. I had only just begun presenting my project as a study of video interpreting systems as social constructions, when I was interrupted by one of the participants. With my background from the Norwegian welfare system and the politics of inclusion there (as described initially), I forgot for a moment that the word "social" has different meanings in the United States than in Norway. While my point as a researcher was to explain that I was not so interested in the technology itself, but that I wanted to study the systems from a social science perspective, my imprecise description of video interpreting as *social* services caused some strong reactions among the participants at the lunch.

They insisted that the video relay service was absolutely not a social service and that is was mandatory for my analysis that I understood this. Immediately, I knew they were right, but their reaction also revealed to me how my background as a Norwegian, raised in a social democratic regime, influenced how the informants related to me and my project. The use of the word *social* marked me as an outsider and as a Scandinavian socialist who really had not understood what the American perception of video relay service and civil rights were all about. I was marked out as an ignorant foreigner, but could at least observe how my clumsy word choice caused a revealing discussion (for me) among some of the informants regarding how they had been successful in establishing VRS as a commercial service.

It would not be an exaggeration to say I was "high on data" when I returned home to Norway a few days later after the workshop at the FCC. Immediately upon my return, a Swedish informant invited me to a meeting hosted by one of the major videophone stakeholders in Sweden, the Swedish Institute for Assistive Technology. This was an annual seminar aimed at the regional officers in charge of providing so-called alternative telephony (including both text-telephones and videophones), developers and manufacturers (who had the regional authorities as their primary market in Sweden). Because of an anticipated change in public tender practice, most of the discussion related to new videophone tenders and distribution processes. A lot of time, however, also was given over to product presentations of both video and text telephones and discussion of the latest technological developments.

Approximately 50 people attended the meeting, and about five of them were deaf, mostly representing regional videophone prescribers and companies specializing in developing and selling videophones. As in the United States, I was introduced as a researcher from Norway and invited to attend a dinner for some of the attendees in the evening. Again, I was engaged in a lively, and this time also a comparative discussion on video interpreting services. At the luncheon after the FCC workshop, the discussion was mostly about issues directly related to the American system, while the Swedes were more curious to learn about the video interpreting systems in other countries. By this time, I was definitely no longer only a researcher gathering data; I also was becoming a provider of information and new perspectives on the work they did every day.

Contrary to the lunch at FCC, nobody raised an eyebrow when they saw the word "social," and my Swedish family heritage had made me familiar with both Swedish Sign Language and Swedish politics. At this stage, I perhaps could have refrained from getting involved in that type of discussion, given that I was no longer only observing a system, but was taking part in it and perhaps also contributing to its development. It was, however, with a feeling of "giving back" that I shared my knowledge with this group of people. Many of them were people I had talked with at earlier stages of the project and from whom I had received much valuable information. It is worth noting that I was one of two deaf people in a group of mostly hearing (and non-signing) people at the dinner, and we communicated by way of Swedish Sign Language interpreters who were provided by the organizers of the workshop. We had a common interest in video interpreting, and the linguistic and hearing differences among us were rendered irrelevant to the situation.

Three weeks after the seminar in Sweden, there was a workshop outside Oslo, primarily directed at interpreter service managers and other officers working in the regional centers for assistive technology to prescribe videophones and other assistive technologies in Norway. Contrary to the United States and Sweden, this meeting was not one among a group of people who already were familiar with the service. Instead, it was a meeting where representatives from the video interpreter services management group informed meeting participants about the possibilities offered by the videophone and the video interpreter service. Some of the participants were familiar with the service before the meeting, but the presenters structured the information to enlighten the audience about the opportunities to use videophones for the regional sign language interpreter services. The dialogue among a variety of actors and organizations that characterized the other two workshops in the United States and in Sweden was not prominently featured at the workshop in Norway.

Another, and quite revealing, difference between the workshop in Norway and the ones in the United States and Sweden was how the organizers and attendees dealt with the presence of a deaf researcher. I had been invited by informants to the workshops in the United States and Sweden, but had to register for the workshop in Norway after learning about it from an external source at the last minute. This took me by some surprise, given that the workshop took place in the very city in which I lived. The organizers had announced they could let representatives from user organizations attend, providing there was enough room. When I made an attempt to registrate as a researcher, the organizers told me they could not guarantee a spot for me at the conference. They explained that they were not sure they would be able to find a Norwegian Sign Language interpreter for me. Again, I was surprised, because I had not requested an interpreter from the organizers and had planned to bring my own. They obviously knew I am deaf, and this suddenly became a difference that mattered in a way it had not in the United States or in Sweden. A sense of paranoia struck me—did they not want me to attend because they saw me as a (deaf) user of the video interpreter service and wanted to discuss the service without the involvement of the users? Or, did they not want the scrutiny of a researcher there and used "lack of accessibility" as an excuse to thwart my attendance? I eventually was allowed in, only to find out that interpreters already had been reserved for the workshop from the beginning. A deaf assistant at a regional interpreter center and a deaf representative from a user organization also were attending. The concern the organizers had expressed regarding my attendance seemed to be without any foundation, and I have never asked them if they had any other motivation to not let me attend. Nevertheless, their response fueled my thinking about my multiple positions in the field. Further, it became a reconfirmation of how the Norwegian system of video interpreting affirmed Buckmaster's (2009) critique of the ambiguity embedded in the inclusion concept, namely, that it continues to reproduce a group of excluded people. My double role as a deaf person and a researcher did not fit into this scheme. I wondered if this was why they had some trouble letting me in, given the impossibility of separating these two roles.

The workshop in Norway is the last of the three events described here. The way the organizers questioned my attendance confirmed what I already had started to observe and what would become a main message from the research project. In Norway, the video interpreting service was a service provided by the national interpreter service for deaf people, with a declared goal of enhancing inclusion in the labor market through increasing access to interpreter services. The interpreter services are, however, organized as a service exclusively for a group of people who are defined as disabled and do not demand changes in structures or systems that remain quite inaccessible. In the United States, the service was constructed within the structure of the telecommunication market and was considered one of several telecommunication services. Organizing the service as a telecommunication service made telecommunication services in general more accessible. The Swedish system represented a hybrid of these two approaches, with its emphasis on how technology could be used to increase access for deaf people, and how both public welfare and telecommunication agencies could be involved in developing the service. The various constructions and scopes of the video interpreting services in the three countries revealed that organizing a service targeted at a group of disabled people external to the system it is intended to give access to reinforces and maintains material and social exclusion mechanisms (Haualand 2014).

CONCLUSION

To me, my experiences as a deaf researcher (some of which have been described here) helped to "illuminate the cultural practices of groups and categories who define themselves as the normal ordinary populations against which other categories are seen as deviant in some way" (Lien & Melhuus 2011:140). The fieldwork had been a search for connections in bundles of technologies, disability, and politics, where I tried to resist taking the categories they represented for granted. I did not pursue a top-down approach to see how disabled people enter or leave the labor market, or how they are given or denied access to particular technologies, etc. Neither did I pursue a bottom-up approach that also took the social categories as facts, possibly with a negative sign indicating that the existing structure oppresses large groups in a society. Being a deaf researcher with multiple positions became a tool by which I could "study across" rather than up or down. Studying across meant that the analysis was framed in "ways that not only focus on this or that particular group, but in a way that catches the dynamic connections between people and institutions with or without power" (ibid, 138). This would not be possible without an active reflexion process wherein I also took responsibility for my positions within the field (Berger 2015). Only then was I able to take advantage of these positions, and acknowledge the effect I had on the informants, the data collection, the analysis, and the outcomes of the research process. I shall not claim that another researcher (whether deaf or hearing, or of another nationality) could not have reached the same conclusions as I, but the experience of being included in some ways while simultaneously being excluded, but always in different ways at different places, was effective and eventually indispensable to catching the dynamic connections across the field.

REFERENCES

Berger, R. (2015). Now I see it, now I don't: Researcher's position and reflexivity in qualitative research. *Qualitative Research, 15*(2), 219–234. doi:10.1177/1468794112468475

Berven, H. M., & Blanck, P. D. (1999). Assistive technology patenting trends and the Americans with Disabilities Act. *Behavioral Sciences & the Law, 17*(1), 47–71.

Buckmaster, L. (2009). *Social inclusion and social citizenship towards a truly inclusive society.* Parliament of Australia.

England, K. V. L. (1994). Getting personal: Reflexivity, positionality, and feminist research. *The Professional Geographer, 46*(1), 80–89. doi:10.1111/j.0033-0124.1994.00080.x

Esping-Andersen, G. (1990). *The three worlds of welfare capitalism.* Cambridge: Polity Press.

Foucault, M. (1967). *Madness and civilization: A history of insanity in the age of reason.* London: Tavistock/Routledge.

Foucault, M. (1971). Orders of discourse. *Social Science Information, 10,* 7–30.

Friedner, M., & Kusters, A. (Eds.) (2015). *It's a small world: International deaf spaces and encounters.* Washington DC: Gallaudet University Press.

Goodin, R. E. (1996). Inclusion and exclusion. *European Journal of Sociology, 37*(02), 343–371. doi:10.1017/S0003975600007219

Hacking, I. (1999). *The social construction of what?* Cambridge, MA: Harvard University Press.

Haraway, D. J. (1991). *Simians, cyborgs, and women: The reinvention of nature.* London: Free Associations Books.

Haualand, H. (2011). Interpreted ideals and relayed rights—Video interpreting services as objects of politics. *Disability Studies Quarterly, 31.*

Haualand, H. (2012). *Interpreting ideals and relaying rights* (Unpublished doctoral dissertation). Universitetet i Oslo, Oslo. Retrieved from https://www.duo.uio.no/bitstream/handle/10852/37639/dravhandling-haualand.pdf?sequence=1

Haualand, H. (2014). Video interpreting services: Calls for inclusion or redialling exclusion? *Ethnos, 79,* 287–305.

Kusters, A., De Meulder, M., Friedner, M., & Emery, S. (2015). On "diversity" and "inclusion": Exploring paradigms for achieving Sign Language Peoples' rights (MMG Working Paper 15–02). Göttingen: Max Planck Institute for the Study of Religious and Ethnic Diversity.

Latour, B. (1993). *We have never been modern.* New York: Harvester Wheatsheaf.

Law, J. (2004). *After method: Mess in social science research.* London: Routledge.

Lien, M. E., & Melhuus, M. (2011). Overcoming the division between anthropology "at home" and "abroad." *Norsk antropologisk tidsskrift, 22,* 134–143.

Miller, D. (2005). *Materiality.* Durham, NC: Duke University Press.

Mol, A. (2002). *The body multiple: Ontology in medical practice.* Durham, NC: Duke University Press.

Moser, I. (2003). *Road traffic accidents: The ordering of subjects, bodies and disability.* Det humanistiske fakultet. Universitetet i Oslo, Oslo.

Nav. (2010). Sum anrop. In J. Hansen (Ed.), (E-mail ed.). Oslo: NAV.

Norges forskningsråd. (2008). Funksjonshemmedeforskning—Prosjektkatalog. Oslo: Norges Forskningsråd.

Oliver, M. (1990). *The politics of disablement: A sociological approach.* New York: St. Martin's Press.

Ott, K., Serlin, D., & Mihm, S. (2002). *Artificial parts, practical lives: Modern histories of prosthetics.* New York: New York University Press.

Powers, S. (2002). From concepts to practice in deaf education: A United Kingdom perspective on inclusion. *Journal of Deaf Studies and Deaf Education,* 7(3), 230–243. doi:10.1093/deafed/7.3.230

Schein, J. D. (1989). *At home among strangers: Exploring the deaf community in the United States.* Washington, DC: Gallaudet University Press.

Shakespeare, T. (2006). *Disability rights and wrongs.* London: Routledge.

Solvang, P. (2000). The emergence of an us and them discourse in disability theory. *Scandinavian Journal of Disability Research,* 2(1), 3–3.

Strauss, K. P. (2009). *Transparency and Functional Equivalency: Core Principles of U.S. Relay Policy.* Paper presented at The Impact of the United Nations Convention on the Rights of Persons with Disabilities on the work of the ITU-T Geneva.

Söder, M. (2009). Tensions, perspectives and themes in disability studies. *Scandinavian Journal of Disability Research,* 11(2), 67–81.

Sørensen, E. (2010). Producing multi-sited comparability in Scheffer, T. og J. Niewöhner (eds.) *Thick comparisons - reviving the ethnographic aspiration.* Leiden & Boston, Brill.

Tøssebro, J. (2004). Introduction to the special issue: Understanding disability. *Scandinavian Journal of Disability Research,* 6, 3–7. doi:10.1080/15017410409512635

Tøssebro, J. (2009). En innsiders skråblikk på funksjonshemming og velferdsforskning. In B. R. Nuland, B. S. Tranøy, & J. Christensen (Eds.). Oslo: Universitetsforl.

14

Negotiating Language Practices and Language Ideologies in Fieldwork: A Reflexive Meta-Documentation

Lynn Y-S Hou

For the most part, the documentation of sign languages and the social lives of deaf and hearing signers in rural communities across the world from Mexico to Israel to Thailand has been conducted by hearing researchers. This is not a unique trend. Hearing researchers predominate in sign language linguistics and other deaf-related disciplines (Baker-Shenk & Kyle 1990). Deaf people were instrumental in developing these fields, particularly sign language linguistics, as language consultants, research assistants, and scholars (albeit few and far between). The existence of deaf people is the linchpin of all scholarship concerning their sign languages, lives, and communities (Ladd 2003). Only in recent decades have a small handful of deaf researchers conducted linguistic and anthropological fieldwork with deaf people in rural signing communities (Dikyuva, Escobedo Delgado, Panda & Zeshan 2012, Kusters 2012). One outcome of deaf-led research in these communities is the production of reflexive discourse about research methods, ethics, and collaboration through the positionalities of researchers of diverse backgrounds (Boland, Wilson & Winiarczyk 2015, Cooper & Nguyen 2015).

What does it mean to be a deaf person researching the lives and/ or sign languages of other deaf people in rural signing communities? In Dikyuva et al. (2012) and in Kusters (2012), two common themes emerge: the researchers developed a deep bond with their participants on the basis of shared experiences of being deaf and demonstrated a willingness, facilitated by prior sign language experience, to learn their participants' sign language. Kusters and Friedner (2015) conceptualized this bond "DEAF-SAME" that pertains to the feeling of sameness between deaf people of diverse backgrounds when they encounter one another in transnational spaces and communicate through an array of semiotic resources, national signed languages, gestures, and International Sign. The ease of communication "produces a desired and imagined deaf geography in which differences between deaf people are rendered minimal" (Kusters & Friedner 2015:x).

Although the DEAF-SAME concept seemingly transcends any extant differences between deaf people, this does not necessarily erase them (ibid). In the case of fieldwork, the intersectional positionality of deaf researchers posed some challenges and conflicts. Kusters's status as a white foreigner in an African community shaped the interactions between her and her participants to the extent that she received "special" treatment as a guest of the deaf people. Yet the deaf researchers did not develop the same bond with hearing participants who could sign and had less sustained interactions with them. The discourse of being deaf generated a critical introspection about fieldwork practices and how they were shaped by the ontology of being deaf, intersected with gender, race, ethnicity, nationality, and other social variables that emerged as differential markers between the researchers and their participants. More crucially, the discourse revealed how the involvement of deaf researchers in rural signing communities impacted their research in many ways they did not anticipate.

The practice of documenting sign languages and the social lives of the signers in rural communities recently became a widespread phenomenon. First, in 1960, William Stokoe, a hearing English professor at Gallaudet College, published a monograph, presenting a linguistic analysis of American Sign Language (hereafter, ASL). His analysis demonstrated how ASL was a full-fledged language with its own grammar, not an elaborate manual derivative of English as previously thought (Stokoe 1960). In 1965, Stokoe and his two deaf colleagues, Carl Croneberg and Dorothy Casterline, published *A Dictionary of American Sign Language on Linguistic Principles* (Stokoe, Casterline & Croneberg 1965). These publications heralded the beginning of a paradigmatic shift in the academia of the 1960s and led to the birth of a new academic discipline, namely, sign language linguistics (McBurney 2012). Second, sophisticated technological advances enabled researchers to record, annotate, and store large amounts of video data, greatly facilitating sign language documentation in the late 20th century. Third, the discipline of sign language linguistics has recently expanded and diversified to include the study of little-known, small-scale varieties of sign languages, including rural and emerging sign languages (Zeshan & de Vos 2012, Nyst 2012, Meir, Sandler, Padden & Aronoff 2010).[1] The

---

[1] Rural sign languages are interchangeable with "village" sign languages that may be young or old. Examples of rural sign languages include Adamorobe Sign Language (Ghana), Kata Kolok (Indonesia), and Al-Sayyid Bedouin Sign Language (Israel). Emerging sign languages are young sign languages that arise in a village or an institutional context such as a school for the deaf; they include Al-Sayyid Bedouin Sign Language and Nicaraguan Sign Language (Nicaragua).

general practice of documenting sign languages is rather contemporary compared with the practice for endangered indigenous spoken languages, given that anthropologists and linguists have been documenting those since the beginning of the 20th century (Woodbury 2011). Few publications explicitly discuss research methodologies for fieldwork in rural sign languages, especially for and by deaf researchers (Nyst 2015).

This chapter aims to contribute to the existing discourse about deaf-led research in rural signing communities with a reflexive analysis of the research methodology used for my doctoral research, a language documentation project of an emerging sign language in Mexico. Following the introduction, the chapter begins with the story of the circumstances that led me to develop my doctoral thesis. Next, I discuss how I started producing "reflexive meta-documentation" (Austin 2013). This is the documentation of the documentation project itself, with a focus on my positionality vis-à-vis that of the deaf participants and their families. I discuss negotiating the web of local language practices, attitudes, and ideologies in the community among my participants, my collaborators, and myself. The result of the negotiation is that the research methodology of my project was transformed, and informed, by my ontology as a person of intersectional identities. What emerged from this transformation was the value of a diverse and flexible approach to sign language documentation and fostering collaboration with hearing researchers in the field.

MY STORY IN A NUTSHELL, OR HOW I WOUND UP DOING FIELDWORK

When I entered graduate school in the Department of Linguistics at the University of Texas at Austin, I intended to specialize in deaf children's acquisition of American Sign Language (ASL). What I did not expect was a chance meeting with Dr. Emiliana Cruz and Dr. Hilaria Cruz. They would unwittingly, or very willingly, play a crucial role in shaping my future research trajectory. At that time, the two sisters were doctoral students in anthropology and linguistics, respectively, at UT Austin. They are native Chatino speakers. The term "Chatino" refers to both a family of indigenous Mesoamerican languages and an ethnic group that traditionally inhabits a small part of a mountainous area in southwestern Oaxaca in Mexico. The Cruz sisters extended me an invitation to visit their village, Cieneguilla, and another nearby village, San Juan Quiahije (hereafter, Quiahije) located about eight hours away from the capital of Oaxaca. The sisters knew a few deaf people, from their extended family, who developed their own signs to communicate with their families and thought I would be interested in meeting them. I accepted the invitation with enthusiasm. In 2010, we arranged for me to accompany Hilaria to the villages for two weeks, which would be purely social on my part.

Quiahije and Cieneguilla, situated three kilometers apart, share the same language, a variety of Chatino known as San Juan Quiahije Eastern Chatino (Cruz & Woodbury 2014). Most people acquire and speak Chatino as their first and dominant language. Younger people speak Spanish as their second language with varying degrees of fluency. Chatino occurs in all aspects of daily life except for schools, where Spanish is the formal language of instruction. Chatino is not taught as a subject. There are only 11 deaf people (five of them children) out of a combined population of 3,628 in both villages. This is not a statistically high rate of hereditary deafness in a given population compared with the rates reported for the overall population of most villages in which rural sign languages arise (Nyst 2012). Nevertheless, my meeting the deaf people and their families left me the initial impression that the deaf people participated in many aspects of the community's life, and their participation paved the way for the creation of a new sign language.

This impression eventually led to a collaborative pilot study with my hearing research partner, Kate Mesh, for a preliminary documentation of the sign language. In 2012, we received a small grant and conducted two months of fieldwork, after which I did a follow-up visit for one month. We have termed this rural sign language San Juan Quiahije Chatino Sign Language (hereafter, SJQCSL) in academic discourse. This sign language is currently in its second generation and is used primarily in the homes of families with deaf people—deaf children of hearing caregivers with at least one deaf adult relative and hearing children with one deaf caregiver and at least one deaf adult relative (the caregivers are not necessarily the biological parents of children). This rural sign language has had no discernible contact with Mexican Sign Language (LSM), the national sign language used by many deaf people in Mexico. The pilot study also inspired the topic of my doctoral thesis. The topic was an ethnography of communication, describing everyday communicative practices of deaf and hearing children and their families, through a year of intensive fieldwork from 2014 to 2015. The goal was to describe and examine how children and their families become "signers" through participating in interaction, and, in turn, understand how interaction contributes to the emergence of SJQCSL (Hou 2016). This would be an ethnographic approach to the language documentation project of an emerging sign language: a combination of documentary linguistics and sign linguistics with a focus on child language acquisition.

THE STORY OF RESEARCHING SAN JUAN QUIAHIJE CHATINO SIGN LANGUAGE

When the pilot study of SJQCSL started in 2012, all the hearing scholars I knew who worked on rural sign languages relied on hearing interpreters and research assistants for interpretation, translation, and transcription of linguistic data via a spoken contact language. In documentary linguistics of spoken languages, this is a common approach for fieldworkers when they begin studying and analyzing a language (Bowern 2008). This was not a feasible option for me, given that I speak neither intelligible Spanish nor Chatino. In documenting a rural sign language, Chican Sign Language, used in a Mayan village, one deaf fieldworker wrote notes in Spanish with literate hearing interpreters to facilitate communication between himself and deaf and hearing participants, particularly in lexical elicitation tasks (Dikyuva et al. 2012). This was not a feasible option for me either. All 11 deaf Chatinos are monolingual in their sign language. Hearing Chatino signers involved in my research do not know any other sign language and are not comfortable with writing in Spanish. The practice of literacy is not common in the community. Younger hearing Chatinos learn to read and write Spanish in school, but many do not acquire full proficiency in the language and are not accustomed to the practice of literacy as part of their daily lives. There is no standard orthography for Chatino; one has been developed recently, but it is not yet widespread or implemented in schools (Cruz & Woodbury 2014). Considering the social context of the community, taking a primarily monolingual approach felt like the best option, which is, in fact, advocated by some documentary linguists (Everett 2001). The monolingual approach requires fieldworkers to immerse themselves in the targeted language and its community of speakers (or signers) so as to acquire the language and study it holistically, instead of using an intermediary language as a starting point of fieldwork (ibid.). I learned SJQCSL by immersing myself in the language environment with the signing families, which enabled me to communicate with them directly. I acquired sufficient SJQCSL to the point where the signing families allowed me to visit them alone after the first month of my intensive fieldwork.

Communicating with signers directly hinged on my ontology of deafness being deaf and intersected with the variables of gender, race, ethnicity, education, mobility, and citizenship. As a self-identified Asian American Deaf woman, who is acquiring a doctorate in linguistics and has the privilege and experience of traveling around the world with a U.S. passport, my background impacted my fieldwork in virtually all aspects. As I describe later, I engaged in an ongoing negotiation over multiple congruencies and conflicts between my own language practices and ideologies about signed and spoken languages and their signers and speakers, and those of the community. The negotiation was an ongoing process that became integral to the methodology of the documentation project. Originally, I envisioned a systematic approach for documenting and analyzing samples of spontaneous interaction between children and their families. I would be a silent observer, hiding behind the camera and videotaping the interactions, without partaking in them. Instead, I became an active participant in the interactions. The deaf adults preferred to talk to me instead of to their children. The children expected me to play with them, after I well intentionally initiated the conversation with them. Consequently, I formed a substantial part of the data collection. As a way of reflecting on the circumstances that led to the "unsystematic" approach of language documentation from the perspective of sign linguistics, I started documenting the changes and progress in my field notes. This kind of documentation constituted "meta-data" or data about data itself. This is a practice that I acquired from documentary linguistics, known as reflexive "meta-documentation" or "meta-documentary linguistics" (Austin 2013).

PRODUCING REFLEXIVE META-DOCUMENTATION

Meta-documentation pertains to the "observation and documentation of the methods, processes, and outcomes of language documentation projects" (Austin 2013:4). Meta-documentation involves recording meta-data, or additional information about the data collected for a language documentation project in order to facilitate the management, identification, retrieval, and understanding of the data (ibid). The meta-data can include personal information on the participants, the methods used for collecting the data, the circumstances in which the data was collected, and the system for labeling and organizing data. Arguably, part of meta-documentation addresses reflexivity, or a critical self-introspection of the researcher's role in the research. The call for reflexive meta-documentation harks back to contemporary reflexive ethnography, a topic that has been heavily discussed and dissected in anthropology since the 1960s (Robben & Sluka 2012).

Reflexivity generally refers to social science researchers constantly reflecting and (re)assessing their own positionality in the research and the ways in which their position affects the whole process of conducting research, including how they select, construct, and produce knowledge (Clifford 1988, Salzman 2002). Reflexivity is a concept developed and expanded in research and now occupies a significant place in contemporary anthropology discourse, particularly in ethnography (see also Haualand, this volume). Conducting an ethnography involves a close examination of individual peoples, cultures, and societies, and frequently also involves immersion in a community or even communities (Bernard 2011). For many researchers, the process of extended participant observation in the targeted community leads to reflexivity when they become aware of the connection between themselves and their research. They see themselves as observers and participants who are situated in their research in ways that require an interpretive lens. For studying language practices, researchers reflect on the meaning of language choices, attitudes, and ideologies as manifested in their behavior and that of their research participants (Austin 2013).

The reflexivity of language occurs in both reflexive meta-documentation and reflexive contemporary ethnography. One crucial difference between the disciplines, however, is that the former explicitly privileges language whereas the latter does not always privilege language. Linguists and linguistic anthropologists primarily focus on the usage of language in context. For my doctoral study, the production of reflexive meta-documentation centers on the theme of language as the primary object of inquiry, the resource of obtaining data about language, and the source of data itself. Other social scientists doing an ethnography focus on other aspects of the social life of a community such as marriage, foraging and hunting, or witchcraft; they do not focus on language as the primary object of inquiry.

Three linked themes of reflexive meta-documentation, as suggested in Austin (2013), are addressed here: (1) the biographies of the project, which refers to the background knowledge, training, and research familiarity of the researcher, participants, and collaborators; (2) the researcher's relationships with the participants, collaborators, and their surrounding speech community, with respect to everyday language practices; (3) the language attitudes and ideologies of the researcher and those of the participants toward their languages, the researcher, and the documentation project. The last two themes are closely interlinked, given that language practices and attitudes together form language ideologies.

Language attitudes pertain to evaluative judgments of language(s) and their users. There are a handful of language attitude studies regarding urban and national Western sign languages, especially ASL and its varieties, from a sociolinguistic framework (Lewis, Palmer & Williams 1995, Burns, Matthews & Nolan-Conroy 2001, Hill 2012, 2013).[2] Language attitudes often form part of language ideologies, though sociolinguistics and linguistic anthropology tend to utilize different methodologies for investigation. Language ideologies pertain to a linguistic anthropology theoretical paradigm that investigates the awareness of how individuals, groups, and nation-states of speakers (or signers) understand, perceive, and use their languages, which may be explicitly expressed and/or embodied in communicative practices (Kroskrity 2004). Although academic studies about spoken language ideologies have received extensive attention, studies about signed language ideologies are rather sparse. A few studies examined language ideologies

---

[2] Urban and national sign languages, in contrast to rural sign languages, emerge in large communities of deaf users where a school for the deaf and/or an urban network of deaf signers exists.

of rural sign languages, Adamorobe Sign Language (Kusters 2014) and Ban Khor Sign Language (Nonaka 2014); the studies examined the status of the language by itself, and in comparison with spoken languages and/or other sign languages. This paper is the first study to examine the impact of language ideologies on the research process of a project.

There are many approaches to studying language ideologies, and the research focus and scope can vary, hence there is no single, all-encompassing definition. Here, I adopt the following definition: "[a] ubiquitous set of diverse beliefs, however implicit or explicit they may be, used by speakers of all types as models for constructing linguistic evaluations and engaging in communicative activity" (Kroskrity 2004:497). The definition captures the varying degrees of awareness of local language ideologies about signing, speaking, and writing, and also serves as a critical means of understanding the interaction of multiple language beliefs and practices between me, my participants, and their families. The language ideologies are not arbitrary. Rather, they are grounded in social experience, and the experience goes back to the ontology of deafness, which was subsequently shaped by our differential life trajectories.

The Biographies of the Project

I am the only deaf person in my family, a U.S.-born child of Taiwanese immigrants of Chinese descent. As an adolescent, I started attending a mainstream program full-time and functioned well enough academically to advance to university. I learned ASL over time through interacting with other deaf people sporadically outside of school, but I only started interacting with them regularly in university. My training is largely rooted in the linguistics of signed languages, with specialization in child language acquisition and linguistic anthropology. Prior to starting extensive fieldwork for my doctoral research, my previous fieldwork experiences were limited to Deaf communities in urban parts of the United States and a short pilot study in Quiahije. To train myself better in the methods of linguistic fieldwork and prepare for ethnographic research, I explored documentary linguistics. At the University of Texas at Austin, I sat in on a field methods class. The class was oriented toward spoken languages, so I tried envisioning how some of the methods could apply to signed languages. I studied written Spanish on my own, because I could not participate in Spanish language classes like a hearing person by acquiring the language through listening and speaking. I acquired a little academic knowledge of Chatino and read previous ethnographic literature about the Chatinos.[3] I developed an

---

[3] Academic knowledge of a language is studying and understanding the grammatical structure of the language. Functional knowledge of a language is knowing how to use it for communicative purposes—speaking/signing, reading, and/or writing.

elaborate plan for executing a successful doctoral study that would exploit and combine the strengths of deaf and hearing researchers, collaborators, and participants.

The doctoral project involved collaboration from a transnational team of several community members from Quiahije and academic colleagues. Dr. Emiliana Cruz and Dr. Hilaria Cruz served as the "gatekeepers" and cultural brokers to the community. They facilitated my access to the village authorities for official permission to conduct research there as well as access to the families for recruitment. Emiliana served as a committee member for my dissertation, providing advice for certain logistics of the project. Hilaria assisted me with the writing of interview scripts in Spanish. She also transcribed and translated some interviews recorded with hearing people in Chatino, Spanish, and English, on ELAN, a multimedia annotation program. The interviews were sent via e-mail and post mail during fieldwork. In reviewing the interviews, Hilaria collaborated with my interpreter and interviewer, Mrs. Epifania Mendez, over the telephone in Chatino to modify the interview protocol, and also advised me separately for providing Epifania constructive feedback. Epifania is a retired preschool teacher from Cieneguilla. She has a local reputation for maintaining a neutral stance on village politics, which facilitates her relationships with many people. She speaks Chatino fluently as her native language and additionally speaks, reads, and writes Spanish. She worked as an interpreter, translator, and interviewer between written Spanish, spoken Spanish, and spoken Chatino for the project.

Ms. Kate Mesh was a graduate student in linguistics at UT Austin. She is hearing, grew up speaking only English, and learned Spanish in high school to fulfill a foreign language requirement. She learned ASL, out of curiosity about signed languages, in graduate school, and acquired enough proficiency for extended conversations. Later, she acquired enough Chatino to conduct a basic conversation with the villagers. We developed individual doctoral research topics to cover more ground on the ongoing documentation of the San Juan Quiahije Chatino Sign Language. Our fieldwork schedules overlapped by six months. For her doctoral study, Kate focused on comparing pointing gestures of hearing Chatinos with pointing gestures of deaf Chatinos; however, she was not conducting ethnography. From her time in the field, she started to acquire Chatino Sign Language and spoken Chatino. Her hearing status also shaped her relationships with deaf signers and their families. Most deaf signers treated me as their conversational partner, whereas they prompted her to talk with their hearing families.

The main participants of my doctoral study were the deaf children of hearing caregivers and hearing children of deaf–hearing caregivers and their families, which totaled six signing families. There are no pairs of deaf caregivers. The cause of deafness is either congenital or early childhood illness. The deaf Chatino adults are monolingual. They only know their own sign language, which grew out of home signs and gestures they produced among themselves and their families. They are first-generation signers. They have not acquired any Chatino or Spanish. Some deaf adults have attended school but never finished and only learned to write letters and numbers by rote. Their hearing families sign with them, but they speak Chatino with other hearing people. Two families use Spanish in the house for occasional practice with their hearing children or for communicating with people who do not speak Chatino.

Most deaf Chatinos are acquainted with one another, but they do not purposefully seek one another out for social interaction. If they live in close proximity, they tend to be from the same extended family and can interact with one another regularly. They reported no sustained interactions with other deaf persons outside of their community. Few have traveled outside of Juquila, the Spanish-speaking commercial center in the Chatino region. Fewer have visited Oaxaca City. Only one deaf person had worked abroad in the United States, as part of the ongoing mass migration of Chatinos that started in the late 1990s and consists of crossing the U.S. border under perilous circumstances and without documentation (H. Cruz 2014). At least one member of each deaf person's family has worked or is currently working abroad in the United States. The villages of Quiahije and Cieneguilla are part of a larger trend of transnational migration to the United States from indigenous Latin American communities in southern Mexico (Cohen 2004).

Given the diverse biographies of all the persons involved in my project, there were interesting and often unanticipated implications for the relationships between the researcher, collaborators, and participants, in the context of everyday language practices and ideologies. Of special interest is how communication between the participants and me led to the change of the research methodology of the project, shifting it away from what was originally envisioned. I discuss the changes in the next section.

Language Practices, and Language Attitudes and Ideologies

For all deaf Chatinos, their knowledge and understanding of deafness, communication, and sign language were shaped exclusively by their own experiences. In their sign language, they refer to themselves as "people who cannot talk" and as members of a tight-knit indigenous Mesoamerican community. For most hearing Chatinos, their knowledge and understanding of these topics were shaped exclusively by their direct experiences with the deaf people from their own community. In their Chatino language, a deaf person is referred to as "one who cannot talk." Bilingual Chatino-Spanish speakers typically refer to a deaf person as *no puede hablar* in Spanish, which is a loan translation from the

Chatino phrase. They also refer to a deaf person as *sordomudo* or "deaf-mute." They assume that the ability to talk is a prerequisite for completing school, given that most deaf people have never attended it. Prior to my arrival in Quiahije, most Chatinos had never met a deaf person who used a different sign language, including Mexican Sign Language (LSM), or a deaf person who was studying in university. Moreover, the very idea of studying deaf people with the aim of documenting their sign language, instead of providing them medical treatment or teaching them literacy was also a novelty, and a baffling one for them. Linguistic and anthropological research is not new in the Chatino region, including Quiahije and Cieneguilla, but the focus has been exclusively on spoken languages and their speakers (H. Cruz 2014). Some families with deaf children have had limited interaction with general practitioners, indigenous healers, ear-nose-and-throat doctors, and audiologists for medical treatment options. A few families even sought out special education teachers in vain. But none had met a sign linguist before.

Working with Caregivers

Originally, I envisioned the original research methodology to consist of filming everyday language practices of the signing families with the researcher participating as a silent observer. This was the type of data targeted for my doctoral topic, but in reality, this goal was nearly unachievable. Deaf caregivers believed that one or two filming sessions of them chatting with their hearing children alone were sufficient. They also insisted that if more filming was to occur, I should wait until their hearing children were older and would be more suitable conversational partners. They claimed that their children were too young to be signing a lot and thus could not participate in extended conversations for more than a few minutes. Sometimes the caregivers attempted to prompt their children to talk, but when they felt the prompting was not productive, they sent the children away. The caregivers understood that I paid them for allowing me to document their lives, but they felt there was no reason to film them and their children signing, unless the adults and I were signing to each other. They were very interested in me and my life and wanted to chat with me, while discouraging their children from interrupting our conversations. My recurrent visits created and reinforced the expectation that when I showed up, we, the adults, would chat and occasionally film ourselves. The expectation prevented me from being a silent observer and filming many spontaneous conversations between the deaf adults and their children.

By contrast, most deaf caregivers did not have the same expectations from Kate. Because she could talk (she is hearing), they expected her to talk to their hearing family members, including their children. They believed that because their hearing children could hear and thus could already talk, there was no reason why Kate could not talk to them and vice versa. They did not always remember that most of their relatives did not speak Spanish fluently and Kate did not speak Chatino fluently, and she had to remind them. If she wanted to film deaf people and their families signing, she had to make an explicit request from them. They did not expect her to film them, because it was not a frequent event compared with my filming them.

The hearing caretakers of deaf children expected that I would play an interventionist role in the lives of the deaf children, such as teaching them some signs and/or how to carry on a conversation. I only became aware of this after Epifania and I conducted ethnographic interviews with them. I was surprised, because the village authorities already had explained my research project to the families. The expectations hinted that the caregivers perceived their existing sign language to lack some vocabulary and/or their children to be lacking conversational skills. In response to the caregivers, through the interpretation of Epifania, I politely clarified what my intentions were and pointed out that the primary sign language I used was not the same language as they used. After this, the caregivers continued expecting me to intervene in their children's lives, believing that the intervention was part of my research project. Such a discrepancy in the expectations of the researcher and those of the community is very common in linguistic fieldwork (Bowern 2008). The caregivers' behavior during my visits and those of Kate revealed their beliefs about their children's signed and spoken language abilities. In the eyes of the deaf caregivers, their hearing children lacked sign language proficiency partly because they were too young and because they could already talk. Hearing caregivers felt their deaf children would benefit from my "teaching" them more sign language because the children needed to enrich their vocabulary and conversational skills.

Another aspect of the original research methodology did not materialize. This would have involved a type of ethnographic interview that consists of reviewing samples from videos of spontaneous conversations with the families for translation of certain signs and for interpretation and discussion of interactional behavior and other related topics (Bernard 2011). Nobody was interested in this task, nor did they have time and training for examining interaction on a microanalytical level. The deaf adults were far more interested in chatting with me, showing me around the mountainous landscape, and introducing me to other people. This led to the development of an intimate relationship that opened a door into their social lives. They allowed me to accompany them on their visits to the residences of their extended family members, to their ranches, to annual festivals, and to various sightseeing spots in the mountains. They extended the invitation to Kate for similar field trips, but they still expected her to chat with their hearing families when the opportunity arose.

Becoming acquainted with the meaning and context of the social lives of the deaf adults allowed me to gain greater proficiency in their sign language and understand cultural associations with many signs. Part of this was due to the ethnographic methodology of fieldwork. Learning more about the lives of the deaf adults facilitated my ability to gloss, translate, and annotate videotaped conversations independently at a later stage of research. At the same time, my production of the scripts of the videotaped conversations was based almost entirely on my own interpretations informed by the ethnographic fieldwork. Becoming acquainted with their lives also allowed me to access and assess their social networks by meeting many people with varying degrees of sign language proficiency *and* willingness to sign, and by observing their interactions.

My socialization as a deaf friend of the deaf adults and their families enabled me to gauge the size and scope of the signing community, a theme that was not initially part of the original research methodology. My gender status as a woman constrained my capacity to participate in all social aspects of the lives of the deaf men. I could not accompany the deaf men if they went out to fraternize with other men. Chatinos have social rules for behavior in public and private spaces. Women and men do not generally mingle for the sake of friendship, unless they consider one another kinfolk or they have a professional relationship. Were I a man, I would have had more access to various social spaces exclusively associated with deaf men and less access to those associated with deaf women. Yet, being a woman was an advantage for working with the children, because they tend to spend much of their time in the company of their female caregivers.

Working with Children

My field observations led me to believe that Chatino adults do not generally play with their children as peers, although some may engage in child-directed speech and baby talk. The role of playmate falls on mixed-age siblings, cousins, and other young relatives who inhabit the same family compound, and perhaps on the neighboring children. Hearing children socialize with their classmates in school and may form friendships, but such non-kin friendships are not central to the social lives of the children. Peer interactions outside of a child's extended family circle are not universal across all cultures (Gaskins 2006). Prior to my arrival, most children, both deaf and hearing, had very minimal experience interacting with strangers, especially non-Mexicans, and deaf children even less. My presence created a disturbance. Not every day does a foreign researcher show up, loaded with video-recording equipment, on the front step of a house in a Chatino village. Visiting deaf children frequently in their homes was essential for them to get accustomed to my presence without being afraid. This took several months. To bond with the children, I talked to them, bought them snacks, and played with them, between periods of silent observation. My actions bore little resemblance to how their caretakers and other adults interacted with them, given that adult-child interactions vary across cultures (Rogoff 2003). Interacting with the hearing children was doubly challenging, because their deaf caregivers expected to talk to me and constantly advised me to come back when the children were older and would know how to sign more for longer conversations.

Gradually, the children treated me as an interactant who would and could play with them, which led them *and* the adults to expect such behavior from me. The expectations of my behavior made it challenging for me to observe spontaneous interactions between the children and their families, but the novelty of my presence wore off. The children frequently played with one another, often without paying attention to me, but they were receptive to participating in most activities I suggested without the intervention of an adult. The adults trusted me to accompany children on short trips to stores for buying food and to the residences of other relatives for company. Accessing and assessing the social networks of the deaf children required more time than it did for deaf adults. Achieving this, however, involved not conforming to local language practices and ideologies of the caregivers and interjecting my own instead.

Community Perspectives of Deaf and Hearing Researchers

In working with deaf children and adults, I occupied a similar position of having minimal access to spoken linguistic input. Because I cannot carry on an extended conversation with a person in either Chatino or Spanish, the majority of my interlocutors in the community and I relied on signs and gestures to communicate. This exposed a greater range and depth of manual communicative functions and practices than what Kate experienced, because the hearing people always spoke to her in Spanish and/or basic Chatino. Thus, being a deaf person allowed me to learn and experience events and meanings of daily social life in ways that approximate, but do not replicate, the deaf Chatinos' experiences. We shared the experience of being sighted deaf people who primarily rely on visual stimuli for communication. Yet, my outsider status meant that I lacked native roots and connections to the community. Hearing people treated me very differently with respect to communication from how they treated deaf people from the same community. Hearing people who were part of a deaf person's social network would greet the person accordingly, joke around, and chat about familiar topics related to their lives, but they would either ignore me, ask me about myself, or ask me for favors and discuss traveling to the United States and working there. Moreover, if a hearing person knew how to write in Spanish, he or she would initiate the conversation through writing notes.

Furthermore, Kate and I received differential treatment from some hearing community members and even some family members of deaf people. Sometimes we received conflicting and disproportionate information about deaf people and their families from the community. The treatment was not exclusively based on our hearing status. My salient physical appearance earned me a nickname from the hearing people: *la china* or "the Chinese woman" in Spanish, due to my salient physical appearance, despite my self-identification. They called Kate *la güera* or "the light-skinned (white) woman" in Spanish and *nepi* or "turkey person" in Chatino (because white people resemble turkeys by virtue of pale skin and tall necks), but they never called me *nepi,* only *la china.* The deaf people assigned me a name sign that referred to the shape of my eyes and referred to Kate by the shape of her eyes, her tall height, or her short hair. Unlike Kate, I did not fit the image of a person from the United States. To them, the United States is largely populated by white people whose ancestors have lived there for many generations, and they believe that Chinese people in the United States are immigrants from China even when they were born in the United States. They did not experience the complex reality of the racial and ethnic diversity of U.S. demographics as we did. Many deaf and hearing people viewed Kate as more knowledgeable about the mainstream culture, language, and politics of the United States and asked her about it more than they asked me. They connected my physical appearance to Chinese people, culture, and language. In the United States, some Chatinos worked in restaurants, managed and owned by Chinese immigrant employers, in rural and suburban parts of the southern and eastern United States. Furthermore, they often experienced discrimination from their employers and staff (H. Cruz 2014). Their marginalization as undocumented indigenous Latin American laborers, along with their relatively short stays, usually lasting several years, formed their experiences and shaped an understanding of the United States fundamentally different from my own. On some occasions, we noticed that some Chatinos would only interact with Kate while ignoring me, but we did not know if the behavior could be attributed to my hearing status, my race and ethnicity, and/or language barriers. It was impossible to disentangle multiple social variables that factored in the differential treatment toward me and Kate, but we worked this to our advantage by comparing our field notes, and sharing and cross-referencing information for a more complete description of the signing community of Quiahije and Cieneguilla.

Literacy Practices and Choices for Communication

Only a handful of community members were comfortable writing in Spanish with me. The practice of literacy is not the norm in the community (Cruz & Woodbury 2014). Few people acquire Spanish as their first and/or dominant language and few also know how to write Chatino. Those who could write with me were older children who were actively practicing literacy in school; a few young and middle-aged bilingual Chatino-Spanish speakers, predominantly male; schoolteachers; some members of the village authorities, mainly the secretaries; and *mestizos* (people of mixed European and indigenous origin) who migrated to Quiahije because they married into a Chatino family or they worked there. Many hearing non-signers and I were doubly disadvantaged at spontaneous, extended communication. There were times when some hearing family members of deaf people wanted to ask complicated questions or convey very specific details. Extended communication required a bilingual and *literate* Spanish-Chatino speaker on-site. If such a person, either an adolescent of school age or a young adult, was available, we wrote notes to each other. The person also would serve as an on-site interpreter, transmitting messages between me and other persons. This approach did not always guarantee clear communication. Proficiency in Spanish varied considerably among young Chatinos, especially among those who did not practice the language on a daily basis in a nearby Spanish-speaking community. Some wrote Spanish with a strong Chatino influence; their Chatino grammar influenced the Spanish grammar. The communication was hampered further by my lack of native proficiency in Spanish and Chatino, but as time passed, my knowledge of both languages improved. Nevertheless, I felt our language differences consistently filtered the writing conversations to the extent that there was always a possibility of not understanding and/or misunderstanding each other, but it was difficult to confirm this.

Interpreting Practices

In some cases where there was no bilingual and literate Spanish-Chatino speaker on-site, I utilized the interpreting services of Epifania for extended communication. Her presence changed the dynamics of communication between me and an interlocutor, because she accompanied me to the residences of the families infrequently. Written conversation is laborious, constrained, and time-consuming compared with spoken and signed conversations. If the people knew Epifania personally, they were interested in chatting with her and she reciprocated, and later, she would summarize the conversations through writing. If they did not know her, she did not initiate conversation without my participation. For setting up interviews with hearing participants, the complicated logistics of conducting them required scheduling coordination, making phone calls via Epifania, and substantial reviewing and discussing of the interview scripts with her in advance. All of this materialized through writing notes back and forth. Early on, I learned that asking meta-linguistic questions in interviews was difficult. Epifania lacked the knowledge of the local sign language and sign languages in general, and the conduct of the interviews in Chatino either discouraged or distracted the interviewees from gesturing and signing. It was necessary to provide explicit examples with demonstrations of signs themselves, with which the deaf adults often assisted, since the interviewees were more accustomed to their style of signing than mine.

The deaf adults believed that my literacy skills could fill in what they perceived as communication gaps between ourselves and their hearing interlocutors. A few believed that in some situations when we did not fully understand one another, their hearing kinfolk, if available, could translate for me via writing. Others believed that I could communicate better with their hearing kinfolk through writing than I could through signing, regardless of whether they were accustomed to the practice of literacy, because their hearing kinfolk may not be skilled or willing signers. Some hearing adults and older children took the initiative of writing to me. It is likely that they felt they could not understand my signs, which were distinctly marked with an ASL accent, or they could not express themselves proficiently enough, or we could not communicate certain issues more in-depth through signs. When a hearing person read my writing and there were other hearing persons around, my writing was spontaneously read aloud and subsequently translated to Chatino, but seldom to signs. My literacy privilege, that is, my proficient ability to write and read, altered the communicative dynamics between the deaf adults and their families, because the deaf adults could not access the conversation. I tried to limit the written conversations, because the deaf could not "oversee" them and freely participate in them. The deaf adults did not object to the written conversations but actually encouraged me to write. They were content with me summarizing the conversations in sign.

The deaf Chatinos and I also had different ideologies about participating in spoken Chatino conversations. When hearing people, whether signers or non-signers, appeared to be engaging in an extended conversation with each other exclusively, deaf people told me that they did not participate because they could not talk, and they did not expect hearing people to sign to include them in the conversation. Sometimes they asked for a summary of the conversation, but more often, they did not. Their expectations ran counter to my belief about the value of deaf people being able to access and being included in conversations with signing and non-signing hearing people. The deaf Chatinos also believed interrupting spoken conversations was inappropriate and rude. They commanded me to wait until the conversation was over, when an early visual cue indicated that the interlocutors had stopped talking and had detached from the conversation. I believed interrupting was not a problem, because H. Cruz (2014) demonstrated how conversations were frequently marked by overlaps and interruptions. But because the structure of conversations, such as verbal turn-taking cues, were not visually accessible to me and the deaf Chatinos, and because I did not know how the hearing Chatinos would interpret my interrupting them, I complied with the deaf Chatinos' expectations most of the time. On the several occasions I did interrupt the hearing Chatinos—by waving at them and/or by passing them notes, at the consternation of the deaf Chatinos—passed without incident. The struggle of reconciling my own language practices and ideologies with those of the deaf and hearing Chatinos marked my interactions with my research participants.

CONCLUSION

This chapter details reflexive meta-documentation of the documentation of an emerging sign language, San Juan Quiahije Chatino Sign Language, and its community of signers in rural Mexico. Originally, I envisioned collecting naturally occurring samples of conversation and interaction among signing families while being a silent observer. Instead, I found myself taking on the role of an active interlocutor in most interactions with the signing families and contributing to the conversations on camera. In the interactions, I found myself negotiating language practices, language attitudes, and ideologies of my own, the research participants, and their families. Consequently, the interactions I recorded are not necessarily representative of the interactions of the signing families. Rather, the interactions are representative of the language attitudes and ideologies about the communicative practices of various modalities of speaking, signing, and writing, between myself, a deaf Asian American woman, and the signing families. The dynamics of interactions also shifted between my research partner, Kate, a hearing Caucasian American woman, and the same people. Not all the changes were necessarily a consequence of shared deaf ontology. Some of the changes, namely the limitations of collecting naturally occurring data, are also common in language documentation projects of spoken languages (Bowern 2008). My reflexive meta-documentation presents a record of how deaf (and hearing) ontologies, intersected with gender, race and ethnicity, education, mobility, and citizenship impact research methodologies for sign language documentation. This entails far-reaching implications for research on/of rural sign languages and their communities of signers. Involvement and collaboration of both deaf and hearing researchers contribute far more to the research than either group alone. In my case, the collaboration produced a more complex depiction of an emerging rural signing community and their language by showing how deaf and hearing ontologies shape interactions between the researchers and their participants, unearthing language practices of, and attitudes and ideologies about signed, spoken, and written languages, in the process.

ACKNOWLEDGMENTS

This work was supported by the Endangered Language Documentation Programme under grant SG0186, the National Science Foundation Dissertation Improvement under grant BCS-1348497, and the National Institute on Deafness and other Communication Disorders of the National Institutes of Health under award number F31DC1397202. The content is solely the responsibility of the author and does not necessarily represent the official views of the National Institutes of Health.

REFERENCES

Austin, P. K. (2013). Language documentation and meta-documentation. In M. Jones & S. Ogilvie (Eds.), *Keeping languages alive: Documentation, pedagogy and revitalization* (pp. 3–15). Cambridge, UK: Cambridge University Press.

Baker-Shenk, C., & J.G. Kyle. (1990). Research with Deaf people: Issues and conflicts. *Disability, Handicap & Society, 5,* 65–75.

Bernard, H. R. (2011). *Research methods in anthropology: Qualitative and quantitative approaches.* Walnut Creek, CA: AltaMira Press.

Boland, A.S., Wilson, A.T., & Winiarczyk, R.E. (2015). Deaf international development practitioners and researchers working effectively in deaf communities. In M. Friedner & A. Kusters (Eds.), *It's a small world: International deaf spaces and encounters* (pp. 239–248). Washington, DC: Gallaudet University Press.

Bowern, C. (2008). *Linguistic fieldwork: A practical guide.* New York: Palgrave Macmillan.

Burns, S., Matthews, P.A., & Nolan-Conray, E. (2001). Language attitudes. In C. Lucas (Ed.), *The sociolinguistics of sign languages* (pp.181–216). Cambridge, UK: Cambridge University Press.

Clifford, J. (1988). *The predicament of culture: Twentieth-century ethnography, literature, and art.* Cambridge, MA: Harvard University Press.

Cohen, J. H. (2004). *The culture of migration in southern Mexico.* Austin, TX: University of Texas Press.

Cooper, A., & Nguyen, T. T. T. (2015). Signed language community-researcher collaboration in Việt Nam: Challenging language ideologies, creating social change. *Journal of Linguistic Anthropology, 25,* 105–128.

Cruz, H. (2014). *Linguistic poetics and rhetoric of Eastern Chatino of San Juan Quiahije.* (Unpublished doctoral dissertation). University of Texas at Austin, Austin, Texas.

Cruz, E., & Woodbury, A. (2014). Collaboration in the context of teaching, scholarship, and language revitalization: Experience from the Chatino Language Documentation Project. *Language Documentation & Conservation, Special Issue: Language Documentation in the Americas, 8,* 262–286. Retrieved from: http://nflrc.hawaii.edu/ldc http://hdl.handle.net/10125/24607.

de Vos, C., & Zeshan, U. (2012). Introduction: Demographic, sociocultural, and linguistic variation across rural signing communities. In U. Zeshan & C. de Vos (Eds.), *Sign languages in village communities: Anthropological and linguistic insights* (pp. 2–23). Berlin: De Gruyter Mouton.

Dikyuva, H., Escobedo Delgado, C.E., Panda, S., & Zeshan, U. (2012). Working with village sign language communities: Deaf fieldwork researchers in professional dialogue. In U. Zeshan & C. de Vos (Eds.), *Sign languages in village communities: Anthropological and linguistic insights* (pp. 313–344). Berlin, Germany: De Gruyter Mouton.

Everett, D. (2001). Monolingual field research. In P. Newman & M.S. Ratliff, (Eds.), *Linguistic fieldwork* (pp.166–188). New York: Cambridge University Press.

Gaskins, S. (2006). The cultural organization of Yucatec Mayan children's social interactions. In X. Chen, D. French, & B. Schneider (Eds.), *Peer relationships in cultural context* (pp. 283–309). Cambridge, UK: Cambridge University Press.

Hill, J.C. (2012). *Language attitudes in the American deaf community.* Washington, DC: Gallaudet University Press.

Hill, J.C. (2013). Language ideologies, policies, and attitudes toward signed languages. In R. Bayley, R. Cameron, & C. Lucas (Eds.), *The Oxford handbook of sociolinguistics* (pp.680–700). Oxford: Oxford University Press.

Hou, L. Y-S. (2016). *"Making hands": Family sign languages in the San Juan Quiahije community* (Unpublished doctoral dissertation). University of Texas at Austin, Austin, Texas.

Kroskrity, P.V. (2004). Language ideologies. In A. Duranti (Ed.), *A companion to linguistic anthropology* (pp. 496–517). Malden, MA: Blackwell.

Kusters, A. (2012). Being a deaf white anthropologist in Adamorobe: Some ethical and methodological issues. In U. Zeshan & C. de Vos (Eds.), *Sign languages in village communities: Anthropological and linguistic insights* (pp. 27–52). Berlin, Germany: De Gruyter Mouton.

Kusters, A., & Friedner, M. (2015). Introduction: DEAF-SAME and difference in international deaf spaces and encounters. In M. Friedner & A. Kusters (Eds.), *It's a small world: International deaf spaces and encounters* (pp. ix–xxix). Washington, DC: Gallaudet University Press.

Kusters, A. (2014). Language ideologies in the shared signing community of Adamorobe. *Language in Society, 43,* 139–158.

Ladd, P. (2003). *Understanding Deaf Culture: In search of Deafhood.* Clevedon, UK: Multilingual Matters.

Lewis, J., Palmer, C., & Williams, L. (1995). Existence of and attitudes toward Black variations of sign language. In L. Byers, J. Chaiken, & M. Mueller (Eds.), *Communication Forum 1995* (pp.17–48). Washington, DC: Gallaudet University.

McBurney, S. (2012). History of sign languages and sign language linguistics. In R. Pfau, M. Steinbach, & B. Woll (Eds.), *Sign language: An international handbook* (pp. 909–948). Berlin, Germany: De Gruyter Mouton.

Meir, I., Sandler, W., Padden, C., & Aronoff, M. (2010). Emerging sign languages. In M. Marschark & P. Spencer (Eds.), *The Oxford handbook of deaf studies, language and education: Volume 2* (pp. 267–280). New York: Oxford University Press.

Nonaka, A.M. (2014). (Almost) everyone here spoke Ban Khor Sign Language—Until they started using TSL: Language shift and endangerment of a Thai village sign language. *Language & Communication, 38,* 54–72.

Nyst, V. (2015). In E. Orfanidou, B. Woll, & G. Morgan (Eds.), *Research methods in sign language studies: A practical guide* (pp. 105–122). Chichester, West Sussex, UK: Wiley Blackwell.

Nyst, V. (2012). Shared sign languages. In R. Pfau, M. Steinbach, & B. Woll (Eds.), *Sign language: An international handbook* (pp. 552–574). Berlin, Germany: De Gruyter Mouton.

Robben, A.C.G.M, & Sluka, J.A. (2012). *Ethnographic fieldwork: An anthropological reader* (2nd ed.). Malden, MA: Wiley-Blackwell.

Rogoff, B. (2003). *The cultural nature of human development.* Oxford: Oxford University Press.

Salzman, P. (2002). On reflexivity. *American Anthropologist, 104,* 805–811.

Stokoe, W.C. (1960). Sign language structure: An outline of the visual communication system of the American Deaf. *Studies in Linguistics Occasional Papers, 8.* Buffalo, NY: University of Buffalo.

Stokoe, W.C., Casterline, D., & Croneberg, C. (1965). *A dictionary of American Sign Language on linguistic principles.* Washington, DC: Gallaudet College Press.

Woodbury, A.C. (2011). Language documentation. In P.K. Austin & J. Sallabank (Eds.), *The Cambridge handbook of endangered languages* (pp.159–186). Cambridge: Cambridge University Press.

Zeshan, U., & de Vos, C., (Eds.) (2012). *Sign Languages in village communities: Anthropological and linguistic insights.* Berlin, Germany: De Gruyter Mouton.

15

Authenticating Ownership: Claims to Deaf Ontologies in the Global South

Erin Moriarty Harrelson

This chapter examines contemporary claims to representation and political recognition being made on behalf of deaf[1] people, most of whom are located in the global South (such as in Cambodia), by other deaf people geospatially situated outside or on the periphery of these groups (such as in the United States). To better understand the (mis) representation of deaf people and signed languages, I ask: How are deaf communities talked about and by whom? How can we account for various claims to authority, including lived experience, insider/ outsider positionalities, professional expertise, and academic training? What forms of authority are endorsed or legitimated and by whom?

Based on my observations and conversations with other deaf academics and transnational political actors, there seems to be a growing number of deaf individuals who are citizens or permanent residents of countries located in the global North making formal and informal claims to represent the sociopolitical interests of deaf people in countries in the global South. Deaf people who are members of a diaspora, such as the Cambodian, Caribbean, Iranian, and Somalian diasporas, have recently authored some of the contemporary political claims on the behalf of deaf people in the countries of their familial origin (J. Hochgesang, personal communication, August 21, 2015; K. Rashid, personal communication, August 21, 2015). Other claims have been authored by tourists, former development workers, teachers, expatriates, and researchers. These claims are made before transnational bodies such as the World Federation of the Deaf (K. Rashid, personal communication, August

---

[1] My usage of d/D is contextual. I use Deaf when referring to categories and concepts originating in the global North such as the concept of a Deaf community. I use "deaf" when discussing deaf people in locations where a Deaf identity (as it is understood in the global North) is not used by indigenous deaf people as a category of self-identification.

21, 2015), in university classrooms (J. Hochgesang, personal communication, August 21, 2015), on social media with political commentary or seemingly apolitical representations (such as photographs of tourist landmarks or videos of deaf people using indigenous signed languages). The disparate activities described above are all connected through claims to authority based on discourses of sameness and difference, lived experience, identity, geospatial knowledge (e.g., "being there"), academic training, and professional expertise. Unfortunately, these acts of representation sometimes obliterate the voices of the people they are supposed to represent because they are not a part of the discussion.

A long history of transnational deaf networks and more recently, connections on social media, especially Facebook, between deaf people in disparate countries and settings shows that deaf people are often curious about and interested in deaf people in other parts of the world (Murray 2007, Kusters & Friedner 2015). Often, this interest, compounded by a sense of responsibility, inspires deaf people in the global North to intervene, socially and politically, in the lives of deaf people in other parts of the world. The ability to physically cross nation-state borders is an inherent privilege that many deaf people in the global North possess because they are able to more easily access the material and social resources needed for transnational mobility (Kusters & Friedner 2015). Another form of privilege is the ability to represent other deaf people because of access to literacy in a written language, especially English.

Inequities in deaf (and hearing) mobilities and literacies has allowed for discourses and concepts originating in the global North, such as deaf education pedagogies and methodology, signed language ideologies, and frameworks for deaf emancipation projects and development to have enormous, often devastating, impacts on deaf people living in the global South and on indigenous signed languages (see Branson & Miller 2004 on the effect of imported deaf education pedagogies on the linguistic competence of deaf students in Bali, Indonesia; see Moges 2015 for the impact of religious missions on Eritrean Sign Language).

In this chapter, I analyze claims to deaf similitude and difference, the experience of "being there," as well as the deployment of nationalist and racialized discourses as *technologies of ownership* to establish *discursive authority over certain spaces and bodies.*[2] By discursive authority, I mean claims of representation based on imagined similitudes, which then function as technologies of discursive ownership over other bodies and spaces. These claims often fail to account for the complex,

---

[2] My gratitude to Audrey Cooper for her observation that claims of similitude can function as "technologies of ownership."

shifting intersections of gender, race, ethnicity, class, and geography and by doing so, reify the social hierarchies they purport to challenge. I also examine *fast social justice*, by which I mean the desire to enact quick fixes to social, political, and economic inequities with little investment in and/or understanding of the context, which carries with it the danger of obfuscating situated voices and perspectives. As such, this chapter foregrounds some of the core dilemmas about power and (mis)representation. It raises salient points for discussion about research and other encounters between deaf people located in the global North and the global South.

Going forward, I use case studies to illustrate some of the epistemological dilemmas and challenges surrounding ethics and representation of deaf people, especially deaf people in the global South. Using ethnographic data collected in Cambodia, the United States, and the virtual spaces where these two ideological and geopolitical territories overlap, this research examines the deterritorialized claims made by deaf people situated outside of the country and the claims of deaf people in the local context with respect to issues of ownership, representation, and power.

MY ROUTE INTO THE FIELD, AND BLOGGING DURING FIELDWORK

I became interested in Cambodia in the beginning of my doctoral studies when I read a newspaper article, "Cambodia's Deaf Wait for Words of Their Own." It claimed that "until recently, Cambodia's deaf population had no language at all" (Melamed 2005). It explained that one of the nongovernmental organizations (NGOs) working with deaf people in Cambodia, Deaf Development Programme (DDP) was promoting the formation of a Deaf community in Cambodia by creating spaces where deaf Cambodians could meet, interact, and (re)create their own sign language.[3] The article also explained that another NGO, Krousar Thmey, which provides formal deaf education from the primary school level to the secondary school level, had imported American Sign Language in 1997 for its teachers to use with deaf students. I was struck by the vast difference in philosophies and approaches to deaf people and signed languages adopted by the two NGOs. I also found the claim of deaf people "having no language" very difficult to process

---

[3] I use (re)create because development workers (deaf and hearing) who worked with deaf people in Cambodia claim that there was no evidence of a shared, national signed language in Cambodia until they started bringing deaf people together in the late 1990s. In fact, during fieldwork in 2015, an interviewee explained that he was in a deaf program that used sign language in 1969 and brought me to the site in January 2016, contradicting NGO and development narratives.

intellectually, given my own lived experiences as a deaf person in the United States.

This became my research focus and I developed a long-term relationship with various people and institutions in Cambodia that continues to this day. I visited Cambodia for the first time in 2009 for a brief stay when I visited Southeast Asia to explore the feasibility of Cambodia and Thailand as research sites. I returned in 2012 to do preliminary fieldwork for a month in Kampot and Phnom Penh. This laid the foundation for my subsequent visits to Cambodia for three months in 2013 and ten months in 2014–2015 as a Fulbright–National Geographic Digital Storytelling Fellow. After the completion of my fellowship in June 2015, I returned to Cambodia in January 2016 for a month to conduct follow-up interviews and to share my initial data analysis/results. As a result of my sustained commitment to Cambodia and deaf Cambodians, I developed close relationships with people of various positionalities such as deaf garment workers, hearing Cambodian Sign Language (CSL) interpreters, deaf and hearing teachers, professionals working with deaf people, NGO funders and administrators, Cambodian and expatriate, which allowed me to understand better the various factors that shaped the complex situation of deaf people in Cambodia.

My research project examines how NGO projects, such as the Cambodian Sign Language development and documentation project, and development discourses naturalize certain identities and political rationalities. A prerequisite for the Fulbright-National Geographic Digital Storytelling Fellowship was to tell the stories of the people I encountered throughout the course of this research on a dedicated National Geographic blogging platform. My goal for my Fulbright–National Geographic project was to tell the stories of deaf people in Cambodia to spotlight the structural inequalities that deaf people face, especially for government policymakers and deaf educators in Cambodia. For this reason, I worked with the United States Embassy in Cambodia to have each blog post translated into Khmer script and I agreed to be interviewed by English- and Khmer-language media outlets as a way of raising awareness of issues important to deaf people in Cambodia. I also produced videos in which I, or one of my Cambodian co-researchers, translated the content of the blogs into Cambodian Sign Language.

The practices I undertook toward transparency and accessibility presented a dilemma—how to protect the confidentiality of my research collaborators as I discuss their everyday experiences working through the structural inequities they faced as deaf people in Cambodia? I also worried about how to present complex issues to a popular audience without oversimplifying or essentializing the people and practices I encountered during fieldwork. In short, I worried about how to *do* public anthropology well. To define public anthropology, I adopt the following:

Public anthropology demonstrates the ability of anthropology and anthropologists to effectively address problems beyond the discipline—illuminating the larger social issues of our times as well as encouraging broad, public conversations about them with the explicit goal of fostering social change. It affirms our responsibility, as scholars and citizens, to meaningfully contribute to communities beyond the academy—both local and global—that make the study of anthropology possible. (Borofsky, in McGranahan 2006:257).

The practice of public anthropology was an integral part of my academic training in anthropology at American University. As with my colleagues at American University, my scholarship is guided by the goal of effecting social change based on ethnographic findings. I hoped that my scholarship in Cambodia would challenge hegemonic discourses regarding Cambodian deaf history and the use of signed language.

Before going into the field, I thought that one of my biggest challenges would be writing for a nonacademic audience, without being sensationalistic, about the often harrowing experiences people shared with me; however, a situation toward the end of my fieldwork in 2015 brought to the forefront core issues that many anthropologists grapple with in their work before, inside, and after the field—positionality, power, and (mis)representation. As a deaf researcher and member of the U.S. deaf community, I was brought to account on social media by another deaf person living in the United States for working in Cambodia, based on my ethnicity and nationality. I first became aware of concerns about me conducting research in Cambodia after I posted a story on the National Geographic blog about deaf–hearing marriages in Cambodia to illustrate the inequalities deaf people in Cambodia experience in the familial sphere. I wrote this post with the intention of leveraging my privileged position and the power of the National Geographic brand to amplify the perspectives of several deaf Cambodians who told me that their parents encouraged, and sometimes forced, them into arranged marriages with hearing people based on the belief they would be provided for by their spouses.[4]

After this blog post ran, a woman living in the United States, a member of the Cambodian diaspora born and raised in the United States and self-identifying as a "Deaf Khmer" (the majority ethnic group in Cambodia[5]) posted on my Facebook page linking to my blog that my representations were not accurate and that as a Deaf Cambodian, she

---

[4] This post can be found at http://voices.nationalgeographic.com/2015/04/06/deaf-hearing-marriages-in-cambodia/

[5] It is important to note that not all people in Cambodia identify as Khmer. Khmer is the majority ethnic group and the name of the national spoken language but Cham and Chinese are also significant group designations in Cambodian society. As Keat Sokly, a hearing NGO

was hurt and upset by my representations. Concerned that I had misrepresented deaf people in Cambodia, I responded in this post's comment thread, asking if she would be willing to share with me what she perceived as inaccurate in my blog post. We engaged in a brief dialogue on my Facebook wall in which she explained that she had the lived experience of being a Deaf Cambodian and that these stories needed to be told by a Deaf Cambodian. She also commented that I was being celebrated as a white savior and that it reinforced the perception that Deaf Cambodians were not capable of telling their own stories, a concern that I understood. I appreciate this important reminder to remain vigilant of my power and privilege. This experience led me to think about the various ways that deaf people from different backgrounds (such as diaspora members, researchers, activists, and tourists), mostly positioned in the global North, assert discursive ownership on behalf of deaf people in other parts of the world.

Discursive authority is most often made possible by the possession of social and material capital, such as literacy in a written language and the ability to engage in transnational political projects. Based on my experience in Cambodia, I believe it is accurate to say that in some global South contexts, it is more difficult for deaf people to participate in transnational academic and activist discussions because of a lack of social capital and material resources. Limited opportunities to become literate in written languages make deaf people in the global South especially vulnerable to misrepresentation, especially in popular media, such as newspapers, and/or in academic scholarship, most of which is written in English. In the Cambodian context, only 14 deaf students are enrolled in higher education, as of this writing, and the first high school diplomas were issued in 2006. Limited opportunities to participate in educational settings with teachers who are fluent signers trained in deaf education pedagogies make it especially difficult for deaf learners to acquire fluency in written languages. Disfluency in a written language, however, should not be taken to mean that deaf people are mystified, which I mean in the Marxist sense, as for example, incapable of critically recognizing the social dynamics in which they are engaged.

In an example of an assumption of mystification, the blogger I mentioned earlier posted on her wall (in response to a video the U.S. State Department asked me to make describing my experiences as a deaf Fulbright fellow that circulated widely on social media), "I'm returning to Cambodia and decolonize MY DEAF KHMERS from YOU"

---

administrator in Cambodia, put it, "Khmer are Cambodian, Cham are Cambodian, Kouy are Cambodian, Phnong are Cambodian, Chino-Khmer are also Cambodian. This means that all Khmer are Cambodian but not all Cambodians are Khmer." Finally, there is no evidence of the usage of the capitalized Deaf, as it is used in the United States, among deaf people in Cambodia.

(emphasis hers).⁶ She also wrote a blog post titled, "My Journey of Resistance with Deaf Khmers in Cambodia in the Decolonization Against U.S. White ASL Globalization."⁷ The misrecognition of deaf people in the global South as unaware of the social dynamics they are entwined within and a sense of imagined similitude in various forms (e.g., deaf–deaf same, national origins, nationality, a shared ethnicity, and/or religion) is a strong motivator for deaf people in more privileged positions to engage in acts of representation and fast social justice on the behalf of other deaf people. This is an understandable sentiment, but it problematically reinforces the impression that deaf people in the global South are incapable of enacting their own indigenous resistance projects and need to be "decolonized" by a Deaf person situated in the global North.

EXPRESSIONS OF AUTHORITY AND OWNERSHIP OF CAMBODIA ON SOCIAL MEDIA

I will now discuss a situation that I observed from afar. In 2012, I was very surprised to see a public page appear on Facebook for the Cambodia Association of the Deaf (CAD). As far as I knew, deaf people in Cambodia had not officially established an association of the deaf. This page had several items of interest about deaf people in Cambodia, such as a post congratulating "*our* Deaf Khmer," (emphasis mine) named Ot Veasna, for being featured in the *Phnom Penh Post* with his art, as well as a post congratulating "4 Deaf Khmers" for their graduation from secondary education and entrance into university. In addition to posts promoting the visibility and achievements of deaf people in Cambodia, this page also included items encouraging deaf people in Cambodia to participate in transnational and regional deaf events and experiences, such as football tournaments in Italy and Thailand.

On February 21, 2012, the administrator of this page posted a photo of a Cambodian couple in wedding clothing with the caption, "The 1st-ever DEAF wedding in the province of Kampot and probably is the 2nd-ever DEAF wedding in the country of Cambodia! Congratulations!" It is not clear on what basis this claim was made but a long-time hearing teacher at the Deaf Development Programme disputed this claim in the comments section, stating that there were others, many others, before this particular wedding. As I previously had discussed in my

---

⁶ This quote is from the commenter's Facebook wall. At the time, we were Facebook friends so I was able to see the comments she directed at me. I am quoting her directly because based on her blog posts about this issue and calls for "community accountability" from members of the Deaf community in the United States, I believe she wanted this issue to become as public as possible and to spark a community-wide discussion.

⁷ This blog can be found at this address: http://findingmylight.squarespace.com/

blog, parental resistance to deaf–deaf weddings in Cambodia is prevalent and deaf–hearing arranged marriages are common because of societal attitudes toward deaf people. This is probably why the expatriate administrator of the CAD page celebrated this particular wedding as a milestone for deaf people in Cambodia.

In a different but related post on the same page from the same day, a hearing CODA[8] from Australia, who had previously worked at the Deaf Development Programme from approximately 2001 to 2006, posted this question: "Hi! I am just wondering and curious who set this page up?" The creator and administrator of this page, a white deaf man from North America living in Cambodia, explained that he "set this up for the Deaf Cambodia communities with the hope that one day, they will take over and lead this association/club. Once a few clubs are set up, then a national association can be created. At least, it's a start but a long journey ahead! (smiley face)." The former development worker then responded, "Thanks (name) for your reply. Do you live in Cambodia? What's your background? I'm curious because I worked with the Cambodian Deaf Community for 5 years." The expat's domestic partner then responded in this same thread that, yes, they lived in Cambodia. The dialogue ended there; this page then disappeared from Facebook. In this example, two people with different geospatial knowledges of Cambodia, one a CODA former international development worker, the other a Deaf expatriate running a business, established their familiarity with Cambodia by referring to their lived experience in Cambodia and their connections with deaf people there. They both deployed the experience of having been "there" in order to establish discursive authority based on different capacities, for example, authority as an expatriate who lived there as opposed to authority derived from professional experience.

In an example of fast social justice, a white, deaf expatriate took the initiative to delineate a sociopolitical space for deaf people in Cambodia on their behalf, with the hope that eventually they would "take over and lead." Problematically, he used terminology of ownership, for example, "our Deaf Khmer," as well as temporally based expectations of a linear sociopolitical organization in Cambodia, as in, "It's a start but a long journey ahead!" By framing political work in Cambodia as a "journey," he applied organizing principles and advocacy strategies that originated in the global North to the local context, overlooking existing indigenous political projects and indigenous ways of managing conflict. As a person situated in transnational deaf political networks, he looked to organizing schemes—intertwined with global North discourses and practices of political recognition and social justice—which

---

[8] CODA denotes a Child of a Deaf Adult and refers to people with deaf parents.

were successful in a very specific context and time, as a blueprint for deaf Cambodian political activity.

Blueprints for deaf liberation projects are based on the expectation that deaf emancipatory practices develop alongside a politicized deaf identity (in addition to other politicized identities, such as ethnicity, race, or nationality). The focus on a Deaf identity as a basis for emancipation overlooks local forms of political activity. These forms of political activity are "hidden transcripts," a subtle form of contesting power by deploying roles and language, such as sarcasm, rumor, gossip, linguistic tricks, metaphors, euphemisms, folktales, passivity, purposeful misunderstandings, avoidance, and anonymity (Scott 1990). In his chapter, "Behind the Official Story," Scott (1990) reminds us that people strategically misrepresent themselves to other people who may help or harm them in some way. Political activity among deaf people, especially in Southeast Asia, is not limited to dramatic or visible activities such as demonstrations, marches, revolution, or other forms of organized, collective confrontation. (See Wrigley 1997 and Reilly & Reilly 2005 for examples of the hidden transcripts of deaf organizing in Thailand.) In Cambodia, "hidden transcripts" of resistance among deaf people include intracommunity sharing of knowledge in the form of warnings to "beware" of certain people, foreign and Cambodian alike, because they are "known" to have engaged in acts of theft or sexual violence against other deaf people. Other forms of more overt resistance include the use of the "thumbs down" feature on Facebook, such as in the case of the Khmer language videos I discuss later in this chapter, along with the posting of photos of particular people on social media with a big red "X" over their faces.

In the Cambodian context, the individual is enmeshed within a structure of hierarchical relationships based on class, gender, and social status (Hughes 2001). This framework shapes how individuals manage conflicts with others and the strategies they deploy to secure their goals (Hughes 2001). For example, several deaf people in Cambodia have asked me (and other deaf/hearing foreigner staff) to bring their concerns, frustrations, and conflicts to the hearing people in positions of authority at an NGO. When I asked them if it would be better for them to speak to those people in positions of authority themselves, they shook their heads and signed, "No, we must respect authority figures. They are the bosses. It is wrong for me to approach them myself. They would think I am behaving beyond my status." After several of these incidents over multiple years, I realized that this indirect approach is one of the "hidden" strategies some deaf people in Cambodia use to address conflict. This indirect approach does not necessarily mean that these deaf people are disempowered or unable to speak for themselves. This is a strategy that is available and was used in this specific context to achieve their political ends.

Abu-Lughod writes, "rather than seeking to 'save' others (with the superiority it implies and the violences it would entail) we might better think in terms of (1) working with them in situations that we recognize as always subject to historical transformation and (2) considering our own larger responsibilities to address the forms of global injustice that are powerful shapers of the worlds in which they find themselves" (2002:1). Unfortunately, good intentions or not, the claims to representation I discuss in this section problematically erase the contingency of particular historical contexts, such as processes of nation-state formation, the establishment and development of deaf education and signed language(s), as well as the various subjectivities of the deaf people in that context and how these subjectivities give form to strategies for political action. They misrecognize the subtle but powerful forms of agency and indigenous deaf political activity that already may be present in the contexts in question.

LANGUAGES AS A DOMAIN FOR CONFLICT

Signed languages are another domain where issues regarding authority, ownership, and representation bubble to the surface. As I will show with the case studies in this chapter, the notion of deaf people outside of North America and Europe as being "linguistically colonized" by ASL is a recurrent theme in narratives about deaf tourism, development work, and signed language documentation projects. These narratives reveal a great deal about tensions in deaf communities regarding the spread of dominant signed languages and signed language sovereignty (Moriarty Harrelson 2013, Cooper 2015). In this section, I will discuss notions of morality regarding signed languages and the neocolonial agendas they reveal.

In 2012, I attended a workshop on Deafhood at a conference hosted by Deaf and Hard of Hearing in Government (DHHIG), an interest group for deaf U.S. government employees that I attended in my capacity as a federal employee. Deafhood is a nebulous term coined by Paddy Ladd to encapsulate a deaf person's progression toward a Deaf identity.[9] After the workshop, I fell into a conversation with a white man who is a prominent member of the deaf community in the United States. I mentioned that I had recently returned from fieldwork in Cambodia and explained that I had been there partly because of the signed language context, a context wherein American Sign Language was imported wholesale in 1997 for use in deaf education while at the same time, there is an ongoing NGO-led effort to invent, then

---

[9] Deaf scholars have criticized the concept of Deafhood as universalizing and essentialist (see Kusters & De Meulder 2013).

document, Cambodian Sign Language. After I explained the linguistic context in which I was working, he was visibly taken aback. Shaking his head, he signed, "That is why I am so careful not to bring ASL with me when I travel! When I travel, I use THEIR sign language. I won't use ASL because I don't want to contaminate their language."

In a more recent instance, I had a discussion with a deaf linguist and university faculty member who was supporting the design of a signed language documentation project in a country located in the Caribbean. She explained that a member of that country's diaspora, a first generation U.S.-born citizen, had recently criticized an element of the project design that proposed to bring people from that country to the university language lab, instead of documenting signs in situ, to be able to use technology at the university. This diaspora member said, "You can't do that. If you bring them to the United States, it will contaminate them!"

The idea of "contamination" is based on the idea of "matter out of place," a spatial taxonomy that organizes what belongs where (Douglas 2002). Notions of pure and impure, clean and unclean, contamination and untouched establish social hierarchies and serve as symbolic boundary maintenance (Douglas 2002). Discourses on linguistic contamination and purity as deployed by deaf people in the global North work to maintain boundaries and serve as organizing principles to categorize deaf people. Based on my observations of discourses on Facebook and in personal conversations with deaf tourists, there seems to be a widespread sense of concern among Deaf people in the United States about the hegemony of ASL and how it could possibly "contaminate" indigenous signed languages. Language contamination and colonization seems to be a recurring theme that appears during discussions about transnational deaf encounters on Facebook and in conversations.

Various people on Facebook reposted the blog post titled, "My Journey of Resistance with Deaf Khmers in Cambodia in the Decolonization Against U.S. White ASL Globalization," that I discussed in the beginning of this chapter. Somebody in the United States posted a commentary responding to this blog in the comments section of someone's reposting of this link. She described experiencing feelings of "sadness" after meeting a deaf Singaporean at a deaf event in London where he had performed a comedy show. She explained that she had easily picked up British Sign Language while in England but the Singaporean "couldn't use BSL" so they conversed in ASL. She asked him why he was using ASL so he explained some of his country's linguistic history. He told her that deaf people in Singapore became accustomed to using ASL because of missionaries who visited from the United States in the 1960s. The commenter goes on to say that she felt embarrassed by her country and that the blog reminded her of her encounter with the Singaporean who "couldn't use BSL." She closes her comment by saying that "Deaf Americans" do not have the right to acquire glory by "saving other cultures and languages" and that they should "respect other cultures' autonomy." She then makes the claim that deaf people in the United States should know this firsthand because of their personal experiences of linguistic oppression by speech-based pedagogies and educational philosophies of total communication.

In this example, the commenter, after an evaluation of the Singaporean's presumed inability to use BSL, connected his use of ASL to a history of signed language imperialism in Singapore. It is not clear from this post what kind of affective subjectivity the deaf Singaporean exhibited (e.g., whether he was angry or neutral about the history of signed language in Singapore), but this commentary discursively establishes a relationship between oppression in the form of communication modality and deaf education pedagogies in the global North to linguistic colonialism and the spread of ASL in the global South.

In numerous cases around the world, deaf people show neutral, or not overly negative, affect regarding the influence of ASL in their signed language history. For example, the presence of ASL in the linguistic history of some countries in Africa, specifically those where Andrew Foster and his disciplines established schools for the deaf, is positively connected with access to formal education. According to Aina (2015), feelings of gratitude are common among deaf people in some of these African countries for their ability to use signed language. Similarly, Friedner (2015) found that deaf people in Bangalore were less concerned with which signed language they were using than with actually communicating. In many of these cases, perceptions of linguistic colonialism are projected on the global South, superseding the thoughts and feelings of the signed language users themselves. Discourses of linguistic colonization sometimes dismiss "neutral" or "grateful" feelings as evidence that deaf people in the global South are mystified, unaware of their own oppression and in need of "decolonization." Discourses of linguistic decolonization, as deployed by persons based in the global North, function as technologies of ownership, by asserting foreign sovereignty over signed languages in other parts of the world, taking away self-determination from the local community of signed language users.

This does not mean, however, that there are not cases where a dominant signed language threatens local signed languages or that the global spread of technologies of deaf education is not located within uneven power structures. The history of the spread of dominant signed language is complex, given that languages are territorialized unevenly in different locations in the world. Feelings of gratitude or neutrality can change, as in the case of the demissionization process in Eritrean Sign Language (Moges 2015).

In an example of local organizing, deaf Eritreans asserted signed language sovereignty by removing the Swedish and Finnish signs imported by missionaries from Sweden and Finland from Eritrean Sign

Language, which Moges (2015) refers to *demissionization*. During the demissionization process, deaf Eritreans mobilized sovereign authority and discourses of authenticity to regain control over language planning. Moges's (2015) ethnography of signed language liberatory projects in Eritrea contests the popular geographical imagining of signed languages and deaf people in the global South as lacking agency to contest hegemonic signed languages. Contrary to the notion of deaf people in the global South as being without agency, there are (and have been) many liberatory projects and instances of translocal deaf organizing (see Cooper 2015, Moges 2015).

Each context is different, with its own complex history and actors. In Cambodia, Krousar Thmey, an NGO providing formal education for deaf and blind children in accordance with the Cambodian national curriculum, imported ASL to provide its teachers a visual modality for teaching deaf children. When I arrived in Cambodia for preliminary fieldwork in 2013 and began learning Cambodian Sign Language, deaf Cambodians affiliated with DDP, upon learning I was from the United States, frequently showed me the ASL signs for "mother" and "father," saying, "These signs are not Cambodian. No. No. They are American," then showed me the CSL signs for "mother" and "father." In this way, they expressed (meta)linguistic knowledge, and asserted agency and linguistic sovereignty in an everyday form. Informal discussions, such as in this example, about signed languages and signed language dictionary projects constitute an important form of translocal and transnational advocacy (Cooper & Nguyen 2015, Moges 2015).

Another important consideration is that the ability to use ASL (or International Sign) can become social capital, such as in the case of the deaf tourism industry in Cambodia (Moriarty Harrelson 2015). The ability to converse with tourists from myriad countries—France, Germany, the Netherlands, Sweden, and the United States— in International Sign or American Sign Language is an asset for deaf Cambodians, because it allows them to access social and material capital. Communication across linguistic and geographical boundaries and the ability to use versions of American Sign Language and International Sign in physical or virtual deaf spaces is related to forms of mobility and the ability to leverage linguistic resources (Ilkbasaran 2015); it is important, however, to be mindful of the history of displacement of some signed languages by dominant signed languages in some contexts. (See Nonaka 2014 for the displacement of village sign language by the national signed language in Thailand.)

More recently, a deaf member of the Cambodian diaspora who was born in a refugee camp on the Thai border and is now living in a country in the global North, posted YouTube videos on Facebook of himself in a dim basement, white PVC pipes visible in the background, explaining English words and grammar using a small white board. He tagged a number of deaf people in Cambodia, presumably his intended students. In addition to these English lessons, he also produced a series of lessons teaching Khmer script and posted these lessons on Facebook, provoking an angry reaction from a few deaf people in Cambodia. The Cambodian diaspora member clearly wanted to support the "development" of other deaf people in Cambodia, but his efforts were not welcomed. I learned about this controversy when a deaf research collaborator in Cambodia asked me whether I had seen these videos, particularly the video where the member of the Cambodian diaspora angrily addressed specific individuals in Cambodia by name, asking why they gave him "thumbs down" on his videos. As we talked about this conflict, my research collaborator explained it to me as, "Khmer is not his language! Why is he teaching us Khmer? It belongs to Cambodians."

Deaf people in Cambodia explicitly asserted their ownership of written Khmer through discourses of language sovereignty, which is another example of how in this particular context, deaf people are concerned about aspects of their language(s). Language sovereignty does not necessarily apply to signed languages only. Assertions of language sovereignty function as markers of group identity in terms of who is an outsider or an insider. This particular case raises salient points for discussion about informal development work, by which I mean small-scale efforts by deaf people conducted on an individual basis to "better" the circumstances of deaf people located in the global South, such as "empowerment" presentations and English/Khmer lessons on YouTube.

Given the history of linguistic colonialism, signed hegemony language and the dominance of certain deaf education technologies, as well as the contemporary processes of gaining or having gained sign language recognition in many countries, it is not surprising that deaf people in the global North have such visceral reactions to projects located in the global South. The history of linguistic colonialism among deaf people, rooted in the belief that indigenous signed languages are inferior, sets the stage for the politicization of deaf identities (Lutalo-Kiingi & De Clerck 2015). Deterritorialized claims to authority often are made based on various identities and geospatial locations. Many of these claims rest on a "politics of recognition" based on specific social identities (Englund 2004); however, notions of deaf oppressions and emancipations are produced within particular cultural, historical, and temporal contexts. (See Nakamura 2006 for a description of intergenerational conflict regarding Japanese Sign Language in Japan.) They are not objective truths universally experienced in the same way by all deaf people in diverse contexts. (See Friedner & Kusters 2014 for a discussion of how concepts of deaf "heavens" and "hells" are deployed to justify interventions by deaf people located in the global North.)

ETHICS IN DEAF COMMUNITY RESEARCH IN THE GLOBAL SOUTH

As I previously discussed in this chapter, the discursive practices of deaf people in the global North often frame deaf people in the global South as nonagentive and vulnerable to Northern influences, especially where signed languages and language contact is concerned. In this section, I first examine issues of authority, representation, and positionality with a brief discussion of my own position and how it influenced some of the ethical and methodological decisions I made in the field. I also discuss how deaf corporeality informs deaf researchers and their work in deaf communities in the global South, as well as the experiences of deaf research participants. Finally, I discuss the (co)production of deaf research spaces and the potential of research to support translocal liberatory projects.

My position as a Fulbright–National Geographic Fellow in Cambodia had its advantages and problems. The United States Department of State, with support from the National Geographic Society, funded my research fellowship in Cambodia. The Fulbright program is an important part of the Department of State's public diplomacy efforts. Cambodia and the United States have a fraught history, dating to the years the United States conducted a secret war in Cambodia as part of its larger geopolitical mission in the region. Between 1969 and 1973, U.S. B-52s carpet-bombed Cambodia, devastating the countryside and causing sociopolitical upheaval that eventually led to the installation of the genocidal Pol Pot regime, which killed approximately one quarter to one third of Cambodia's estimated eight million citizens in a little under four years (Hinton 2005, Tyner 2012). Given this history, my situatedness as a white citizen of the United States most certainly had some kind of impact on how I was recognized by people in Cambodia. I was (and remain) conscious of my positionality as an academic who is a white, deaf woman from the United States with English as my first language. Throughout my fieldwork, I remained conscious of how my status as a fluent, yet non-native Cambodian Sign Language user and a "foreigner" in Cambodia could possibly impact how deaf people in Cambodia interacted with me.

Recently, anthropologists have begun to examine how ideologies of deaf similitude can either foreground or obscure power differentials, especially in situations where deaf people from the global North and South come into contact (e.g., Friedner & Kusters 2014, Kusters & Friedner 2015, Moriarty Harrelson 2015). It could be argued that the corporeal experience of being a deaf person in a world that is largely structured by hearing primacy and its attendant societal barriers creates an affinity among deaf people who use signed language; however, the assumption of a common experience among deaf people with disparate subjectivities (class, gender, race, nation-state citizenship, etc.) has sometimes led to notions of *deaf universalism* (Friedner & Kusters 2014). According to Kusters and Friedner (2015), deaf universalism is the belief in an automatic deep connection felt between deaf people in disparate social and geographic locations in the world—a connection that transcends class, cultural, geographical, historical, and religious differences. Their critique troubles the assumption that deaf people in various locations throughout the world have the same lived experience and experience forms of oppression in the same way.

Notions of deaf universalism have led some scholars and activists to view "deaf" as an identity and use it as a point of analysis. Using identity as a category does not offer much in terms of analysis and at worst, can constitute a form of violence toward the people identified (Bourdieu & Wacquant 1992, Branson & Miller 2002, Brubaker & Cooper 2005, in Pine 2009:4). Building on previous work on subjectivity, I consider being "deaf" to be a subjective experience, rather than a reified identity, to avoid the essentialization of specific subject positions. Subjectivities are "embodied experiences within a hierarchy of power" (Pine 2009:12). I argue that "deaf" should be understood as an embodied subjectivity—one of many subjectivities—constructed and authenticated through intersubjective encounters with societal barriers, other deaf people, and signed languages. Examining deaf subjectivities as embodied experiences within hierarchies of power, which change depending on national and cultural contexts, allows for a more flexible understanding of diverse deaf experiences located within frequently overlapping social categories such as class, culture, disability, education, ethnicity, geography, history, linguistic competency, race, and religion.

In her discussion of a deaf leadership program in Nigeria, Rashid (2015) illustrates how problematic issues still cropped up despite the familiarity the trainers had with the region. Three of the trainers were Nigerian-born but had lived in the United States for decades. Rashid shows how, despite having a shared heritage background with the participants and the shared corporeal experience of being deaf, differences in status and lived experiences resulted in friction. Rashid wrote, "They viewed us as "other" because of our differences in status, our role as experts, and our advocacy of new ideas" (2015:157). Rashid concluded that the notion of DEAF-SAME should be used sparingly, if at all. Extending Rashid's argument, I argue that claims to deaf similitude in any form (such as claims based on nationalist or racialized terms) should be considered very carefully before being deployed because of the complexity and variety of individual lived experiences, especially in terms of material and social capital.

To understand complex lived experiences better, the ethnographic authority of "being there" has its own important purpose as a research methodology. In her case study of deaf people in Cameroon, De Clerck (2011) proposes the concept of indigenous deaf epistemologies as an analytical tool to understand better the diverse lives and experiences of deaf people. The ethnographic immersion into ways of life allows for the learning of different indigenous deaf competences, political aims, and processes for deaf emancipation. As Kusters, De Meulder, and O'Brien (this volume) discuss, many deaf scholars are now exploring how the embodied experience of being deaf informs researchers' positionalities and their relationships with deaf research participants. In some instances, deaf researchers will experience some of the same deaf-specific barriers the people they work with experience, such as my own experience in Cambodia of relying on hearing people to make phone calls and the inability to attend public events or lectures readily because of a lack of ASL interpreters and limited availability of Cambodian Sign Language interpreters.

There are examples of deaf researchers experiencing an intuitive connection with other deaf people, both in national and transnational contexts, and their deaf research participants have expressed similar sentiments, possibly because of their embodied experiences of being deaf signed language users (see Kusters 2012). This connection, however, does not obscure power differentials such as race, class, nationality, and religion. In her discussion of "insider" and "outsider" perspectives in a research setting, Kusters points out that it was "impossible to disentangle the influences of my deafness from those of my white skin or outsider/visitor status" (2012:36). She did, however, note that deaf people in Adamorobe were more likely to complain to her about hearing people, compared with the experience of a hearing linguistics researcher, Nyst, who had previously conducted fieldwork in the same village, evidencing a sense of solidarity among deaf people where hearing people and societal barriers are concerned.

Hou (this volume) discusses how her background impacted her fieldwork. Hou's project in Mexico is an intriguing example of how being deaf can enhance research methodology. In her chapter, Hou also discusses how an ongoing process of negotiation about language practices and ideologies shaped her methodology. Differing epistemologies between community members and researchers sometimes result in different expectations and understandings of the research process. For example, hearing people in the community Hou worked with had very different expectations for her, a deaf researcher, as compared with her hearing co-researcher. Some of the hearing community members Hou worked with expected her to assume specific roles, such as being a signed language model, for the deaf children. In her chapter, Hou also discusses the importance of reflexivity; to conduct ethical research, it is critical to consider how positionalities such as citizenship, gender, race, ethnicity, education, able-bodiedness, and sexuality impact encounters between people in the global North and South.

Research (and other encounters) with deaf people involves complex power differentials, especially related to education, language, literacy, and various forms of knowledge. Informed consent is another complicated issue. Research ethics mandate informed consent from project stakeholders and signature forms are typical. Ensuring that consent is truly informed can be complex, however, given different epistemologies between the researcher and project stakeholders. To ensure people in Cambodia understood why I was there and to explain my methodology, I had one-on-one conversations with individuals, discussed consent before the filming of interviews, and had group meetings. At the end of my fieldwork in 2015, I presented my research to the public at the Deaf Development Programme Deaf Community Center in Phnom Penh. In an effort to explain why I was in Cambodia, I would show my co-researchers books and copies of other deaf anthropologists' dissertations. Using these as visual aids, I explained what I hoped to do with the information they shared with me during interviews and with my notes from participant observation. I found this process to be particularly effective, an effectiveness validated when I saw how deaf people in Cambodia introduced me to other people in their networks by signing the following, in various ways but with the same message, "This is (name sign, Erin) from America. She will ask you questions, then go to America and write a book. I encourage you, talk to her."

As a deaf researcher, I was very conscious of issues related to access to information, literacy, and language use. In an effort to address the power differentials in my research, especially given the public nature of the National Geographic blogging platform and historical inequalities in terms of literacy, I had my blogs translated from written English into Cambodian Sign Language and written Khmer. At first, I made videos of myself translating my blogs into Cambodian Sign Language, and then I began filming deaf Cambodian volunteers. Unfortunately, I had to give up on video production because of time and technology constraints, but I tried to compensate for this by holding public "town halls," where I used a projector to project my blogs onto the wall and translated each post into CSL. Using my laptop, I also would translate the posts for people individually or in small groups. Ensuring that my work is accessible and useful for deaf people in Cambodia is an important consideration in my work as a public anthropologist. Other deaf anthropologists have done similar things. De Clerck (2011) discussed her findings with deaf leaders and key informants, as did Kusters (2012), who also had a town hall meeting prior to entering her fieldsite.

Kusters (2012) discusses the (co)production of deaf research spaces. In coproduced research spaces, there is great potential for emancipation. Cooper and Nguyen (2015) made two important points: (1) indigenous deaf political activity of some form is always present and (2) research with deaf people and signed language often requires some kind of advocacy work because of ideologies about the capabilities of signed languages and deaf people. Cooper and Nguyen productively examine deaf community–researcher collaborations, pointing out several significant issues in deaf community research, specifically, the impact of asymmetrical power relationships and the importance of community–researcher "epistemological equity" (De Clerck 2011).

As Cooper and Nguyen noted, "When researchers leverage expert privilege to facilitate deaf people's participation in and leadership with institutional elites, deaf constituencies may use such opportunities to represent their own interests" (2015:5). During De Clerck's fieldwork in Cameroon, some of the deaf people she worked with asked her to use her research to educate the government. They told her, "You are white, you can do that" (2011:1423). The deaf people in Cameroon, far from being the constrained "developing country" constituency deaf people in the global North imagine them to be, purposefully leveraged De Clerk's whiteness and academic privilege to achieve their political ends.

At the midpoint of my fieldwork, the head of Krousar Thmey in Cambodia invited me to present my preliminary findings to government officials from the Ministry of Education and other stakeholders in the field of inclusive education, such as teachers and administrators from Krousar Thmey, an NGO-run deaf school. I used that opportunity to discuss the implications of "inclusive education" for deaf people in Cambodia. Inclusive education for deaf students, as practiced in Cambodia, means sitting in a classroom without a Cambodian Sign Language interpreter, copying other students' notes into notebooks. Many of the deaf Cambodians who experienced this commented that they did not understand anything nor did they learn very much. I presented this data with the full understanding that I only had this high-level access to present to policymakers and government officials in Cambodia because I am a white deaf researcher from the United States with academic credentials. I was cognizant of using my academic credentials and expert privilege to communicate the concerns of deaf people in Cambodia to government officials, including the Minister of Education, Youth and Sport, Dr. Hang Chuon Naron. At the end of my presentation, numerous people stood up during the Question and Answer session and commented that they had never seen an academic presentation in signed language. This led to a positive discussion in the room about the importance of signed language and many of the policymakers and teachers expressed interest in learning Cambodian Sign Language.

As noted by Cooper, a hearing researcher from the United States, and Nguyen Tran, a deaf researcher from Viet Nam, academic credentials and expert privilege can be used to support translocal and transnational liberatory projects (Cooper & Nguyen 2015). Anthropologists—and other social science researchers—can and should contribute to informed decision-making processes and policy discussions concerning signed languages and deaf people on the national and transnational level, remaining mindful of local ownership of deaf emancipation projects.

CONCLUSION

This chapter is an effort to address recent trends among deaf people in the global North to rely on frameworks developed in a very specific context for their social justice projects. I raise these issues not to undermine efforts to challenge the very real hegemonic structures that oppress people, but to point out that the discursive practices and political concerns deaf people in the global North engage in are specific to their particular political and social contexts. I argue that the strength of emotional reactions to perceived practices of exploitation or oppression are rooted in anxieties about deaf identity/identities and the perception that the politicization of deaf communities is necessary for deaf emancipation.

Encounters between deaf people in the global North and South can be especially fraught because of the structural inequalities inherent in the North and South divide; however, this does not necessarily mean deaf people in the global South need to be rescued or "decolonized." There is a very real misperception that deaf people in the global South are mystified and unable to recognize the structural violence that shapes their lives. Recent discussions and interventions regarding deaf people in the global South are based on one-dimensional understandings of power and authority, which result in acts of fast social justice that overlook situated agentive projects. This is one way in which public anthropology can be of benefit—by carefully and thoughtfully deploying "expert" privilege to amplify the viewpoints of deaf people who may not have access to these conversations because of literacy issues. Amplifying these viewpoints does not necessarily mean representing or "speaking" for others. By amplification, I mean using ethnographic data such as the concepts, words, drawings, or signs that deaf people have used themselves in interviews and conversations, as I did in my blogs for National Geographic.

I hope that my discussion of the positionalities of Deaf researchers, development workers, and other types of "outsiders" vis-à-vis the population they are working with; essentialized notions of sameness and difference as deployed by deaf people; and claims to various similitudes or differences will contribute to a model for deaf research premised on social activism and collaborative research. With this chapter, I hope to contribute to a discussion about the ethical, methodological, and theoretical issues involved in encounters between deaf people situated in the global South and North. I argue that relationships among signed language communities, observers, participants, and researchers cannot be reduced to simple audiological, racialized, and nationalist equations, but it remains critical to examine these issues reflexively. Ultimately, any discussion on reflexivity in research cannot be reduced to essentialized dichotomies of race, nation, and hearing status. To do so is a disservice to scholarship and to the deaf people who are situated in the local context.

ACKNOWLEDGMENTS

At various stages of this project, from research to write-up, many people have generously their time, energy, and expertise shared with me. Thank you for your assistance: Arlinda Boland, Audrey Cooper, Joseph Murray, and, especially, Rezenet Moges. As always, gratitude and affection for the people in Cambodia, who welcomed me into their lives and asked me to share their stories.

REFERENCES

Abu-Lughod, L. (2002). Do Muslim women really need saving? Anthropological reflections on cultural relativism and its others. *American Anthropologist, 104*(3), 783–790. Retrieved from http://search.proquest.com/docview/198217752?accountid=8285

Aina, G. (2015). Andrew Foster touches eternity: From Nigeria to Fiji. In M. Friedner & A. Kusters (Eds.), *It's a small world: International deaf spaces and encounters* (pp. 127–239). Washington, DC: Gallaudet University Press.

Bourdieu, P., & Wacquant, Loic J. D. (1992). *An invitation to reflexive sociology.* Chicago, IL: University of Chicago.

Branson, J., & Miller, D. (2002). *Damned for their difference.* Washington, DC: Gallaudet University Press.

Branson, J., & Miller, D. (2004). The cultural construction of linguistic incompetence through schooling: Deaf education and the transformation of the linguistic environment in Bali, Indonesia. *Sign Language Studies, 5*(1), 6–38.

Cooper, A. (2015). Signed language sovereignties in Viet Nam: Deaf community responses to ASL-based tourism. In M. Friedner & A. Kusters (Eds.), *It's a small world: International deaf spaces and encounters* (pp. 29–111). Washington, DC: Gallaudet University Press.

Cooper, A. C., & Nguyễn, T. T. T. (2015). Signed language community-researcher collaboration in Việt Nam: challenging language ideologies, creating social change. *Journal of Linguistic Anthropology, 25*(2), 105–127.

De Clerck, G. (2011). Fostering Deaf peoples' empowerment: The Cameroonian Deaf community and epistemological equity. *Third World Quarterly, 32*(8), 1419–1435.

Douglas, M. (1966/2002). *Purity and danger.* London: Routledge Press.

Englund, H. (2004). Introduction: Recognizing identities, imagining alternatives. In H. Englund & F.B. Nyamnjoh (Eds.), *Rights and the politics of recognition in Africa* London: Zed Books.

Friedner, M., & Kusters, A. (2014). On the possibilities and limits of "DEAF DEAF SAME": Tourism and empowerment camps in Adamorobe (Ghana), Bangalore and Mumbai (India). *Disability Studies Quarterly, 34*(3), 1–22.

Friedner, M. (2015). *Valuing deaf worlds in urban India.* New Brunswick, NJ: Rutgers University Press.

Hinton, A. (2005). *Why did they kill? Cambodia in the shadow of genocide.* Berkeley: University of California Press.

Hochgesang, J. (2015). Personal communication, August 21, 2015.

Hughes, C. (2001). *An investigation of conflict management in Cambodian villages.* Phnom Penh, Cambodia: Centre for Peace and Development, Cambodia Development Resource Institute.

Ilkbasaran, D. (2015). Social media practices of deaf youth in Turkey: Emerging mobilities and language choice. In M. Friedner & A. Kusters (Eds.), *It's a small world: International deaf spaces and encounters* (pp. 112–125). Washington, DC: Gallaudet University Press.

Kusters, A. (2012). Being a deaf white anthropologist in Adamorobe: Some ethical and methodological issues. In U. Zeshan & C. de Vos (Eds.), *Sign languages in village communities: Anthropological and linguistic insights* (pp. 27–52). Berlin, Germany: Ishara Press.

Kusters, A., & De Meulder, M. (2013). Understanding Deafhood: In search of its meanings. *American Annals of the Deaf, 158*(5), 428–438.

Kusters, A., & Friedner, M. (2015). Introduction: Deaf-same and difference in international deaf spaces and encounters. In M. Friedner & A. Kusters (Eds.), *It's a small world: International deaf spaces and encounters* (pp. ix–2). Washington, DC: Gallaudet University Press.

Lutalo-Kiingi, S., & De Clerck, G. (2015). Deaf citizenship and sign language diversity in Sub-Saharan Africa: Promoting partnership between sign language communities, academia, and NGOs in development in Uganda and Cameroon. In A.C. Cooper & K.K. Rashid (Eds.), *Citizenship, politics, difference: Perspectives from Sub-Saharan signed language communities* (pp. 29–63). Washington, DC: Gallaudet University Press.

McGranahan, C. (2006). Introduction: Public anthropology. *India Review, 5*(3–4), 255–267.

Melamed, S. (2005). *Cambodia's Deaf Wait for Words of Their Own.* The Cambodia Daily, retrieved from http://www.parish-without-borders.net/ddp/resources/sign%20lang%20article.htm, accessed June 7, 2013.

Moges, R. T. (2015). Challenging sign language lineages and geographies: The case of Eritrean, Finnish and Swedish sign languages. In M. Friedner & A. Kusters (Eds.), *It's a small world: International deaf spaces and encounters* (pp. 83–94). Washington, DC: Gallaudet University Press.

Moriarty Harrelson, E. (2013). "Cambodia Deaf Await Words of Their Own": Competing compassionate sovereignties in the development of Cambodian Sign Language. Paper presented at The Future of NGO Studies conference, Chicago, Illinois, November 2013.

Moriarty Harrelson, E. (2015). SAME—SAME but Different: Tourism and the deaf global circuit in Cambodia. In M. Friedner & A. Kusters, (Eds.), *It's a small world: International deaf spaces and encounters* (pp.199–211). Washington, DC: Gallaudet University Press.

Murray, J. (2007). One touch of nature makes the whole world kin: The transnational lives of deaf Americans, 1870–1924 (Unpublished doctoral dissertation). University of Iowa, Iowa City.

Nakamura, K. (2006). *Deaf in Japan: Signing and the politics of identity.* Ithaca, NY: Cornell University Press.

Nonaka, A.M. (2014). (Almost) Everyone here spoke Ban Khor Sign Language—Until they started using TSL: Language shift and endangerment of a Thai village sign language. *Language & Communication, 38,* 54–72.

Pine, A. (2009). *Working hard, drinking hard: On violence and survival in Honduras.* Berkeley: University of California Press.

Rashid, K. (2015). Personal communication, August 21, 2015.

Rashid, K. (2015). A deaf leadership program in Nigeria: Notes on a complicated endeavor. In M. Friedner & A. Kusters (Eds.), *It's a small world: International deaf spaces and encounters* (pp. 150–159). Washington, DC: Gallaudet University Press.

Reilly, C.B., & Reilly, N.W. (2005). *The rising of lotus flowers: Self-education by deaf children in Thai boarding schools.* Washington, DC: Gallaudet University Press.

Scott, J. (1990). *Domination and the arts of resistance: Hidden transcripts.* New Haven, CT: Yale University Press.

Tyner, J. (2012). *Genocide and the geographical imagination: Life and death in Germany, China, and Cambodia.* Lanham, MD: Rowman and Littlefield.

Wrigley, O. (1997). *The politics of deafness.* Washington, DC: Gallaudet University Press.

Afterword
Paddy Ladd

I am honored to be asked to write an Afterword for a book that is both historically important and qualitatively significant. I hope that Deaf and hearing readers alike will feel proud of the multigenerational collective achievement that has brought us all to this moment in history.

Although it is a tragedy (some would say a disgrace) that the University of Bristol's Centre for Deaf Studies (CDS) was forced to close, it is personally rewarding to see that some of the seeds that were planted by its master's and doctoral programs have flowered in this way. Deaf-focused centers such as the CDS create a nurturing environment for both Deaf and hearing students coming from a wide range of disciplinary backgrounds, who might otherwise be isolated in a hearing university, to both meet and learn from one another.

The importance of master's programs for the development of Deaf Studies cannot be overestimated. Traditionally, the discipline has focused on first degrees, which by their nature do not allow for sustained in-depth discussion and analysis of Deaf issues, and on doctoral students who often have to operate in relative isolation. Master's programs are a vital bridge between the two, a plateau that encourages collective reflection, along with the development of many useful dissertations, as springboards for further research (see De Meulder this volume) and future collaboration. It is from just such a spirit of collaboration and discussion among academics that this book has emerged.

Among the many exciting features of the work produced here are the wide range of subjects and disciplines covered, from theology to bioethics to literature; the determination to engage with other disciplines whose practices can actually empower Sign Language Peoples (SLPs); the commitment to have SLP communities be the subjects, not the objects of research; the commonalities that can be found across these papers, which give us a strong sense of underlying cultural collectivities even as we problematize ideas about "DEAF-SAME"; and perhaps most important of all, the strong sense of commitment to those communities, something that has very rarely been found in other Deaf Studies texts. Through these achievements the editors have created a benchmark against which future research, by both Deaf and hearing academics, can be measured.

Although my interests and writings span a range of academic disciplines, I write this from the perspective of what might be termed cultural studies. I apologize for writing mainly from a Western/Northern perspective, and also for not engaging with some of the new concepts presented in the book, for example, the D/d and intersectionality discourses. This is because of lack of space, and because I want to emphasize the need to understand cultural perspectives more thoroughly.

The original impulse that led to the studying and reporting of Deaf cultures, and the use of ethnography, especially critical ethnography, to do so, was that it could enable the "voices" of our Deaf peoples to be heard, as far as possible in their own ways and on their own terms. This was not only important for understanding ourselves, but also so that we could demonstrate to those holding power over us that we should not be confined to the medical or social models, given that we led collectivist lives based on culturally transmitted values, beliefs, and norms. In setting down these perspectives we asserted that those with power should thereby heed the views that political activists express on behalf of our peoples. This culturo-linguistic turn was intended to be the first step toward decolonization—that is, SLP communities being able to take control of their own interactions with the governing bodies and other organizations that rule their lives. We initially had thought that the work of sign linguists would be enough to achieve that aim, but it became clear that this was not the case—we still were seen merely as individuals who happened to sign.

One of the ironies of my 2003 book, *Understanding Deaf Culture—In Search of Deafhood,* with its interweaving of UK Deaf history, culture, and class, was that it was intended to offer a framework from which both UK Deaf people and those in other countries could go on to set down their own cultural histories. I felt this to be of urgent importance, because we were coming to the end of the "era" of traditional Western Deaf cultures rooted in Deaf schools and Deaf clubs, and the number of informants left alive to describe and explain our traditions was rapidly decreasing. There exists plenty of academic and informal "data" about "traditional" Deaf–hearing issues, such as education and employment, but very little about Deaf–Deaf interaction, and the cultural and sociological relationships of social class, gender, Deaf families, generational differences, ethnicity, and sexuality.

Without an informed academic understanding of these differences, and the creation of opportunities to present the findings to Deaf communities for them to reflect on and develop, we risked moving away from Quantz's valuable perspective that "culture is better understood as a contested terrain" (1992:483). That is (to oversimplify for ease of understanding) that the totality of a society's culture is made up of various "groups" who contest the values, norms, and beliefs of that society, so that if one moves to another society, one has to learn about all these differences in order to properly understand that culture at any one moment in time. Without this recognition of cultures as dynamic and constantly changing, we risked falling back on oversimplified generalizations about "being Deaf." And, indeed, this is still very much the case when it comes to teaching about Deaf cultures. Further, this made it very likely that we would experience the continuation of the problems caused by overclaiming of the epistemic privilege of being "Deaf." I was concerned that, in an era where more opportunities to gain positions of power and influence were opening up, denying ourselves the tools to analyze our own communities, and perpetuating the idea that simply being Deaf (whatever that was construed by its users to mean) was sufficient qualification for the rebuilding tasks ahead, would be counterproductive, in the same way that it has been for other decolonizing entities.

So, the cultural turn has not yet really taken place. Instead, people became fascinated with the concept of Deafhood, which was used in the book as a way of problematizing and challenging existing Deaf cultural beliefs and values by pointing out a number of ways in which they had become diminished or compromised by the colonization process. The spread of the Deafhood concept has been very exciting and heartening and has led to all manner of positive developments that I could not have envisaged at the time of writing. But to all intents and purposes, most Deaf and hearing people still have very little understanding of how Deaf cultural processes work—their traditional origins (insofar as we can use such a term, given that we have experienced the huge effects of Oralism, and its disruption of our 19th-century cultural traditions) and thence how the social changes of the past 40 years have affected those cultures. And it is probably now almost too late to recover those traditional cultural patterns.

So, it looks instead as if we will have to rely on refining the work that is being developed through the Deafhood concept, the related turn toward intersectionality and so on, if we are to ensure that we as Deaf academics do not perpetuate the kind of elitist divisions that characterize much of academia in general. How might we approach this task?

One strategy is reflexivity, and it is heartening to note how many of the authors in this volume are concerned to engage with this concept. This is especially important given that the rapid erasure of Deaf schools means that many future Deaf academics will come from a mainstreamed background. The editors cite the position of hearing academics as "[They] can go up to the fence and look through, but . . . cannot cross," and how this "could equally apply to the current generation of often mainstreamed deaf scholars, who may not be able to fully understand or appreciate the ontologies following from a deaf school background, often the background of those people who are considered to be more traditional or core members of deaf communities." De Meulder's and O'Brien's chapters offer valuable routes for more detailed cultural research that will assist the reflexivity process.

That process can be reinforced by another vital strategy—to develop a better understanding of, and respect for, those who form the majority of our communities, without whom there would not be communities to join. We should note especially that our Deaf ancestors (the vast majority of whom were nonprofessional Deaf people) were forced to transmit our sign languages and cultures subversively down each generation. In developing that understanding of those we term "Deaf subaltern" and Deaf "grass-roots," we also need to problematize the important (if unfortunately named) term "monolingual Deaf people." The term was very valuable when it first emerged in that it acknowledged the dangers of elitism, but now paints too black and white a picture of Deaf language practices. Clearly a continuum exists, but if we are to prevent this becoming a chasm as more Deaf mainstreamed Deaf academics appear, we must address this through financing of Deaf-centered research that actually seeks to identify Deaf subaltern experiences of, degrees of fluency in, engagement with, and strategies for, negotiating majority language situations. This, in turn, will enable us to develop cultural strategies that will enable our communities to feel more engaged in what, after all, is a collective task of gathering and presenting Deaf ontologies and epistemologies.

There are three "groups" of Deaf scholars, whose situations need to be addressed in this respect. Firstly, as the editors rightly point out, "many deaf scholars cease their research work after receiving their PhD, never publish their PhD dissertation in articles or books, and end up teaching sign language and Deaf Studies rather than investing their time, through choice or not, into research and publication." From my experience, this is partly because the immense number of hours one has to put in to survive and function in a neoliberal academic environment works against a key requirement of many Deaf cultures—to socialize in those communities to the extent required to maintain cultural acceptance, in order to fulfil important responsibilities to those communities. Faced with this double-bind, many Deaf academics opt for a less labor-intensive academic path. But also, again from my experience, a number of those scholars struggled with English to the extent that the huge achievement required to obtain a PhD was as far as they wished to go in that struggle. Yet many of these were people I learned the most from, was most inspired by, in our sign language conversations, especially those from a subaltern background.

The second example comes from my experience of teaching the Deafhood master's degree at the Bristol CDS. Some of my Deaf students, especially those from a subaltern background to whom academic English did not come easily, produced valuable dissertations on a range of subjects. But they have not been able to get these published in current

Deaf Studies journals because they were unable in the eyes of the editors and referees to demonstrate a sophisticated literature review, or the English skills needed to engage fully with highly complex academic concepts, which are, of course, also beyond the vast majority of hearing people. As a result, their valuable findings are at present denied to us all.

The third example is the work of Deaf Studies scholars from non-English-using countries. I am awed by the authors here and elsewhere who have developed such highly proficient English. But as the editors note, they were unable to offer financial aid for translating work to English and thus could not include several contributions. This is more of a problem in respect to the flow of Deaf cultural information than, for example, sign linguistics (which is mainly led by hearing academics, whose English is often better than their signing skills). As yet, we are unable to benefit from a wealth of Deaf historical and sociological information in other languages. And, of course, this is even more of a problem for non-English-using Deaf academics from those countries, for whom we have as yet created few means of making our own work accessible.

One of the things I find most striking (and impressive) about this book is the very intense nature of much of the academic writing. At times, it feels almost as if we have to prove ourselves by using the same jargon-intensive registers as hearing social sciences. This is very similar to the way I felt I had to approach my own book. But this placed it out of reach not only of most Deaf people but also of many hearing students. Thankfully, numbers of people in several countries, notably the Deafhood Foundation in the United States, have taken up the slack in giving workshops, courses, and filmed sign translations. But more could be done to produce our material in more informal English registers. For my part, having "proved" myself with that book, I was freed up to ensure that my forthcoming book on Deaf educators would move toward those registers, and I hope current and future Deaf academics also will experience the same freedom.

These kinds of concerns have a more severe impact in the social science disciplines than in the humanities, where writings in history and literature use more informal registers. So, it is also important that we explore social science innovations that validate the use of more informal English, such as those found in Narrative Theory and (to a certain extent) autoethnography.

The increasing pressure to "publish or perish" in academic journals approved of by government-driven neoliberal agendas also works against both Deaf and other minority academics. Although we need to keep proving ourselves and disseminating valuable information in a wide range of journals, we also need to return to recreating publications like the UK's *SignPost* (and to a certain extent, *Sign Language*

Studies and *Deaf Worlds*), which encouraged a range of writing styles, including opinion-editorials (Op-Eds), interviews, and articles that summarized research findings. This would greatly encourage all three aforementioned "groups" to present their work to the public. And their work would in the process become much closer to being accepted as "admissible data," which could then be cited.

"Admissible data" is a vitally important issue for communities whose voices have been ignored. One of the major difficulties I faced when doing the initial research for my book was the immense amount of "cultural data" being expressed informally in the UK community, which had (and still has) never been committed to print, making it, therefore, "inadmissible data" in conventional academic eyes. Hence the need to find more ways in which that valuable information can be "validated" in printed form, given that, sadly, this is the criteria by which most of academia is measured.

An important related issue, especially for minorities, is the challenge of validating such data and how issues around typicality then raise questions about how communities should be involved and represented in validating data. If we have not developed sociological and cultural analyses of our own SLP communities, how can we be sure that our findings are appropriately situated in terms of representation? Further, if, like the Maori, we wish to have greater control over who conducts research "on" or with us, who should our community representatives be, and how should their "qualifications" be evaluated? Deafhood theory begins to address these kinds of issues, but it is indeed just a beginning.

Finally, strategies are, of course, also required to find more ways of communicating our findings in sign languages themselves, for apart from anything else, they are the key marker of our cultures. And the greater the imbalance between English use and sign languages in academia, the more we reinforce impressions of elitism. The Internet has opened up immense possibilities for visual peoples, and we need to think creatively in this respect.

It is also worth bearing in mind that the ways in which the Internet already is used are themselves worthy of study. Much can be learned from studying existing forums about our social and class issues, and how these intersect with particular beliefs about sign languages, Deaf cultures, and Deaf political activities. For example, there are significant differences in discourse registers between sites that operate only in English and others where sign language postings are enabled. Together with the highly important development of vlogs, such cultural "content" can thence be translated into English and become admissible data.

Understanding and appreciating Deaf cultural collectivism (as well as the individualist forces acting on us) is well illustrated by the manner in which the book's introduction was developed. As the edi-tors say, "there is something 'deaf' about the process." This leads me to another important strategy. Other minorities (as O'Brien illustrates with the Kaupapa Maori example) are often collectivist and even egali-tarian in their intent. But one of the ongoing weaknesses of Deaf Studies is that we have not critically engaged with other minorities, have not felt the need to understand their own dynamics, and thus realize the extent to which SLP communities share some profound commonali-ties with those minorities. Until we do this, Deaf Studies and work on both Deafhood and intersectionality will be missing important clues in respect to discovering new dimensions for the field.

To give two examples, work in African American Studies and Postcolonial Studies offers a depth and breadth of writing, not only about scholars' own research, but also the issues that affect their own struggles with positionality and commitment to their own peoples. Understanding the histories and power relationships within minority studies would not only help us appraise and frame our own critique of hearing-dominated studies of SLP communities and individuals, but would enable us to assess our own readiness to take up positions of power and influence. Finally, in turn, familiarity with such work would assist in the much-needed development of far more research with and by minority Deaf peoples, which would, in turn, inform our apprecia-tion of intersectionality.

If we are to achieve the kind of Deaf Studies many of us wish to see, the huge imbalances of funding and research among disciplines need to be addressed more directly. Until we attempt this, we will not know the extent to which resources can be directed away from disci-plines whose concept of us is rooted in the "Other," whether these be reactionary ones such as medicine, technology and education, or liberal ones such as sign linguistics, and re-channeled into agendas that we ourselves develop for the long-term welfare of our peoples, as seen in the Kaupapa Maori model.

Such explorations also would help us identify which of our hearing colleagues are willing to engage in reflexivity and reciprocity, and act as allies in coalition-building for the struggle to convey SLP communi-ties' views to those in power. We especially need to assess how these qualities can best be formally evaluated, thus minimizing emotive reac-tions from both parties. It is noticeable also that some of our hearing colleagues who most wish to see active coalition building feel that they must wait for Deaf leadership, lest they repeat the paternalistic patterns of the past. Because in many countries Deaf academics have yet to form ongoing national organizations, this leaves a vacuum for those who are less scrupulous to continue those patterns.

Given that we are not yet ready to assume significant control of Deaf Studies, not least because the need to balance between the murderous pace of life involved in running departments in the neoliberal era works against our need to remain "at the coalface," we all need to evaluate what our roles should be.

And one of the most important achievements of this book is that, in effect, it begins to make the case for Deaf academics to take "intellectual ownership" of the field of Deaf Studies. If pursued, this might enable us to devise strategies together with those hearing colleagues who are busy spinning wheels and plates to keep the departments going.

Finally, as Bhabha (1994) has it, "the state of emergency in which [minority cultures] live is not the exception, but the rule." And there is no better illustration of this than the burgeoning eugenics movement. At present, I am engaged in writing a history of Deaf educators—something that has not been attempted before. As many people know, the period between 1880 and 1900 (which I term the "Resistance Era") saw intense international battles against Oralism and eugenics.

The parallels with our own era are very stark, and one wonders whether we now have more social and cultural capital to fight these battles for the future generations of Deaf children. In writing that history, it became very clear to me that the roles played by academics, both Deaf and hearing, were more limited than the opportunities we have today. Conversely, the eugenics movement is in a much stronger position than before. So the need to engage with both the powers that be and the general public in illustrating and celebrating SLP diversity, as well as our value to societies in general, has become too serious for any academic to opt out of it. This book and its implications for future research directions and praxis illustrate clearly how that duty also can be rewarding and stimulating, even as we accept our responsibility to maintain the existence of the peoples who have so enriched our lives.

REFERENCES

Bhabha, H. (1994). *The location of culture*. London: Routledge.
Quantz, R. (1992). Critical ethnography. In M. LeCompte, W. Millroy, & J. Preissle (Eds.) *Handbook of qualitative research in education*. San Diego, CA: Academic Press.

Index